Assessment of Polymeric Materials for Biomedical Applications

This book initiates with an introduction to polymeric materials, followed by various classifications and properties of polymeric implant material including various development methods of polymeric materials and their characterization techniques. An overview of various toxicology assessments of polymeric materials and polymeric materials for drug delivery system is also included. Design and analysis of polymeric material-based components using Ansys software along with polymeric materials for additively manufactured artificial organs are also discussed.

Features:

- Addresses assessment of polymeric materials in biomedical sciences, including classification, properties, and development of polymeric implants.
- Covers various topics in the field of tissue regeneration.
- Discusses biocompatibility, toxicity, and biodegradation of polymeric materials.
- Explores wide-scale characterization to study the effect of inclusion size on the mechanical properties of polymeric materials.
- Reviews limitations and future directions on polymeric material with emphasis on biocompatibility.

This book is aimed at graduate students and researchers in biomaterials, biomedical engineering, composites, and polymers.

Emerging Materials and Technologies

Series Editor:
Boris I. Kharissov

The *Emerging Materials and Technologies* series is devoted to highlighting publications centered on emerging advanced materials and novel technologies. Attention is paid to those newly discovered or applied materials with potential to solve pressing societal problems and improve quality of life, corresponding to environmental protection, medicine, communications, energy, transportation, advanced manufacturing, and related areas.

The series takes into account that, under present strong demands for energy, material, and cost savings, as well as heavy contamination problems and worldwide pandemic conditions, the area of emerging materials and related scalable technologies is a highly interdisciplinary field, with the need for researchers, professionals, and academics across the spectrum of engineering and technological disciplines. The main objective of this book series is to attract more attention to these materials and technologies and invite conversation among the international R&D community.

Functional Biomaterials
Advances in Design and Biomedical Applications
Anuj Kumar, Durgalakshmi Dhinasekaran, Irina Savina, and Sung Soo Han

Smart Nanomaterials
Imalka Munaweera and M. L. Chamalki Madhusha

Nanocosmetics
Drug Delivery Approaches, Applications and Regulatory Aspects
Edited by: Prashant Kesharwani and Sunil Kumar Dubey

Sustainability of Green and Eco-friendly Composites
Edited by Sumit Gupta, Vijay Chaudhary and Pallav Gupta

Assessment of Polymeric Materials for Biomedical Applications
Edited by Vijay Chaudhary, Sumit Gupta, Pallav Gupta, and Partha Pratim Das

Nanomaterials for Sustainable Energy Applications
Edited by Piyush Kumar Sonkar and Vellaichamy Ganesan

Materials Science to Combat COVID-19
Edited by Neeraj Dwivedi and Avanish Kumar Srivastava

Two-Dimensional Nanomaterials for Fire-Safe Polymers
Yuan Hu and Xin Wang

For more information about this series, please visit: www.routledge.com/Emerging-Materials-and-Technologies/book-series/CRCEMT

Assessment of Polymeric Materials for Biomedical Applications

Edited by
Vijay Chaudhary, Sumit Gupta,
Pallav Gupta, and Partha Pratim Das

CRC Press
Taylor & Francis Group
Boca Raton London New York

CRC Press is an imprint of the
Taylor & Francis Group, an **informa** business

First edition published 2024
by CRC Press
6000 Broken Sound Parkway NW, Suite 300, Boca Raton, FL 33487-2742

and by CRC Press
4 Park Square, Milton Park, Abingdon, Oxon, OX14 4RN

CRC Press is an imprint of Taylor & Francis Group, LLC

ISBN: 9781032333243 (hbk)
ISBN: 9781032333250 (pbk)
ISBN: 9781003319139 (ebk)

DOI: 10.1201/9781003319139

Typeset in Times
by codeMantra

Contents

About the Editors...vii
List of Contributors..ix

Chapter 1 Recent trends and future potential for polymeric materials
(natural and synthetic)..1

*Sushil Kumar Singh, Yusuf Jameel, Ravi Kumar Goyal and
Anshuman Srivastava*

Chapter 2 Characterization of polymeric materials for biomedical
applications..13

Barnika Chakraborty

Chapter 3 Toxicology assessment of polymeric material
for implants..33

*Neeraj Kumar Shrivastava, Devendra Singh, Sunil Kumar
Verma, Anay Pratap Singh and Anshuman Srivastava*

Chapter 4 Molecularly imprinted polymer-based materials for
biomedical applications...55

Necla Yucel and Pinar Cakir Hatir

Chapter 5 Polymeric materials for drug delivery systems.................................73

Aszad Alam

Chapter 6 Analysis of polymeric composite material-based components
using ANSYS workbench...93

Sajith T. A., Ajay Vasudeo Rane and Krishnan Kanny

Chapter 7 Anti-microbial activities of nano-polymers for biomedical
applications..101

Sawna Roy

Chapter 8 Tribological performance of polymeric materials for
biomedical applications...121

Tannu Garg, Gaurav Sharma, S. Shankar and S. P. Singh

Chapter 9   Aspects of dynamic mechanical analysis in
polymeric materials.. 139

*Milanta Tom, Sabu Thomas, Bastien Seantier, Yves Grohens,
P. K. Mohamed, S. Ramakrishnan and Job Kuriakose*

Chapter 10 Additive manufacturing of artificial organs using
polymeric materials.. 155

*Asit Behera, R. R. Behera, S. K. Mohapatra, P. Jha,
K. K. Joshi, Rahul, P. Sahu and S. K. Ghadei*

Chapter 11 An investigation of polymeric materials for hip joint 181

Ranjeet Kumar Singh, Swati Gangwar and D. K. Singh

Index..205

About the Editors

Dr. Vijay Chaudhary is currently working as an Assistant Professor (Grade-II) in the Department of Mechanical Engineering, Amity School of Engineering and Technology (A.S.E.T.), Amity University Uttar Pradesh, Noida (INDIA). He completed his B. Tech. in 2011 from the Department of Mechanical Engineering, Uttar Pradesh Technical University, Lucknow, India and then completed M. Tech. (Hons.) in 2013 from the Department of Mechanical Engineering, Madan Mohan Malviya Engineering College, Gorakhpur, India. He completed his Ph.D. in 2019 from the Department of Mechanical Engineering, Netaji Subhas University of Technology, University of Delhi, India. His research area of interest lies in the processing and characterization of polymer composites, tribological analysis of bio-fiber-based polymer composites, water absorption of bio-fiber-based polymer composites, and surface modification techniques related to polymer composite materials. Dr. Chaudhary has over eight years of teaching and research experience. He has published more than 50 research papers in peer-reviewed international journals as well as in reputed international and national conferences. He has published 16 book chapters with reputed publishers. More than 25 students have completed their Summer Internships, B.Tech. Projects, and M.Tech. Dissertations under his guidance. Currently, he is working in the fields of bio-composites, nanocomposites, and smart materials. Dr. Chaudhary has h-index of 07 and i10-index of 07 as per Google Scholar indexing.

Dr. Sumit Gupta is presently working as an Assistant Professor (Grade-III) in the Department of Mechanical Engineering, Amity School of Engineering and Technology, Amity University Uttar Pradesh, Noida, India. Prior to this, he has also served as an Assistant Professor in the School of Engineering, G. D. Goenka University, Gurugram, India. He graduated in Mechanical Engineering from the University of Rajasthan in 2008 and earned Master's as well as Doctorate degree from the Malaviya National Institute of Technology, Jaipur, India in 2010 and 2016, respectively. His areas of research are sustainable manufacturing, lean manufacturing, reverse logistics, sustainable product design, and sustainable supply chain management. Dr. Gupta has over ten years of teaching and research experience. He has published over 70 research papers in peer-reviewed international journals as well as in reputed international and national conferences. A large number of students have completed their Summer Internships and B.Tech. Projects under his guidance. He has guided ten M.Tech. Dissertations and is presently guiding two Ph.D. Scholars as well. He is Reviewer of various national and international journals. He is a member of various international and national professional societies.

Dr. Pallav Gupta is presently working as an Assistant Professor (Grade-III) in the Department of Mechanical Engineering, Amity School of Engineering and Technology, Amity University Uttar Pradesh, Noida, India. He completed his B.Tech. (Honors) from the Department of Mechanical Engineering, Integral University,

Lucknow, India in the year 2009, Qualified GATE in 2009 with AIR-3291, and then completed his M.Tech. (Honors) from I.I.T. (B.H.U.), Varanasi, INDIA in 2011 followed by Ph.D. in 2015 from I.I.T.(B.H.U.), Varanasi, India. His area of research includes material processing; composite materials; mechanical behavior, and corrosion. He also has a good command over teaching subjects like Material Science, Engineering Materials, Manufacturing Processes, Measurement, and Metrology and Composite Materials. Dr. Gupta has over eight years of teaching and research experience. He has published over 100 research papers in peer-reviewed international journals as well as in reputed international and national conferences in India as well as abroad. Apart from this, he has also published 14 chapters in books published by different publishers. A large number of students have completed their Summer Internships, B.Tech. Projects, and M.Tech. Dissertations under his guidance. Three scholars have completed and five are presently registered for their Ph.D. research work under his supervision in the area of "Coatings, Metal Matrix Composites and Polymer Matrix Composites."

Mr. Partha Pratim Das completed his Master of Technology (Materials Science and Metallurgical Engineering) from the Department of Materials Science and Metallurgical Engineering at Indian Institute of Technology-Hyderabad (IITH), India. Currently, he is working in the field of active food packaging to extend the shelf-life of fresh produce with Cellulose and Composites Research Group at IIT Hyderabad. He completed his B.Tech in Mechanical Engineering with first-class distinction in the year 2021 from Amity University Uttar Pradesh, Noida, India. During his B.Tech, he worked on various projects with the Indian Institute of Technology Guwahati and Indian Oil Corporation Limited, Guwahati, Assam. He has presented several research papers at national and international conferences and published a good number of research papers in SCI journals and book chapters to his credit with reputed publishers. He also served as a reviewer in *Materials Today: Proceedings* and *Applied Composite Materials*. In the year 2020, he received the Innovative researcher of the year award. He is also a Certified Executive of Lean Management and Data Practitioner (Minitab and MS-Excel) from the Institute for Industrial Performance and Engagement (IIPE), Faridabad, India. He is a community associate member at American Chemical Society (ACS). His area of research includes natural fiber-based composites, processing and characterization of polymer matrix composites, nano-filler-based composites for various applications and biodegradable food packaging.

Contributors

Aszad Alam
Indian Institute of Technology
Hyderabad, India

Asit Behera
KIIT Deemed to be University,
Odisha, India

R. R. Behera
KIIT Deemed to be University,
Odisha, India

Barnika Chakraborty
Kiel University and Katholieske
University Leuven

Swati Gangwar
Netaji Subhas University of Technology,
Delhi, India

Tannu Garg
AIAS, Amity University,
Noida (U.P.), India

S. K. Ghadei
KIIT Deemed to be University,
Odisha, India

Ravi Kumar Goyal
Nirwan University Jaipur, India

Yves Grohens
Univ. Bretagne Sud, Lorient, France

Pinar Cakir Hatir
Istinye University, Istanbul, Turkey

Yusuf Jameel
University Putra Malaysia, Serdang,
Selangor, Malaysia

P. Jha
KIIT Deemed to be University,
Odisha, India

K. K. Joshi
KIIT Deemed to be University,
Odisha, India

Krishnan Kanny
Composite Research Group, Durban
University of Technology, Durban,
South Africa

Job Kuriakose
Global R&D Centre, Asia, Apollo Tyres
Ltd., Tamil Nadu, India

P. K. Mohamed
Global R&D Centre, Asia, Apollo
Tyres Ltd., Tamil Nadu, India

S. K. Mohapatra
KIIT Deemed to be University,
Odisha, India

S. Ramakrishnan
Global R&D Centre, Asia, Apollo Tyres
Ltd., Tamil Nadu, India

Ajay Vasudeo Rane
Composite Research Group, Durban
University of Technology, Durban,
South Africa

Sawna Roy
Indian Institute of Technology
Guwahati, Assam, India

P. Sahu
KIIT Deemed to be University,
Odisha, India

T. A. Sajith
KMEA Engineering College,
 Kerala, India

Bastien Seantier
Univ. Bretagne Sud, Lorient, France

S. Shankar
ARSD College, University of
 Delhi, India

Gaurav Sharma
AIAS, Amity University,
 Noida (U.P.), India

Neeraj Kumar Shrivastava
Shambhunath Institute of Engineering
 and Technology, Prayagraj, India

Anay Pratap Singh
Shambhunath Institue Of Pharmacy,
 Uttar Pradesh, India

Devendra Singh
B.N. College of Engineering and
 Technology, Lucknow, India

Sushil Kumar Singh
Nirwan University, Jaipur, India

D. K. Singh
Madan Mohan Malaviya University of
 Technology, Gorakhpur, India

Ranjeet Kumar Singh
Madan Mohan Malaviya University of
 Technology, Gorakhpur, India

S. P. Singh
ARSD College, University of
 Delhi, India

Anshuman Srivastava
Shambhunath Institute of Engineering
 and Technology, Prayagraj, Uttar
 Pradesh, India

Sabu Thomas
Mahatma Gandhi University,
 Kerala, India

Milanta Tom
Mahatma Gandhi University,
 Kerala, India

Sunil Kumar Verma
B.N. College of Engineering and
 Technology, Lucknow, India

Necla Yucel
Yildiz Technical University, İstanbul,
 Turkey

Rahul
KIIT Deemed to be University, Odisha,
 India

1 Recent trends and future potential for polymeric materials (natural and synthetic)

Sushil Kumar Singh, Yusuf Jameel, Ravi Kumar Goyal and Anshuman Srivastava

CONTENTS

1.1 Introduction 2
1.2 Synthetic polymers 2
1.3 Synthetic polymers in everyday use 3
1.4 Types of synthetic polymers 3
    1.4.1 Low-density polyethylene 3
    1.4.2 High-density polyethylene 3
    1.4.3 Polypropylene 4
    1.4.4 Polyvinyl chloride 4
    1.4.5 Polystyrene..4
    1.4.6 Nylon...4
    1.4.7 Teflon 4
    1.4.8 Thermoplastic polyurethane 5
    1.4.9 Polylactic acid 6
    1.4.10 Polyhydroxyalkanoates 6
    1.4.11 Polybutylene succinate..7
1.5 Bio-polyethylene 7
1.6 Bio-based natural polymers...8
    1.6.1 Starch 8
    1.6.2 Cellulose 8
1.7 Chitin and chitosan 9
1.8 Current status and future trends 10
1.9 Challenges in biopolymers 10
1.10 Conclusions..11
References..11

DOI: 10.1201/9781003319139-1

1

1.1 INTRODUCTION

Polymer science is the oldest field of science (it has existed since the origin of living cells) and was founded as a separate, well-defined subject less than a century ago—between 1920 and 1930 [1]. Humans used polymer materials with little awareness of how these materials differed from others. Their diversity and quantity continue to grow as a result of the enormous potential given by new synthetic routes and macromolecules feature, which is their chain nature. This permits the creation of wholly new materials with desired properties or the dramatic enhancement of a quality in a previously existing material route [2]. In addition to the numerous advantages of synthetic polymer materials, which make them an appealing and important material, these materials have major drawbacks that have a negative impact on the environment. The microscopic structure of polymer molecules influences a polymeric material's varied qualities. As a result, polymers are classed as either amorphous or semi-crystalline (partially crystalline). Semi-crystalline polymers are slightly coordinated in an organized crystalline structure, whereas amorphous polymers have an incorrect structural arrangement and are randomized. Polymerization and polycondensation are two chemical processes that may be used to synthesize polymers, according to fundamental understanding. Polymer membranes containing synthetic organic macromolecules are becoming increasingly important in terms of technical applications due to their high chemical and physical stability. Nonetheless, scientists have concluded in last 30 years that main synthetic polymers, such as poly(alkylene oxide), poly(vinyl alcohol), poly(acrylic acid), and polyacrylamide, can be replaced by natural and biodegradable polymers, such as starch and cellulosic, which have less negative environmental effects [9]. Practically, materials formed of organic polymers offer various benefits over materials made of metals and inorganic substances, such as simplicity of processing, anti-rust, high strength, and low weight [3]. Metal, for example, has a reasonably high specific strength with no accumulation of colored rust. Nonetheless, exposure to hot and/or cold temperatures, sunshine and/or rain, and being underwater and/or beneath earth may cause polymer materials to breakdown. There are several polymer material uses, such as vibration isolation and damping, weight reduction, heat insulation and coating, and covering. Some can be utilized on outside and inside of a car, plane, train, or ship, while others can be used in residences, structures, construction, housewares, commodities, toys, and electrical equipment. Hydrolysis, oxidation, ultraviolet (UV) radiation, age, chemical effects, swelling, fatigue, the complicated state of respective deterioration, as well as wet and dry cycles, all of which can modify diverse polymer material characteristics over time. The deterioration of polymer materials causes various variations in mechanical strength, depending on polymer material type, condition, manufacture, and additive package [4, 5]. As a result, it is critical to investigate deterioration factor under actual settings using a reproduction test and an artificial aging test [6].

1.2 SYNTHETIC POLYMERS

Synthetic polymers are man-made polymers generated from traditional energy sources such as crude oil and petrochemicals [7, 8]. They are divided into four groups based on their utility: thermoplastics, thermosets, elastomers, and synthetic fibers.

Thermoplastics are polymers that become moldable and bendable after reaching a particular temperature and harden upon cooling. Similarly, thermosets harden and cannot alter shape after they have set; as a result, they are frequently employed in adhesives. An elastomer, sometimes known as rubber, is a kind of flexible polymer. Synthetic fibers, which comprise a vast category of polymers, are made by improving on natural plant and animal fibers.

Poly acrylates are the building blocks for several synthetic polymers, including polythene and polystyrene. They are made up of carbon–carbon bonds, whereas heterochain polymers like polyamides, polyesters, polyurethanes, polysulfides, and polycarbonates have other elements (such as oxygen, sulfur, and nitrogen) introduced along the backbone. Non-covalent bonding allows coordination polymers to have a wide range of metals in their backbone. A wide variety of synthetic polymers with various main chains and side chains are also available.

1.3 SYNTHETIC POLYMERS IN EVERYDAY USE

Nylons in textiles and fabrics, Teflon in nonstick cookware and polyvinylchloride in pipes are examples of household synthetic polymers [9]. PET bottles are constructed of a synthetic polymer called polyethylene terephthalate. Plastic kits and coverings are typically constructed of synthetic polymers such as polythene, whereas tires are made of Buna rubbers. Due to the environmental difficulties caused by these synthetic polymers, which are frequently non-biodegradable and derived from petroleum, alternatives such as bioplastics are being studied; however, bioplastics are frequently more expensive than synthetic polymers.

Many polymers are completely composed of hydrocarbons. This makes them hydrophobic, which means they don't absorb water easily; this is a helpful quality because alternatives—imagine a water bottle that turns soggy when filled with water, for example—could be devastating.

1.4 TYPES OF SYNTHETIC POLYMERS

1.4.1 Low-density polyethylene

One of the most common types of synthetic organic polymers found in houses is low-density polyethylene (LDPE) polymers. LDPE is produced from ethylene under severe polymerization conditions in autoclaves and tubular reactors using free radical-initiated polymerization in high-pressure and high-temperature autoclaves or tubular reactors [10]. It was one among first polymers to be made, and Imperial Chemical Industries produced it in 1933 using a high-pressure process known as free radical polymerization. This is how it is done nowadays. LDPE is frequently recycled, and its recycling sign is #4. Despite competition from more modern polymers, LDPE remains an important plastic grade.

1.4.2 High-density polyethylene

High-density polyethylene (HDPE) or polyethylene high-density (PEHD) is a petroleum-based thermoplastic polyethylene. One kilogram of HDPE necessitates

1.75 kilograms of petroleum (in terms of energy and raw ingredients). HDPE is often recycled, and its recycling indicator is number two.

1.4.3 POLYPROPYLENE

Polypropylene (PP), also known as polypropene, is a thermoplastic polymer used in a wide range of applications, including packaging and labeling, textiles, stationery, plastic parts and reusable containers of various types, laboratory equipment, loudspeakers, automotive components, and polymer banknotes. PP monofilament sutures are made from isotactic polypropylene [10]. It is a strong polymer made from the monomer propylene that is extremely resistant to a variety of chemical solvents, bases, and acids.

1.4.4 POLYVINYL CHLORIDE

After polyethylene and polypropylene, polyvinyl chloride (PVC) is the third most common plastic. PVC is utilized in building because it is less expensive and lasts longer than more conventional materials such as copper or ductile iron. Plasticizers, most common of which are phthalates, can soften and stretch it. This kind of PVC is utilized in clothes and upholstery, electrical wire insulation, inflatable items, and a number of other applications where rubber is substituted [10].

1.4.5 POLYSTYRENE

Polystyrene (PS) is an aromatic polymer made from petrochemical styrene in liquid form. PS is a colorless solid that is used in a variety of applications, such as disposable cutlery, plastic models, CD and DVD covers, and smoke detector housings. Foamed polystyrene is used to make packing materials, insulation, and foam drink cups. Its slow biodegradation is a topic of dispute, and it is commonly found outside, particularly along shorelines and rivers.

1.4.6 NYLON

Wallace Carothers developed nylon, a class of synthetic polymers known generically as polyamides, at DuPont's research center on February 28, 1935. Nylon is a polymer that is widely utilized. Because of its amide backbone, nylon is more hydrophilic than polymers discussed above. Consider how your nylon clothing absorbs water; this is due to the fact that nylon, unlike bulk of plastics, can establish hydrogen bonds with water.

1.4.7 TEFLON

Teflon (Polytetrafluoroethylene or PTFE) is a tetrafluoropolymer with several applications. PTFE is a solid chemical with a high molecular weight that is entirely composed of carbon and fluorine. Because PTFE is hydrophobic, it does not react with water or water-containing chemicals. PTFE is used as a nonstick coating for pans and other kitchenware due to its minimal friction with other compounds. Because of the strength of the carbon–fluorine bonds, it is very non-reactive and is commonly used in containers and pipelines for reactive and corrosive chemicals. When used as a lubricant, PTFE reduces friction, wear, and energy consumption in equipment. Although it is not true that Teflon was developed as a result of NASA space programs, it has been employed by NASA.

1.4.8 THERMOPLASTIC POLYURETHANE

TPU (thermoplastic polyurethane) refers to a kind of polyurethane plastic. It possesses a variety of helpful qualities, including as flexibility, transparency, and resistance to oil, grease, and abrasion. The bulk of these properties are due to fact that TPU is hydrophilic and may react with water. TPU is a thermoplastic elastomer made up of hard and soft linear segmented block copolymers.

Both natural and synthetic polymers have an essential part in comfort and convenience of human existence, as they are responsible for life itself, medication, sustenance, communication, transportation, irrigation, container, clothing, recording history, buildings, highways, and so on. Indeed, it is difficult to imagine human society without synthetic and natural polymers. In our ever-increasing contemporary world, science plays an important part in providing solutions to critical concerns, such as food, clean and abundant water, air, energy, and health. Polymer knowledge and linked literature provide both facts and insights toward their better understanding in our lives. Understanding polymers is facilitated by knowledge gained in basic science lessons. This information contains scientific concepts that are factual, theoretical, and practical. It is beneficial for those who just want to be well-educated as well as those who wish to study medicine, engineering, physics, chemistry, biomedical sciences, law, business, and other fields [9, 2, 3].

In recent years, global interest in bio-based polymers has been spurred by desire and requirement to find non-fossil fuel-based polymers. Figure shows that number of publication citations on bio-based polymers and applications has expanded considerably in recent years, according to ISI Web of Sciences and Thomas Innovations [14]. Bio-based polymers provide considerable advantages by reducing dependency on fossil fuels and resulting in positive environmental consequences such as fewer CO_2 emissions. The regulatory environment is also changing, with initiatives such as European Union's Lead Market Initiative and bio-preferred supporting bio-based goods (USA). As a result, there is a global need to replace petroleum-derived raw materials in polymer manufacture with raw materials sourced from renewable resources. Polymers generated from agricultural feedstocks, such as maize, potatoes, and other carbohydrate feedstocks, were used in the first generation of bio-based polymers. However, due to a desire to shift away from food-based resources and significant advances in biotechnology, focus has shifted in recent years. Bio-based polymers, which are equivalent to conventional polymers, are produced using bacterial fermentation procedures that synthesize building blocks (monomers) from renewable resources such as lignocellulosic biomass (starch and cellulose), fatty acids, and organic waste. Natural bio-based polymers, which include proteins, nucleic acids, and polysaccharides, are other type of bio-based polymer found in nature (collagen, chitosan, etc.). In terms of scientific advancements and commercial uses, these bio-based polymers have seen tremendous progress in recent years.

This research looks at the use of renewable resources, such as lignocellulosic biomass, to create monomers and polymers that can replace petroleum-based polymers like polyester, polylactic acids, and other natural bio-based polymers.

1.4.9   POLYLACTIC ACID

Polylactic acid (PLA) was discovered in 1845 but was not marketed until early 1990. PLA is an aliphatic polyester having lactic acid as its primary constitutional unit. Monomer lactic acid is hydroxyl carboxylic acid produced by bacterial fermentation from maize (starch) or sugars supplied from renewable resources. While alternative renewable resources can be employed, maize has benefit of producing high-purity lactic acid, which is essential for an effective synthesis process. Depending on microbial strain utilized during fermentation process, L-lactic acid or D-lactic acid is produced. PLA is frequently utilized in a variety of commonplace applications.

It is mostly used in food packaging (including food trays, tableware such as plates and cutlery, water bottles, candy wraps, and cups). PLA is inappropriate for use in electrical devices or other technical applications, while having one of greatest thermal and mechanical resistances of any bio-based polymer. NEC Corporation (Japan) recently developed a PLA that is both thermally and flame retardant by incorporating carbon and kenaf fibers. Fujitsu (Japan) created a polycarbonate-PLA mix for computer housings. PLA has lately been employed in automotive and chemical sectors as a membrane material [11].

1.4.10   POLYHYDROXYALKANOATES

PHAs (polyhydroxyalkanoates) are bacterially produced polyesters that have potential to replace hydrocarbon-based polymers. PHAs are naturally found in a wide variety of species; however, microbes may be employed to control their synthesis in cells. In 1926, Maurice Lemoigne discovered polyhydroxybutyrate (PHB), most basic PHA, as a component of bacterium Bacillus megaterium. A variety of bacteria may produce PHA from a range of renewable waste feedstocks. Fermentation, separation, and purification from fermentation broth are all processes in a general bacterial fermentation method for manufacturing PHA. A massive fermentation tank is filled with mineral medium and bacteria from a seed culture. Feedstocks include cellulosics, vegetable oils, organic waste, municipal solid waste, and fatty acids, depending on the amount of PHA required. The carbon source is fed into tank until it is depleted, indicating end of cell growth and PHA formation. Fermentation time should be limited to no more than 48 hours. Cells are concentrated, dried, and extracted with solvents such as acetone or chloroform to isolate and purify PHA. The solid-liquid separation process separates remaining cell debris from dissolved PHA-containing solvent.

After that, PHA is precipitated with an alcohol (such as methanol) and recovered by a precipitation method. More than 150 PHA monomers have been discovered as PHA components. It is feasible to create bio-based polymers with a wide range of characteristics that may be adapted to specific purposes. The first bacterial PHA discovered was poly-3-hydroxybutyrate. It has gotten the most interest for route characterization and industrial-scale manufacture. It has the same thermal and mechanical qualities as polystyrene and polypropylene [15]. However, because to its sluggish crystallization, limited processing temperature range, and tendency to 'creep,' it is unsuitable for a wide range of applications, needing more research to tackle these challenges [16]. To improve the properties of PHAs, many businesses have developed PHA copolymers with 80–95% (R)-3-hydroxybutyric acid monomer and 5–20% of a second monomer.

1.4.11 Polybutylene succinate

PBS (polybutylene succinate) is an aliphatic polyester with comparable properties to PET. PBS is formed through condensation of succinic acid and 1,4-butanediol. PBS can be manufactured from petroleum-based monomers or by bacterial fermentation. Succinic acid can be made from fossil fuels in a variety of ways. Electrochemical synthesis is a typical procedure that produces excellent yields at a low cost. When compared to chemical approach, fermentation synthesis of succinic acid offers several benefits. Fermentation, as opposed to chemical procedures, uses renewable materials and requires less energy. Several companies (alone or in combination) are currently expanding bio-succinate manufacturing technologies that were previously afflicted by low productivity and high downstream processing costs. Mitsubishi Chemical (Japan) has developed biomass-derived succinic acid in collaboration with Ajinomoto to commercialize bio-based PBS. DSM and Roquette are working together to develop a commercially viable fermentation technology for producing succinic acid, 1, 4-butanediol, and PBS. Myriant and Bioamber have developed a method for manufacturing monomers through fermentation. Bioplastics: Products, Markets, Trends, and Technologies (Bioplastics: Products, Markets, Trends, and Technologies, 2010).

1.5 BIO-POLYETHYLENE

Polyethylene (PE) is a widely used technical polymer that is traditionally made from fossil fuels. PE is made by polymerizing ethylene at high temperatures and pressures in presence of a catalyst. Ethylene is traditionally made by steam cracking naphtha or heavy oils, or by dehydrating ethanol. With rise in oil prices, microbial PE, also known as green PE, is currently made by dehydrating ethanol produced by microbial fermentation. The idea of making PE from bioethanol isn't really novel. Braskem produced bio-PE and bio-PVC from bioethanol in 1980s. Low oil costs and limitations of biotechnology techniques, on the other hand, rendered technology unappealing at time. Currently, sugarcane is used to make bio-PE on a large scale from bioethanol. Bioethanol can also be made from biorenewable feedstocks such as sugar beet, maize, wood, wheat, corn, and other plant wastes using a microbial strain and biological fermentation method. Extracted sugarcane juice with a high sucrose concentration is anaerobically fermented to make ethanol in a typical procedure. Ethanol is distilled at end of fermentation process to remove water and produce an azeotropic mixture of hydrous ethanol. Ethanol is then dehydrated over a solid catalyst at high temperatures to create ethylene and, eventually, polyethylene [17].

1.6 BIO-BASED NATURAL POLYMERS

This category includes polymers found in nature, such as cellulose, starch, chitin, and other polysaccharides and proteins. The properties and applications of these materials and their derivatives are diverse. Some natural bio-based polymers and their uses in diverse fields are addressed in this section.

1.6.1 STARCH

Because it exists in nature as distinct granules, starch is a unique bio-based polymer. Starch is a natural carbohydrate-based polymer that is common in nature and may be obtained from a variety of sources including wheat, rice, maize, and potato. It is also end product of photosynthesis in plants. Starch is composed of two polysaccharides: amylose (a linear polymer) and amylopectin (a highly branched carbohydrate). Thermoplastic starch, in particular, is gaining popularity in the industry. Starch's thermal and mechanical qualities are highly variable, depending on elements such as the amount of plasticizer present. The Tg ranges from 50 to110 degrees Celsius, and modulus is close to that of polyolefins. Commercially viable starch plastics have a number of problems. The molecular structure of starch is complicated and somewhat nonlinear, which causes ductility problems. Retrogradation is a natural rise in crystallinity that occurs over time in starch and starch thermoplastics, resulting in increased brittleness. Movement is a market leader in the processing of starch-based goods [12]. Using proprietary blend compositions, the company creates a variety of starch-based goods.

1.6.2 CELLULOSE

Cellulose is most abundant constituent in all plant cell walls. Cellulose is a crystalline carbohydrate with a complicated structure. Cellulose varies from starch in that glucose units are linked by -1,4-glycosidic bonds in cellulose, whereas starch links are primarily -1,4 linkages. Cotton fibers and wood are most common raw materials used in the creation of cellulosic plastics. Plant fiber is dissolved in alkali and carbon disulfide to produce viscose, which is subsequently transformed to cellulose in cellophane form after being dissolved in sulfuric acid and sodium sulfate. To extract cellulose from other wood constituents, two techniques are now used. Sulfite and pre-hydrolysis kraft pulping use high pressure and chemicals to separate cellulose from lignin and hemicellulose, resulting in cellulose purity of better than 97%. cellulose acetate, cellulose esters (molded, extrusion, and films), and regenerated cellulose for fibers are most common cellulose derivatives used in industry. Cellulosic polymers are made by chemically modifying cellulose and are employed in a wide range of applications. Cellulose esters, especially cellulose nitrate and cellulose acetate, are utilized principally in film and fiber industries. A certain bacterium is capable of producing chemically pure cellulose. Bacterial cellulose is distinguished by its great purity and strength. It may be used to create high-tensile-strength objects. Bacterial cellulose's applications outside of culinary and medicinal fields are currently limited because to its expensive cost. Among the various uses are acoustic diaphragms, mining, paints, oil gas recovery, and adhesives.

1.7 CHITIN AND CHITOSAN

Chitin and chitosan are the most common natural amino polysaccharides and key bio-based natural polymers derived from prawn and crab shells, respectively. Chitin and chitosan are presently commercially generated using a chemical extraction technique from crab, shrimp, and prawn wastes. Chitin extraction chemically is a relatively severe method that involves acid demineralization, alkali deproteination, and deacetylation into chitosan. Chitin can also be made by enzyme hydrolysis or fermentation; however, these methods are not widely used since they are not cost-effective. Chitosan is biodegradable, biocompatible, chemically inert, has a high mechanical strength, has strong film-forming properties, and is inexpensive. Chitosan is used in a variety of goods and applications, such as medicines and cosmetics, as well as water treatment and plant protection. Different chitosan properties are required for each application, which vary depending on degree of acetylation and molecular weight. Chitosan can be used with a wide range of physiologically active compounds found in cosmetics. Chitosan has become a particularly intriguing material in such broad applications as biomaterials in medical devices and as a pharmaceutical component due to its low toxicity, biocompatibility, and bioactivity. Chitosan can be found in shampoos, rinses, and permanent hair dyes. In skin care sector, chitosan and its derivatives are also employed. Chitosan can be used to hydrate skin, and because it is less expensive, it may be able to compete with hyaluronic acid in this regard [11].

1.8 CURRENT STATUS AND FUTURE TRENDS

Bio-based feedstocks are not a new notion in the chemical industry. For more than a decade, they have been demonstrated to be industrially feasible on a huge scale. Bio-based products were not emphasized since price of oil was so cheap at the time, and the rise of oil-based products provided so many opportunities. Several causes, including a limited and unpredictable supply of fossil fuels, environmental concerns, and technological advancements, have accelerated the development of bio-based polymers and goods. The fossil fuel-based chemical business took more than a century to develop; however, the bio-based polymer sector is swiftly catching up to the fossil fuel-based chemical industry, which has increased significantly in the past 20 years. It is now feasible to produce bio-based polymers and other compounds from renewable resources because to breakthroughs in white biotechnology. First-generation bio-based polymer technologies were primarily focused on food resources such as maize, starch, and rice. As the food-versus-fuel argument intensified, the focus of technology changed to cellulose-based feedstocks, with a concentration on waste from wood and paper industries, food sectors, and even stems and leaves and solid municipal waste streams. While more of these technologies are being developed to address aforementioned waste streams, generating full spectrum of chemicals based on these technologies might take another 20 years [13].

1.9 CHALLENGES IN BIOPOLYMERS

Raw material management, bio-based material performance, and production cost are all issues that will need to be addressed in the next years. One of primary obstacles for the manufacture of bio-based monomers and bio-based polymers from renewable sources will be economies of scale. Large-scale facilities may be difficult to build due to a lack of expertise with new technologies and forecast of supply/demand balance. To make these technologies economically viable, (1) logistics for biomass feed stocks must be developed, (2) new manufacturing routes must be developed by replacing existing methods with high yields, (3) new microbial strains/enzymes must be developed, and (4) efficient downstream processing methods for bio-based product recovery must be developed. The present goal of bio-based sector is to create bio-versions of existing monomers and polymers. The performance of these objects is well established, and it is very easy to replace existing commodities with bio-versions that function similarly. Many of features of the aforementioned polymers are shared by today's fossil-based polymers. There have lately been several initiatives to create novel bio-based polymers with increased performance and value. Nature Works LLC, for example, has launched new PLA grades with enhanced thermal and mechanical properties. According to reports, the behavior of new PLA-triblock copolymers is comparable to that of a thermoplastic elastomer. Various polyamides, polyesters, polyhydroxyaloknates, and other materials with a wide range of final qualities are presently being developed for use in automotive, electronics, and biomedical applications [11].

1.10 CONCLUSIONS

Bio-based polymers are now closer to replacing conventional polymers than they have ever been. Due to advancements in biotechnologies and public awareness, bio-based polymers are now routinely found in a wide range of applications, from commodity to high-tech. Despite these developments, there are still a few drawbacks that prevent bio-based polymers from being widely commercialized in many applications. This is mostly due to their inferior performance and cost when compared to conventional polymers, which continues to be a key problem for bio-based polymers.

REFERENCES

1. Feldman D. Polymer history. *Des Monomers Polym* 2012;11: 1–15. https://doi.org/10.1163/156855508X292383.
2. Zhang ZP, Rong MZ, Zhang MQ. Polymer engineering based on reversible covalent chemistry: A promising innovative pathway towards new materials and new functionalities. *Prog Polym Sci* 2018;80:39–93. https://doi.org/10.1016/j.progpolymsci.2018.03.002.
3. Selim MS, Shenashen MA, El-Safty SA, Higazy SA, Selim MM, Isago H, et al. Recent progress in marine foul-release polymeric nanocomposite coatings. *Prog Mater Sci* 2017;87:1–32. https://doi.org/10.1016/j.pmatsci.2017.02.001.
4. Soares RMD, Siqueira NM, Prabhakaram MP, Ramakrishna S. Electrospinning and electrospray of bio-based and natural polymers for biomaterials development. *Mater Sci Eng C Mater Biol Appl* 2018;92:969–982. https://doi.org/10.1016/j.msec.2018.08.004.
5. Notario B, Pinto J, Rodriguez-Perez MA. Nanoporous polymeric materials: A new class of materials with enhanced properties. *Prog Mater Sci* 2016;78–79:93–139. https://doi.org/10.1016/j.pmatsci.2016.02.002.
6. Mohanty AK, Misra M, Hinrichsen G. Biofibres, biodegradable polymers and bio-composites: An overview. *Macromol Mater Eng* 2000;276–277:1–24. https://doi.org/10.1002/(SICI)1439-2054(20000301)276:1<1::AID-MAME1>3.0.CO;2-W.
7. Saba N, Jawaid M, Paridah MT, Al-othman OY. A review on flammability of epoxy polymer, cellulosic and non-cellulosic fiber reinforced epoxy composites. *Polym Adv Technol* 2016;27:577–590. https://doi.org/10.1002/pat.3739.
8. Todkar SS, Patil SA. Review on mechanical properties evaluation of pineapple leaf fibre (PALF) reinforced polymer composites. *Compos Part B Eng* 2019;174:106927. https://doi.org/10.1016/j.compositesb.2019.106927.
9. Namazi H. Polymers in our daily life. *Tabriz Univ Med Sci* 2017;7:73–74. https://doi.org/10.15171/bi.2017.09.
10. Kutz M. (Ed.). *Applied Plastics Engineering Handbook: Processing and Materials.* 2011. William Andrew.
11. Babu RP, O'Connor K, Seeram R. Current progress on bio-based polymers and their future trends. *Prog Biomater* 2013;2:8. https://doi.org/10.1186/2194-0517-2-8.
12. Shen L, Haufe J, Patel MK. Product overview and market projection of emerging bio-based plastics PRO-BIP 2009. Report for European polysaccharide network of excellence (EPNOE) and European bioplastics, 243, 1–245.
13. Carus M., Carrez, D., Kaeb, H., & Venus, J. *Level Playing Field for Bio-based Chemistry and Materials.* Nova Institute. 2011: 04–18.
14. Chen, S., & Ravallion, M. More relatively-poor people in a less absolutely-poor world. *Rev. Income Wealth* 2013;59(1):1–28.

15. Savenkova, L., Gercberga, Z., Nikolaeva, V. J. P. B., Dzene, A., Bibers, I., & Kalnin, M. Mechanical properties and biodegradation characteristics of PHB-based films. *Process Biochem* 2000;35(6):573–579.
16. Reis, S. Analyzing land use/land cover changes using remote sensing and GIS in Rize, North-East Turkey. *Sensors* 2008;8(10):6188–6202.
17. Chen, G., Li, S., Jiao, F., & Yuan, Q. Catalytic dehydration of bioethanol to ethylene over TiO2/γ-Al2O3 catalysts in microchannel reactors. *Catalysis Today* 2007; 125(1–2):111–119.

2 Characterization of polymeric materials for biomedical applications

Barnika Chakraborty

CONTENTS

2.1 Introduction 13
2.2 Characterization of polymeric materials based on their sources having
     biomedical applications 14
     2.2.1 Naturally occurring biodegradable polymeric materials 14
           2.2.1.1   Collagen 15
           2.2.1.2   Gelatin... 17
           2.2.1.3   Fibrin... 18
           2.2.1.4   Hyaluronic acid 19
           2.2.1.5   Chitosan 20
           2.2.1.6   Starch 22
           2.2.1.7   Alginate...23
           2.2.1.8   Silk 24
           2.2.1.9   Polyhydroxyalkanoates (PHA)...26
           2.2.1.10 Sundew adhesives 26
     2.2.2 Synthetic biodegradable polymers...27
2.3 Conclusion 28
References...29

2.1 INTRODUCTION

Polymers are large molecules that are composed of simpler and smaller subunits called monomers. Polymers hold the major advantage in being biodegradable and non-toxic. They act as proteinaceous enzymes that date back to the 19th century [1]. However, their efficiency held back their shell life real long to the 21st century and beyond. Over the years, polymers have proven to be more biocompatible than other materials such as alloys, ceramics, and metals [2–3]. Biocompatibility, i.e., the healthy relationship between the foreign polymeric material and the body tissues, is the key. The physical and chemical properties of the polymers provoke such compatibility, thus fitting them into the role. Properties such as molecular weight, solubility,

DOI: 10.1201/9781003319139-2

surface energy, lubricity, shape, reaction with water affect biocompatibility favorably for such operations [4]. Not only with the interaction but also with the metabolism, degradation, and removal from the body, polymeric materials are highly advantageous over other biomaterials. Other factors that contribute to polymers being effective biomaterials are as follows:

1. The degradation time of the biomaterial, i.e., polymeric materials coincide with the degradation/healing time of the body tissues.
2. Materials possess suitable permeability that is expected for biomedical applications.
3. Materials should have enough mechanical strength to regenerate within patient's body.

The diversity of polymeric materials that are ideally significant is immense, with each tailored for specific biomedical applications. Apart from such applications, polymeric materials are also utilized for the development of therapeutic devices, three-dimensional porous scaffolds for tissue engineering, drug delivery, and so on. Biodegradable biomaterials can exhibit a variety of biological and physicochemical properties of different tissues and are thus used as large implants, small implants, porous structures, plain membranes for guided tissue regeneration, and multifilament meshes for tissue engineering [5]. The biodegradable polymeric materials can be used in micro- or nanoscale drug delivery systems as well [6]. We will deal with all such applications in detail.

2.2   CHARACTERIZATION OF POLYMERIC MATERIALS BASED ON THEIR SOURCES HAVING BIOMEDICAL APPLICATIONS

On the basis of source and composition, polymers can be classified majorly into two types:

a. Naturally occurring biodegradable polymeric materials
b. Synthetic biodegradable materials

We will discuss each one of them in detail, with examples of each type specifying their biomedical applications.

2.2.1 NATURALLY OCCURRING BIODEGRADABLE POLYMERIC MATERIALS

Naturally occurring biodegradable polymeric materials can be either proteins, polysaccharides, or a group of polyesters. Proteinaceous biomaterials include collagen, silk, and fibrin, whereas polysaccharides contain starch, alginate, and chitin [7–9]. Polyesters include polyhydroxyalkanoates (PHA), sundew adhesives, and ivy nanoparticles, which also fall under the category of naturally occurring biodegradable polymeric materials. The latter functions as specific nanocarriers in drug delivery [10, 11]. Let us discuss with examples of each kind in detail.

2.2.1.1   Collagen

Collagen has huge utility among animal proteins for the preparation of specific components such as leathers, glue, gelatin, strings of musical instruments, and tennis rackets. It is the most abundant among all animal proteins. To discuss biomedical applications more in detail—primary function—to provide support to tissues, not only for their connection to cells or to each other but also for their specific functions [12]. It acts as the most prevalent, flexible, and dynamic substance that is essential for proper structural and functional components.

Structure: Rod-type polymer (approx. 300 nm)

Molecular Weight: Approximately 300 kDa

Formation: Formed from free amino acids that further undergo transcription, translation, and further modifications in different cells of osteoblasts and fibroblasts. Figure 2.1 showcases the structure of collagen in its helical form.

Diversity of Collagen: A total of 22 types are present, with types I–IV being the most common and type I being highly abundant.

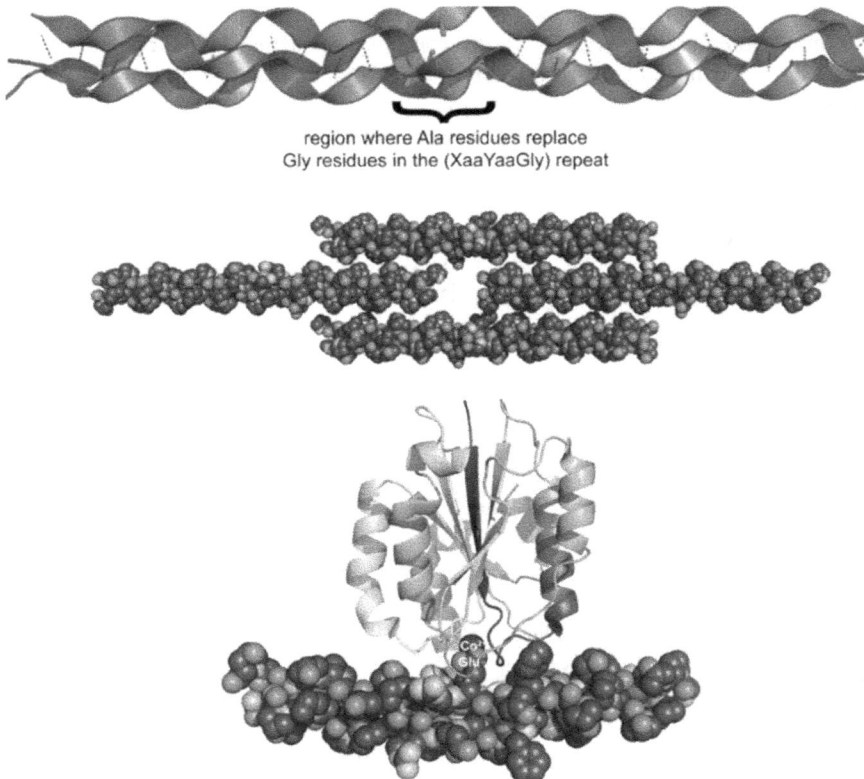

region where Ala residues replace
Gly residues in the (XaaYaaGly) repeat

FIGURE 2.1   Structure of collagen triple helices [13].

Degradation Methods: Degraded easily by several enzymes such as matrix metalloproteinases and collagenases to give further simplified amino acids.

Properties:

  a. Easy Enzymatic degradability
  b. Strong Mechanical Support Providing Ability
  c. High Biocompatibility
  d. Biodegradable and non-toxic upon exogenous application
  e. High tensile strength
  f. Weak antigenicity

Biomedical applications: Collagen has enormous biomedical applications, such as drug delivery systems by forming collagen shields, specifically in ophthalmology [14], can be used as sponges for burns or injuries, utilized as mini-pellets and tablets for protein delivery, helps in gel formulation combined with liposomes for sustained drug delivery, and acts as a controlling material for transdermal delivery. It can also act as nanoparticles for gene delivery, basic matrices for cell culture systems, for tissue engineering including skin replacement, bone substitutes, and artificial blood vessels and valves (Table 2.1).

Among other advantages, there are several other pharmaceutical companies such as Innocoll Pharmaceuticals Ltd. and Biomet that manufacture collagen-based drugs due to their anti-infectious properties [16].

Disadvantage of collagen-based biomaterial: Mild immunogenicity constricts its biomedical application to some extent [17]. Other disadvantages include the cost of collagen, an animal-driven polymer, and the risk of infectious diseases. Hence, some recombinant technologies are popping up in order to do away with the same and only keep positivity intact [18]. This could be brought about by simple modification of amino acid sequences. The issue with such a type of modification lies

---

TABLE 2.1

Biomedical applications of every specific composition and forms of collagen [15]

Composition	Biomaterial form	Applications
Collagen	Gel	Drug Delivery
	Sponge	Wound Healing; Drug Delivery; Skin Replacement
	Hollow fiber tubing	Cell Culture for Nerve Regeneration
	Sphere	Microcarrier for Drug Delivery System
	Membrane	Wound Healing; Dialysis; Tissue Regeneration; Skin patches
	Rigid Form	Bone Repair
Collagen +GAG	Membrane	Tissue Regeneration; Skin Patches
Collagen + Hydroxyapatite	Powder sponge	Bond filling and Repair of Drug Delivery

in the fact that they cannot effectively operate at areas of stability and strength, at more guarded and significant organs, i.e., heart and brain. Here, posttranslational modification is something that is yet to have some light thrown upon.

2.2.1.2 Gelatin

Sources of gelatin: Collagen on hydrolysis under several mediums such as acidic, alkaline, or under the targeted action of any specific enzyme gives gelatin [19]. Considering its origin, it is also figured to have similar properties that makes it a well-defined biomaterial for biomedical applications. The major advantage and additional properties that gelatin possess over collagen is its low-cost, versatility, ability to produce thermoreversible gel, being water permeable, and water soluble. It can also be obtained from porcine skin, bovine skin, and bones. Gelatin, alongside collagen, contributes to more than 30% of the total proteins in most animals. Figure 2.2 showcases the composition of amino acid that are present in gelatin.

Properties favoring biomedical applications: Properties such as biodegradability, non-toxicity, and biocompatibility make it a perfect match for functions mentioned formerly, such as stabilizers in vaccines for measles, mumps, and rubella and micro- and nanocarrier used in broad-scoped drug delivery systems [20, 21]. Owing to its above-mentioned properties, gelatin can contribute as an extremely versatile biopolymer for a wide range of drug delivery systems [22]. Gelatin nanoparticles are effective in cell amplification. They function extra-ordinarily for the brain and also for intravenous delivery [23]. They are contemporarily found to manufacture huge efficiencies for drug delivery and protein-loading.

Another majorly functional form of gelatine is BSA (bovine serum albumin)-loaded microparticles, which can be embedded within scaffolds of polycaprolactone (PCL) and polylactide(PLA). These can favor tissue engineering, bone regeneration, and repair [24]. BSA-loaded gelatin microparticles can be prepared by grinding freeze-dried membranes of gelatin and BSA. Gelatin can act as antifungal applications if they are polyene loaded. They also aid in fighting against skin infections [25]. Gelatins can act as polymeric additives when they are adhesive based. The properties of such a version of gelatin make it quite comfortable for its role. Its characteristics as a bioadhesive and reaction with water make it fit for drug release, bonding via its properties as an adhesive, wound healing like biomedical applications [26]. Figure 2.3 showcases the structural formation of gelatin chemically.

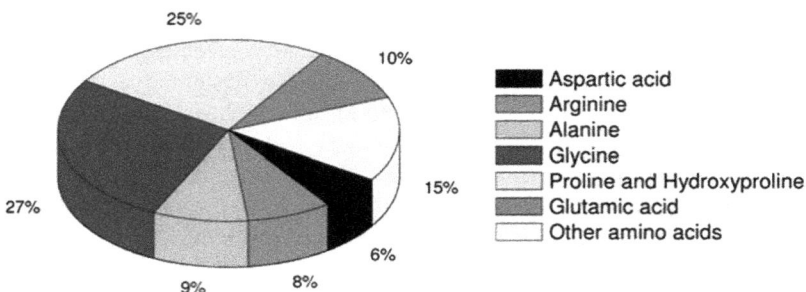

FIGURE 2.2 Amino acid composition of gelatin.

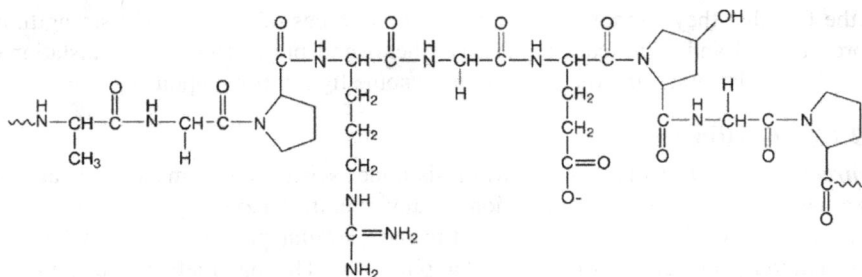

FIGURE 2.3   Basic structure of gelatin [27].

Disadvantages of gelatin: Considering its origin, it is observed to be driven by various religious-related issues, as porcine- and bovine-derived products are forbidden in Judaism and Buddhism [28]. It has had its functions limited due to poor mechanical properties. However, keeping in view the wide use of gelatin in several industries, likely in food and pharmaceuticals, solutions are being sought to do away with the disadvantages. Like always, an effective solution has been the use of recombinant technologies [29].

2.2.1.3   Fibrin

Molecular Weight: 360 kDa
Properties [30]:

    a. biodegradability
    b. Abundantly available
    c. Biocompatibility
    d. High elastic and viscous properties
    e. Excellent deformability

Figure 2.4 showcases the flowchart of the structure of fibrinogen and its conversion to fibrin involving the pathways of dissolution using enzymes and proteins.

Biomedical Applications: It is a highly advantageous biopolymer that helps in blood clotting naturally, advanced cell adhesion, surgical procedures, and reconstructive surgery [32]. Fibrin helps in the generation of a number of tissues, such as heart tissues, tendons, nervous tissue, and respiratory tissues. It can play its role as a drug-carrier vehicle, acting greatly for bioactive molecules acting for drugs, chemotherapy agents, or antibiotics. It is due to its properties of injectability and biodegradability [33]. Fibrin was successfully used against chronic cutaneous wounds recently. It was catered with mixing keratinocytes with fibrin. Fibrin contributes to tissue engineering processes due to its release of growth factors.

Disadvantages: Fibrin-based polymers have specific limitations in sustaining their mechanical ability. They are unstable, and thus, quick degradation of the same occurs even before the targeted mission is achieved. Nevertheless, such advantages can be eliminated by embedding stronger polymers by recombination and using cross-linking techniques at micro- and nanolevels.

Leukocyte $\alpha_M\beta_2$

Fibrinogen

E domain

D domain

D:D

Db

Da

α_2-PI

β_C

Plgn

tPA

XIII

B

A

427

γ'

411

Thrombin

γA

Platelet $\alpha_{IIb}\beta_3$

411

XIIIa XIIIb

427

GEGQQHHLGGAKQVRPEHPAETEYDSLYPEDDL.

γXL

GEGQQHHLGGAKQAGDV.

XIIIa XIIIa

γXL

Ca^{2+}

XIIIa A*

FPA FPB

Plasmin

Fibrin

Heparin
VE-cadherin

Plgn tPA

15

B

β_C

Ee

γ' 17 EA

γ-dimer

α_C PAI-2

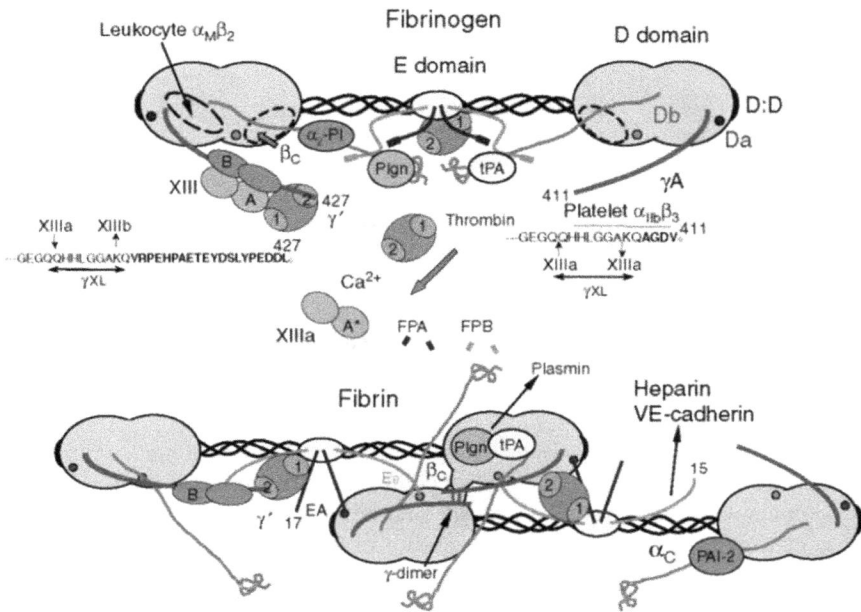

FIGURE 2.4 Diagram of fibrinogen and its conversion to fibrin [31].

2.2.1.4 Hyaluronic acid

Hyaluronic acid (HA) belongs to the GAG family and consists of alternate chain bindings of N-acetyl-d-glucosamine and glucuronic acid. It occurs in abundance in natural sources such as synovial fluids, rooster combs, and bovine vitreous humor. It is present in almost all specified tissues in vertebrates.

Polysaccharides are arranged in a linear manner to contribute to the structure. HA is essential for biomedical applications such as cellular signaling, wound repair, wound dressing, and also for the organization of matrix [34, 35]. HA is currently being discovered to act as building blocks for establishing newer biomaterials that find applications in cell therapy, tissue engineering, 3D cell culture, etc. [36, 37]. The same is found to act as free radical scavenger [38]. They can stimulate angiogenesis and regulate injury-induced inflammation. Additionally, noteworthy properties that can together make it the best fit for tissue engineering include the following:

a. potency immunoneutral
b. cell migration and differential functional activities
c. aqueous solubility making it more porous

Figure 2.5 showcases the chemical structures of monomers constituting the polymer hyaluronic acid (HA). For example, an HA-based product, HYAFF 11 is found to behave as carrier vehicle for growth factors, stem cells, and morphogens. HA-based products are found to play an important role in injectable soft tissue fillers thereby

Hyaluronic Acid (HA) Unit

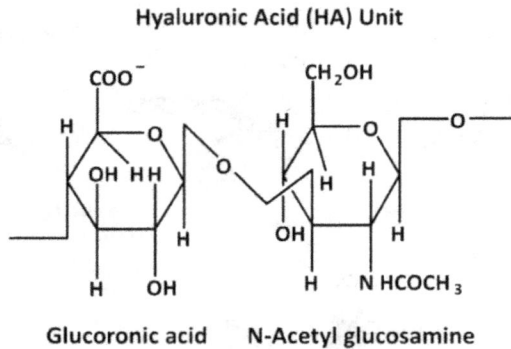

Glucoronic acid   N-Acetyl glucosamine

FIGURE 2.5   Structure of Hyaluronic Acid (HA) [42].

replacing collagen-based materials. Moreover, HA can now act well within complex scaffolds [39]. They can help protect complex eye tissues during surgeries, such as glaucoma, cataract, or corneal transplantation. HA products that are viscous in nature can reduce pain and improve mobility of joint in patients when applied as synovial fluid substitutes [40]. HA can be further modified chemically to give different derivatives, such as esters and HA gels. However, such modifications have failed being promising forever. They, on the other hand, resulted in degraded beneficiary chemical properties due to hydrolytic degradation. Herein lie its limitations in diversification [41].

2.2.1.5   Chitosan

Going forward, among other important naturally derived biodegradable polymers is chitin/chitosan. Chitin is reportedly the second most abundant polymer, and chitosan is a derivative of the former. It occurs naturally among exoskeleton of insects [43]. It is mainly composed of glucosamine and N-acetyl glucosamine combined [44]. However, such linkages can be broken down by human enzyme, e.g., lysozymes. However, the major disadvantage of chitosan over other polymers lies in its low mechanical strength, low tensile strength, and modulus range. Another disadvantage lies in its insolubility in organic solvents, thus making hydrophobic drug delivery difficult. Chitosan shows noteworthy application in tissue engineering and biomedical applications. They are also seen to perform well in complex scaffolds and work in vivo. Figure 2.6 depicts the chemical structure of chitosan and its derivatives. Chitosan can chelate with Calcium and Magnesium ions—a scaffold that helps destroy the bacterial wall and change its permeability [46]. Such properties make it hugely efficient for biomedical applications and tissue engineering. Oral mode of administration allowance is a major advantage.

Chitosan-based scaffolds can now be prepared in nanometre scale making it more conductive, enhancing better tissue formation. Biomaterials based on chitosan participated in cartilage repair due to their similarity with GAGs available within cartilage.

To overcome its limitations and bring to highlight the beneficiary aspects of chitosan, Tamburaci et al. introduced diatomite with chitosan. Improvement was observed

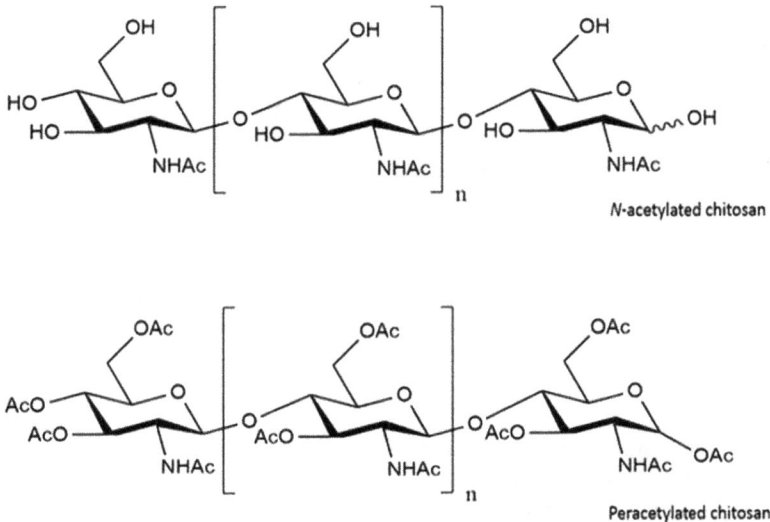

FIGURE 2.6   Chemical structure of chitosan and its derivatives [45].

in the combined scaffold with respect to the surface area, protein adsorption abilities, swelling properties, lesser cytotoxic effect, roughness, and improved biocompatibility. Properties such as proliferation and alkaline phosphate activity were also observed to increase extensively [47].

Similar derivatives like, glutaraldehyde cross-linked collagen chitosan hydrogel, reflected promising results toward adipose tissue engineering. The photopolymerizable hydrogels also act as cell carrier vehicles and make chitosan perfect for tissue engineering. It can also be used for treatment of wounds and burns. Chitosan combined with silver nanoparticles are reportedly observed to perform the following benefits- [48, 49]

a. Form successful scaffolds for healing of wounds.
b. Held anti-bacterial properties when tested against *E. coli.*
c. Blood clotting properties developed.

Apart from such biomedical applications, the most important application finds in its role of acting as drug delivery systems. Among the most significant roles include the following:

a. Carboxymethyl chitin nanoparticles coupled with $FeCl_3$ and $CaCl_2$, proved to be non-toxic to mouse.
b. Controlled drug delivery for HIV.
c. Able to penetrate the blood-brain barrier to deliver drugs and help inhibit HIV replication in neutral bodies.
d. Chitosan nanoparticles can encapsulate the antiretroviral drugs that target HIV cells helping effectively control viral proliferation in target T cells [50].

e. Chitosan nanoparticles make them more visible to immune system, making uptake by phagocytes more efficient [51].
f. Exhibits anticancer activities at optimum pH with controlled drug delivery.
g. Chitosan-based materials can participate in insulin delivery systems making the process better sustained and faster on-demand responses.
h. Helps regulate blood glucose levels.
i. Excellent biodegradability and biocompatibility makes it antiulcer, antiacid properties effectively.

Thus, to summarize, chitosan is an effective polymer that finds excellent applications diversified. Research is going on to do away with its limitations according to ability so on and so far.

2.2.1.6   Starch

Talking of polymers, among the most applicable naturally occurring polymers, comes starch. It is a basic source of energy that is composed of amylose (linear polymer made up of glucose acting as monomers) and amylopectin (branched polymer). The properties of starch depend on the ratio among the monomers, its biocompatible nature, the composition of minerals constituting it, the amount of phosphorous and phospholipid content, and its cell adhesion properties. Properties such as solubility, mechanical strength, surface area, thermal resistance, and digestibility toward enzymes determine their functionality, to be precise, in different forms, such as nanometre-sized particles or hydrogels [52]. Sometimes starch blended with separate scaffolds can help develop better properties. The following Figure 2.7 showcases the biomedical applications of starch, a highly bioavailable and renewable natural polymer.

Starch blended with PCL shows better properties of reduced stiffness and can overcome one of the major limitations of high moisture sensation. Starch-blended products are hugely cost-effective due to the low cost of raw base products [54]. Starch can be also blended with SPCL to give effective tissue engineering properties. Most

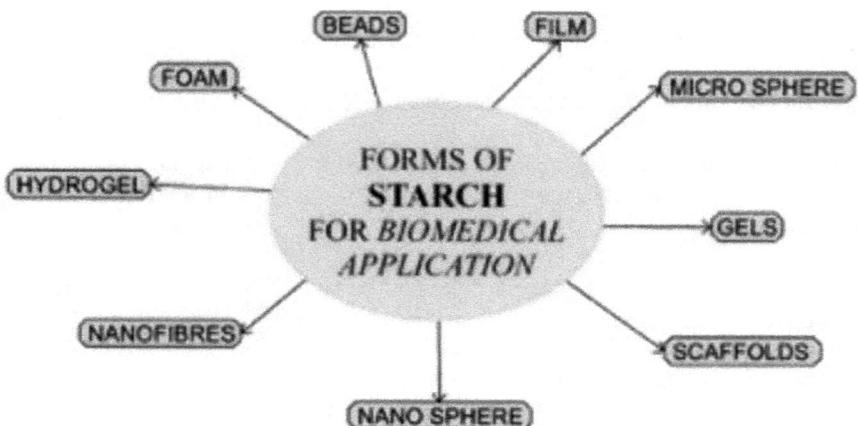

FIGURE 2.7   Biomedical applications of starch [53].

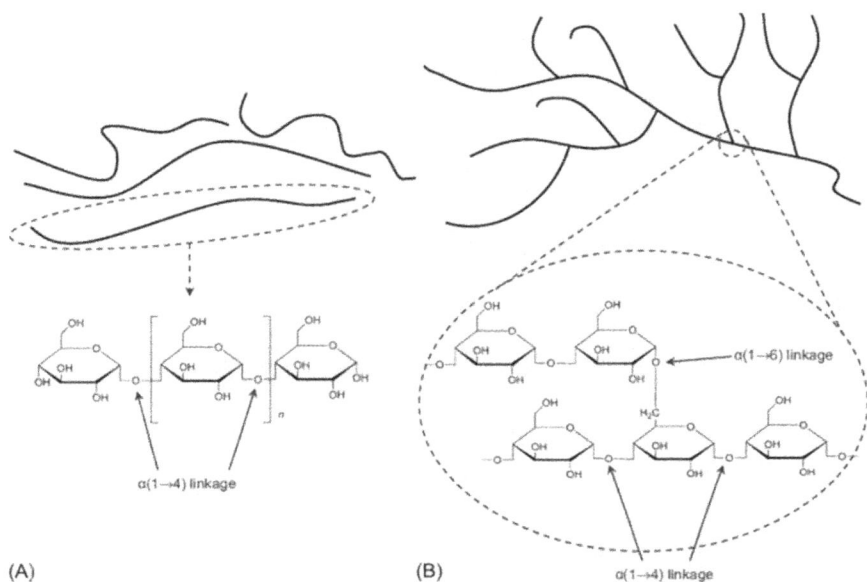

FIGURE 2.8   Structure and bindings of starch [56].

importantly, the drug delivery systems can happen in different forms such as hydrogels. Major advantage lies in their possibility of oral administration and site-specific delivery [55]. Additionally, they can also participate in colon-specific delivery systems due to their properties of thermal stability and less solubility. However, to be practical, not all its theoretical proofs have given promising results when applied practically on a large scale in an industrial level. Research is still going on to get better performance effectively. Physical modifications and derivatives can bring about positivity to certain extent, as believed. Figure 2.8 reflects the structure and bindings of starch.

2.2.1.7   Alginate

The above-mentioned polysaccharide is extracted from the cell wall of brown seaweeds. Due to its availability naturally and in abundance, it can be found at low-cost, making the entire manufacturing process cost-effective. They also occur abundantly extracellularly in bacteria. Properties that make them famous include the following (Figure 2.9):

   a. Biocompatibility
   b. Non-toxicity
   c. Non-inflammatory
   d. Low cost

Applications, like all former polymers, include drug delivery, tissue engineering, and wound healing by sodium alginate, myocardial tissue generation, and clinical applications. However, the major disadvantages still lie in their mechanical strength,

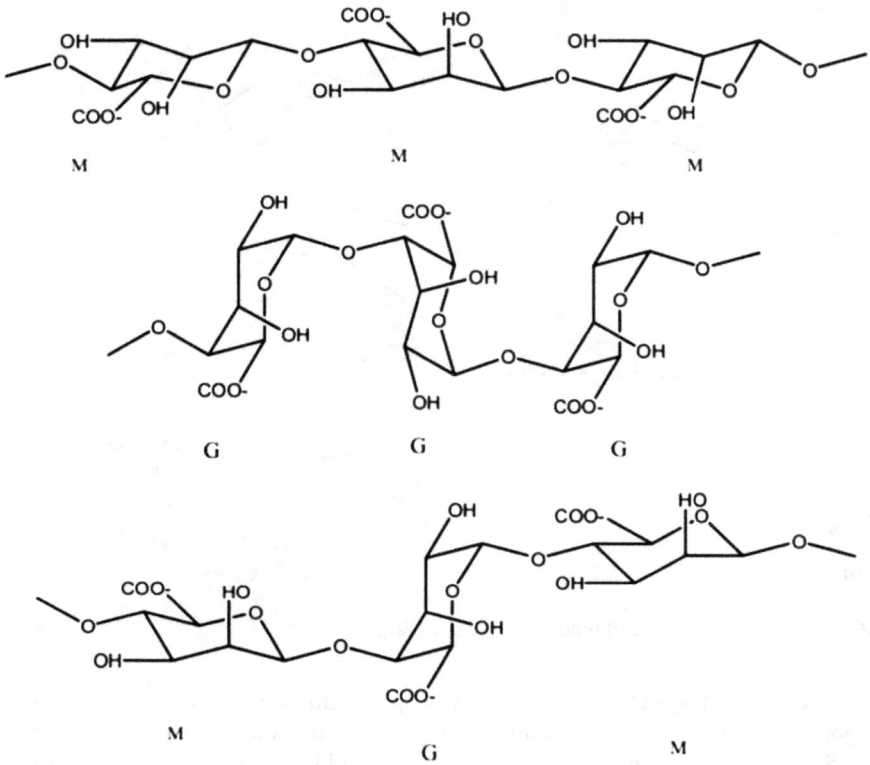

FIGURE 2.9 Structural units of alginate (M = mannuronic acid and G = guluronic acid) [59].

lesser ability to adhere to cells and lack of biodegradability [57]. Such disadvantages are attempted to be taken care of by maintaining complex scaffolds while combining alginate with other polymers such as previously discussed chitosan, hyaluronic acid, or carbohydrate sources such as agarose, gelatin, or by creating collagen/alginate scaffold or even DNA. Another major advantage lies in its negative nature. It helps to get attracted toward positively charged metals to form successful scaffolds [58]. It can operate in different forms such as hydrogels, microspheres, sponges, elastomers, and fibers. Research is still on the process for the effective control over the drug delivery of alginate-based compounds to manufacture its duration and sequencing of delivery to revolutionize the use of such a highly bioavailable polymer.

2.2.1.8 Silk

Silk is a natural fiber that can be obtained from the silkworm *Bombyx mori*. The structure consists of linked proteins [60]. It has been used in biomedical purposes for ages now. The structure consists of two SF proteins that are oriented parallel and can be linked via a layer of silk sericin protein. However, the biocompatibility of silk is still under questionable status [61]. The following figure 2.10 shows the formation of different biomaterials formed from silk and its derivatives.

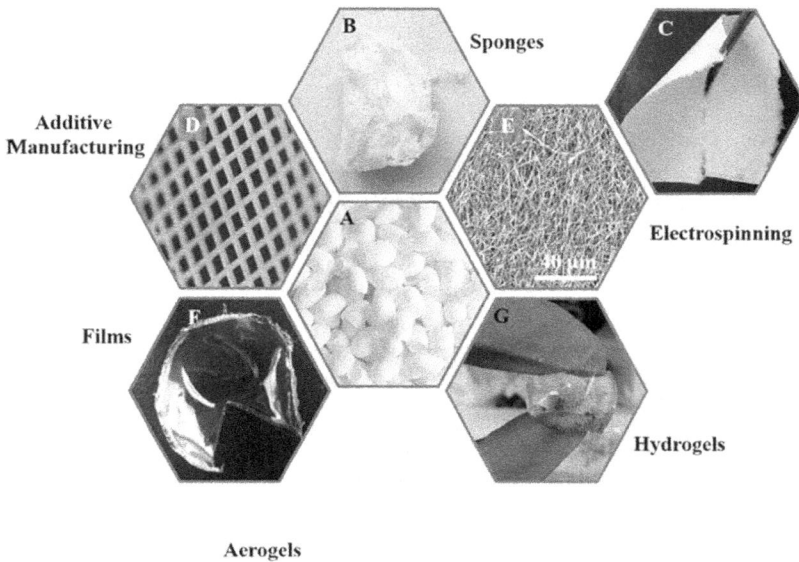

FIGURE 2.10 The different forms of silk and its derivative giving different biomaterials [61].

Effective properties that help silk to behave and form suitable biopolymer include the following:

a. Semi-crystalline structure gives high mechanical properties and has high tensile strength.
b. Elasticity and flexibility shows noteworthy advancement.
c. Ten-fold better strength-to-density ratio than other alloys such as steel [62].
d. Mechanical properties, biodegradability, and lower solubility in acid are quite advantageous.
e. Varieties of noble applications in genetic and tissue engineering.

Silk can find applications in several forms, such as nanofilms, gels, nanofibers, and foam. Fields such as drug delivery, wound repair, bioinking, 3D bioprinting, and clinical practice are all included in its applications. Like all other biopolymers, they also function better on scaffolds. They are advantageous over normal silk fiber, as proved by Shao et al., in the following patterns:[63]

a. The fibers were manufactured by the process of electrospinning, using electrical energy.
b. The modulus and breaking stress increased by an amount of 90-fold and two-fold, respectively, over the initial natural amount.
c. Scaffold portrayed better biocompatibility, proliferation, biomineralization, and cell adhesion, thus apparently removing the disadvantages that it had as a natural fiber.

d. Enhanced mechanical strength and biomimetic properties made the scaffold more promising than ever in the field of tissue engineering, and the list of improvements continues.

Other groups have also demonstrated similar advancements for several other scaffold such as hair keratin blended scaffolds and shidaiyi for skin tissue engineering. For skin, they have developed advanced properties such as the following: [64]

a. Great hemostatic properties
b. Low inflammatory potential
c. High permeability toward oxygen and water vapour.

In drug delivery systems too, silk fibers have better blended properties to help incorporate more sensitive drug into the body. Diverse drugs can be delivered applying this as a vehicle. Its ability to work in adverse pH conditions makes drug release easier. Protein and anticancer molecules fall under the range of deliverable drugs by silk. However, research is still under way to improve the efficiency of functioning of all the applications of SF [65].

2.2.1.9 Polyhydroxyalkanoates (PHA)

Next important natural polymer is polyhydroxyalkanoates (PHA), a polyester which is biodegradable in nature. It is mainly utilized for carbon and energy storage purposes [66]. Figure 2.11 shows the chemical structure of PHA in general.

Like all previous polymers, PHA also has similar mention-worthy properties of being biocompatible, biodegradable, non-toxic to play important roles in similar fields such as tissue engineering, drug delivery, wound repair, and additionally, this time, as a substitute for implantable devices [68]. The disadvantages/limitations have also been pulled up similarly as low mechanical strength, low thermal stability, hydrophobicity at a higher level, slow degradation rate, and so on. Again, derivatives are prepared to do away with the limitations of PHA [69].

2.2.1.10 Sundew adhesives

It is a natural hydrogel obtained from a plant named Sundew Drosera, a carnivorous plant that can prepare this polysaccharide [70]. The stalk of the plant produces adhesives that are highly biocompatible and biodegradable. They allow neuron-shaped cells, fibroblasts, muscle cells, etc. to attach and grow on nanofibers [71]. However, there exists some notable drawbacks, which includes its ability to lose adhesion properties at very low temperature of −20°C to −80°C. A detailed study is yet to be

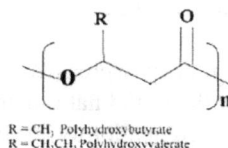

R = CH, Polyhydroxybutyrate
R = CH₂CH, Polyhydroxyvalerate

FIGURE 2.11   General chemical structure of polyhydroxyalkanoates [67].

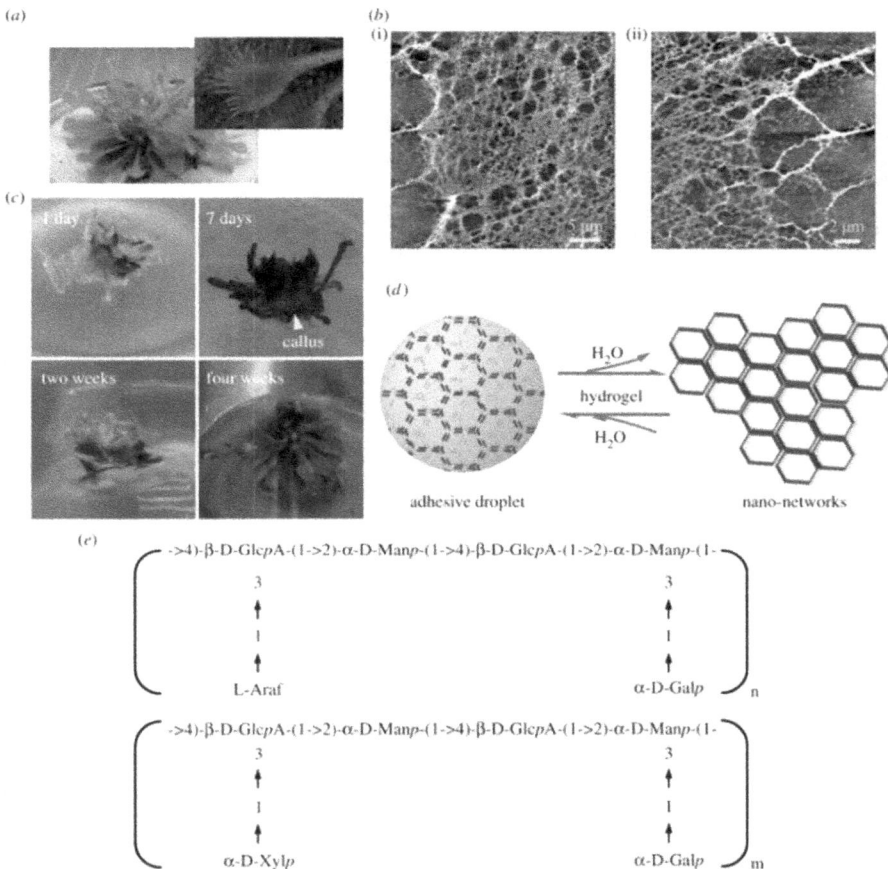

FIGURE 2.12 (a) Images of the plant and its stalks for secretion, (b) AFM images of nano-network architectures, (c) *In vitro* tissue culture of Sundew plant, (d) Schematic diagram of the same hydrogel, (e) Chemical Structure of Sundew Adhesive.

carried out for this process later. Figure 2.12 depicts a structure of Sundew Adhesive, chemically and structurally.

2.2.2 SYNTHETIC BIODEGRADABLE POLYMERS

Natural polymers have been seen to extract out their purpose well except for the few limitations that they already had. So to do away with those or, at least, lessen their effects, a number of synthetic biopolymers, like **saturated aliphatic polyesters**, are used.

A number of saturated aliphatic polyesters such as PGA, PLA, and PLGA copolymers play an important role in tissue engineering [72]. The structures of few of them are as follows (Figures 2.13–2.15):

PGA

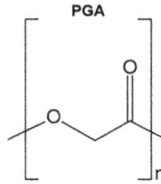

FIGURE 2.13 Structure of PGA.

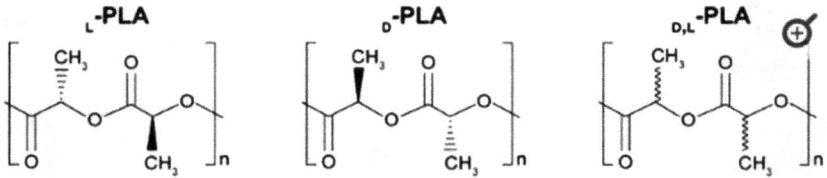

FIGURE 2.14 Structure of PLAs.

PLGA

x = # of units of lactic acid
y = # of units of glycolic acid

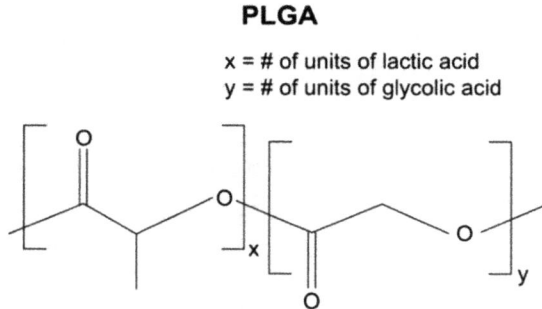

FIGURE 2.15. Structure of PLGA.

Other compounds synthesized artificially include polyanhydrides, polyurethane, and polyphosphazenes. However, the latter ones are quite less productive for market use. They also perform similar functions such as tissue engineering, wound healing but with some modified properties, such as better hydrosolubility and biocompatibility. PGA and PLA are also seen to be used in medical devices for implantation [73]. PGA can also be further used for waste water management, food products, and biological glue making [74]. PGA sheets help reduce post-operative pain and bleeding. Scaffold formation again helps improve properties.

2.3 CONCLUSION

In general, all biomaterials have their own kind of advantages and limitations—both natural and synthetic. We should focus on the advantages and try to develop them. By selecting the positive advantages, we can combine them artificially to obtain a wider horizon of biomedical applications. We can also focus on developing the number of fields polymer-based biomaterials can address.

REFERENCES

1. Barbucci, R. (2002) *Integrated Biomaterials Science*. New York: Kluwer Academic/ Plenum Publishers.
2. Langer, R., Vacanti, J. P. (1993) Tissue engineering. *Science (New York, N. Y.),* **260**(5110):920–926.
3. Vacanti, J. P., Langer, R. (1999) Tissue engineering: the design and fabrication of living replacement devices for surgical reconstruction and transplantation. *Lancet,* **354**(Suppl 1):S32–S34.
4. Kohane, D. S., Langer, R. (2008) Polymeric biomaterials in tissue engineering. *Pediatr Res,* **63**(5):487–491.
5. Vert, M. (2005) Aliphatic polyesters: great degradable polymers that cannot do everything. *Biomacromolecules,* **6**(2):538–546.
6. Gollwitzer, H., Ibrahim, K., Meyer, H., Mittelmeier, W., Busch, R., Stemberger, A. (2003) Antibacterial poly(D, L-lactic acid) coating of medical implants using a biodegradable drug delivery technology. *J Antimicrob Chemother,* **51**(3):585–591.
7. Freyman, T. M., Yannas, I. V., Yokoo, R., Gibson, L. J. (2001) Fibroblast contraction of a collagen–GAG matrix. *Biomaterials,* **22**(21):2883–2891.
8. Marijnissen, W. J. C. M., van Osch, G. J. V. M., Aigner, J. (2002) Alginate as a chondrocyte-delivery substance in combination with a non-woven scaffold for cartilage tissue engineering. *Biomaterials,* **23**(6):1511–1517.
9. Park, H., Choi, B., Hu, J., Lee, M. (2013) Injectable chitosan hyaluronic acid hydrogels for cartilage tissue engineering. *Acta Biomater,* **9**(1):4779–4786.
10. Lenaghan, S. C., Serpersu, K., Xia, L., He, W., Zhang, M. (2011) A naturally occurring nanomaterial from the Sundew (*Drosera*) for tissue engineering. *Bioinspir Biomim,* **6**(4):046009.
11. Huang, Y., Wang, Y. J., Wang, Y. (2015) Exploring naturally occurring ivy nanoparticles as an alternative biomaterial. *Acta Biomater,* **25**:268–283.
12. Gelse, K., Pöschl, E., Aigner, T. (2003) Structure C- function, and biosynthesis. *Adv Drug Deliv Rev,* **55**(12):1531–1546.
13. Shoulders, M.D., Raines, R. T. (2009) Collagen structure and stability. *National Library of Medicine,* **78**:929–958.
14. Lee, C. H., Singla, A., Lee, Y. (2001) Biomedical applications of collagen. *Int J Pharm,* **221**(1–2):1–22.
15. Chattopadhyay, S., Raines, R. T. (2014) Review collagen-based biomaterials for wound healing. *Biopolymers,* **101**(8):821–833.
16. Gruessner, U., Clemens, M., Pahlplatz, P. V., Sperling, P., Witte, J., Rosen, H. R. (2001) Improvement of perineal wound healing by local administration of gentamicin-impregnated collagen fleeces after abdominoperineal excision of rectal cancer. *Am J Surg,* **182**(5):502–509.
17. Koide, T. (2007) Designed triple-helical peptides as tools for collagen biochemistry and matrix engineering. *Philosophical Trans Royal Society B Biol Sci,* **362**(1484):1281–1291.
18. Brodsky, B., Ramshaw, J. A. (2017) Bioengineered Collagens. In: Parry, D. A. D., Squire, J. M., editors. *Fibrous Proteins: Structures and Mechanisms.* Cham: Springer International Publishing, pp. 601–629.
19. Ghasemi-Mobarakeh, L., Prabhakaran, M. P., Morshed, M., Nasr-Esfahani, M.-H., Ramakrishna, S., Poly, E. (2008) Electrospun poly(ε-caprolactone)/gelatin nanofibrous scaffolds for nerve tissue engineering. *Biomaterials,* **29**(34):4532–4539.

20. Burke, C. J., Hsu, T. A., Volkin, D. B. (1999) Formulation stability, and delivery of live attenuated vaccines for human use. *Crit Rev Ther Drug Carrier Syst*, **16**(1):1–83.
21. Gou, Y., Miao, D., Zhou, M., Wang, L., Zhou, H., Su, G. (2018) Bio-inspired protein-based nanoformulations for cancer theranostics. *Front Pharmacol*, **9**:421.
22. Saddler, J. M., Horsey, P. J. (1987) The new generation gelatins. A review of their history, manufacture and properties. *Anaesthesia*, **42**(9):998–1004.
23. Foox, M., Zilberman, M. (2015) Drug delivery from gelatin-based systems. *Expert Opin Drug Deliv*, **12**(9):1547–1563.
24. Ozkizilcik, A., Tuzlakoglu, K. (2014) A new method for the production of gelatin microparticles for controlled protein release from porous polymeric scaffolds. *J Tissue Eng Regen Med*, **8**(3):242–247.
25. Lakshminarayanan, R., Sridhar, R., Loh, X. J. (2014) Interaction of gelatin with polyenes modulates antifungal activity and biocompatibility of electrospun fiber mats. *Int J Nanomedicine*, **9**:2439–2458.
26. Cohen, B., Shefy-Peleg, A., Zilberman, M. (2014) Novel gelatin/alginate soft tissue adhesives loaded with drugs for pain management: structure and properties. *J Biomater Sci Polym Ed*, **25**(3):224–240.
27. Kommareddy, S., Amiji, M., Shenoy, D. (2007) Gelatin nanoparticles and their biofunctionalization. *Nanotechnologies for the Life Sciences*. https://doi.org/10.1002/9783527610419.ntls0011
28. Karim, A. A., Bhat, R. (2009) Fish gelatin: properties, challenges, and prospects as an alternative to mammalian gelatins. *Food Hydrocoll*, **23**(3):563–576.
29. Bigi, A., Cojazzi, G., Panzavolta, S., Roveri, N., Rubini, K. (2002) Stabilization of gelatin films by crosslinking with genipin. *Biomaterials*, **23**(24):4827–4832.
30. Ahmed, T. A. E., Dare, E. V., Hincke, M. (2008) Fibrin: a versatile scaffold for tissue engineering applications. *Tissue Eng Part B Rev*, **14**(2):199–215.
31. Mosesson, M. W. (2005) Fibrinogen and fibrin structure and functions. *J Thromb Haemost*, **8**(3): 1894–1904.
32. Rajangam, T., An, S. S. A. (2013) Fibrinogen and fibrin based micro and nano scaffolds incorporated with drugs, proteins, cells and genes for therapeutic biomedical applications. *Int J Nanomedicine*, **8**:3641–3662.
33. de La Puente, P., Ludeña, D. (2014) Cell culture in autologous fibrin scaffolds for applications in tissue engineering. *Exp Cell Res*, **322**(1):1–11.
34. Toole, B. P. (2004) Hyaluronan: from extracellular glue to pericellular cue. *Nat Rev Cancer*, **4**(7):528–539.
35. El Maradny, E., Kanayama, N., Kobayashi, H. (1997) The role of hyaluronic acid as a mediator and regulator of cervical ripening. *Hum Reprod*, **12**(5):1080–1088.
36. Allison, D. D., Grande-Allen, K. J. (2006) Review. Hyaluronan: a powerful tissue engineering tool. *Tissue Eng*, **12**(8):2131–2140.
37. Burdick, J. A., Prestwich, G. D. (2011) Hyaluronic acid hydrogels for biomedical applications. *Adv Mater*, **23**(12):H41–H56.
38. Prestwich, G. D. (2011) Hyaluronic acid-based clinical biomaterials derived for cell and molecule delivery in regenerative medicine. *J Control Release*, **155**(2):193–199.
39. Eppley, B. L., Dadvand, B. (2006) Injectable soft-tissue fillers: clinical overview. *Plast Reconstr Surg*, **118**(4):98e–106e.
40. Kato, Y., Nakamura, S., Nishimura, M. (2006) Beneficial actions of hyaluronan (HA) on arthritic joints: effects of molecular weight of HA on elasticity of cartilage matrix. *Biorheology*, **43**(3–4):347–354.
41. Lepidi, S., Grego, F., Vindigni, V. (2006) Hyaluronan biodegradable scaffold for small-caliber artery grafting: preliminary results in an animal model. *Euro J Vasc Endovasc Surg*, **32**(4):411–417.
42. Nasr, M. (2008) Intra-articular drug delivery: a fast growing approach. *Recent Pat Drug Deliv Formul*, **2**:231–237.

43. Kumar, M. N. V. R., Muzzarelli, R. A. A., Muzzarelli, C., Sashiwa, H., Domb, A. J. (2004) Chitosan chemistry and pharmaceutical perspectives. *Chem Rev,* **104**(12):6017–6084.
44. Raveendran, S., Rochani, A., Maekawa, T., Kumar, D. (2017) Smart carriers and nano-healers: a nanomedical insight on natural polymers. *Materials,* **10**(8):929.
45. Hao, C., Wang, W., Wang, S., Zhang, L., Guo, Y. (2017) An overview of the protective effects of chitosan and acetylated chitosan oligosaccharides against neuronal disorders. *Mar Drugs,* **15**:89.
46. Ahsan, S. M., Thomas, M., Reddy, K. K., Sooraparaju, S. G., Asthana, A., Bhatnagar, I. (2017) Chitosan as biomaterial in drug delivery and tissue engineering. *Int J Biol Macromol,* **110**:97–109.
47. Tamburaci, S., Tihminlioglu, F. (2017) Diatomite reinforced chitosan composite membrane as potential scaffold for guided bone regeneration. *Mater Sci Eng C,* **80**:222–231.
48. Madhumathi, K., Sudheesh Kumar, P. T., Abhilash, S., Sreeja, V., Tamura, H., Manzoor, K., Nair, S. V., Jayakumar, R. (2010) Development of novel chitin/nanosilver composite scaffolds for wound dressing applications. *J Mater Sci Mater Med,* **21**(2):807–813.
49. Kumar, P. T. S., Abhilash, S., Manzoor, K., Nair, S. V., Tamura, H., Jayakumar, R. (2010) Preparation and characterization of novel β-chitin/nanosilver composite scaffolds for wound dressing applications. *Carbohydr Polym,* **80**(3):761–767.
50. Gu, J., Al-Bayati, K., Ho, E. A., Ea, H. (2017) Development of antibody-modified chitosan nanoparticles for the targeted delivery of siRNA across the blood-brain barrier as a strategy for inhibiting HIV replication in astrocytes. *Drug Deliv Transl Res,* **7**(4):497–506.
51. Ramana, L. N., Sharma, S., Sethuraman, S., Ranga, U., Krishnan, U. M. (2014) Evaluation of chitosan nanoformulations as potent anti-HIV therapeutic systems. *Biochim Biophys Acta,* 1840;**2014**(1):476–484.
52. Kaur, L., Singh, J., Liu, Q. (2007) Starch – a potential biomaterial for biomedical applications. In: Mozafari, M. R., editor. *Nanomaterials and Nanosystems for Biomedical Applications.* Dordrecht: Springer, pp. 83–98.
53. Hemamalini, T., Dev, V. R. G. (2017) Comprehensive review on electrospinning of starch polymer for biomedical applications. *Int J Biol Macromol,* **106**:712–718.
54. Averous, L., Moro, L., Dole, P., Fringant, C. (2000) Properties of thermoplastic blends: starch–polycaprolactone. *Polymer,* **41**(11):4157–4167.
55. Saboktakin, M. R., Tabatabaie, R. M., Maharramov, A., Ramazanov, M. A. (2011) Synthesis and in vitro evaluation of carboxymethyl starch–chitosan nanoparticles as drug delivery system to the colon. *Int J Biol Macromol,* **48**(3):381–385.
56. Nasrollahzadeh, M., Issaabadi, Z. *An Introduction to Green Nanotechnology.* Amsterdam: ScienceDirect Topics.
57. Lee, K. Y., Mooney, D. J. (2012) Alginate: properties and biomedical applications. *Prog Polym Sci,* **37**(1):106–126.
58. Sharma, C., Dinda, A. K., Potdar, P. D., Chou, C.-F., Mishra, N. C. (2016) Fabrication and characterization of novel nano-biocomposite scaffold of chitosan–gelatin–alginate–hydroxyapatite for bone tissue engineering. *Mater Sci Eng C,* **64**:416–427.
59. Homayouni, A., Ehsani, M. R., Azizi, A., Yarmand, M. S., Razavi, H. (2007) Effect of lecithin and calcium chloride solution on the Microencapsulation process yield of calcium alginate beads. *Iran Polym J,* **16**(9):597–606.
60. Altman, G. H., Diaz, F., Jakuba, C. (2003) Silk-based biomaterials. *Biomaterials,* **24**(3):401–416.
61. Cao, T.-T., Zhang, Y.-Q. (2016) Processing and characterization of silk sericin from Bombyx mori and its application in biomaterials and biomedicines. *Mater Sci Eng C,* **61**:940–952.
62. Giesa, T., Arslan, M., Pugno, N. M., Buehler, M. J. (2011) Nanoconfinement of spider silk fibrils begets superior strength, extensibility, and toughness. *Nano Lett,* **11**(11):5038–5046.

63. Shao, W., He, J., Sang, F. (2016) Coaxial electrospun aligned tussah silk fibroin nanostructured fiber scaffolds embedded with hydroxyapatite-tussah silk fibroin nanoparticles for bone tissue engineering. *Mater Sci Eng C Mater Biol Appl,* **58**:342–351.

64. Gil, Eun S., Panilaitis, B., Bellas, E., Kaplan, David L. (2012) Functionalized silk biomaterials for wound healing. *Adv Healthc Mater,* **2**(1):206–217.

65. Hofer, M., Winter, G., Myschik, J. (2012) Recombinant spider silk particles for controlled delivery of protein drugs. *Biomaterials,* **33**(5):1554–1562.

66. Chen, G. Q. (2009) A microbial polyhydroxyalkanoates (PHA) based bio- and materials industry. *Chem Soc Rev,* **38**(8):2434–2446.

67. Priyadarshi, S., Shukla, A., Borse, B. B. (2014) Polyhydroxyalkanoates: role of Ralstonia eutropha. *Int J Biomed Adv Res,* **5**(2): 68–76.

68. Li, Z., Loh, X. J. (2017) Recent advances of using polyhydroxyalkanoate-based nanovehicles as therapeutic delivery carriers. *Wiley Interdiscip Rev Nanomed Nanobiotechnol,* **9**(3):e1429-n/a:e1429.

69. Chen, G. Q., Wu, Q. (2005) The application of polyhydroxyalkanoates as tissue engineering materials. *Biomaterials,* **26**(33):6565–6578.

70. Huang, Y., Wang, Y., Sun, L., Agrawal, R., Zhang, M. (2015) Sundew adhesive: a naturally occurring hydrogel. *J R Soc Interface,* **12**(107):20150226.

71. Zhang, M., Lenaghan, S. C., Xia, L. (2010) Nanofibers and nanoparticles from the insect-capturing adhesive of the Sundew (Drosera) for cell attachment. *J Nanobiotechnology,* **8**:20.

72. Seal, B., Otero, T. C., Panitch, A. (2001) Polymeric biomaterials for tissue and organ regeneration. *Mater Sci Eng Rep,* **34**(4–5):147–230.

73. Mano, J. F., Sousa, R. A., Boesel, L. F., Neves, N. M. (2004) Bioinert, biodegradable and injectable polymeric matrix composites for hard tissue replacement: state of the art and recent developments. *Composit Sci Technol,* **64**(6):789–817.

74. Buescher, J. M., Margaritis, A. (2007) Microbial biosynthesis of polyglutamic acid biopolymer and applications in the biopharmaceutical, biomedical and food industries. *Crit Rev Biotechnol,* **27**(1):1–19.

3 Toxicology assessment of polymeric material for implants

Neeraj Kumar Shrivastava, Devendra Singh, Sunil Kumar Verma, Anay Pratap Singh and Anshuman Srivastava

CONTENTS

3.1   Introduction 34
3.2   Use of old polymers but new composites 34
3.3   Material prerequisites for devices and implants 36
    3.3.1   Materials 37
        3.3.1.1   Polyethylene (PE) 37
        3.3.1.2   Polypropylene (PP) 37
        3.3.1.3   Polyurethane (PU) 38
        3.3.1.4   Polytetrafluoroethylene (PTFE) 38
        3.3.1.5   Silicone, e.g., Parylene, PDMS 38
        3.3.1.6   Polymethylmethacrylate (PMMA) 39
        3.3.1.7   Polyamide (PA) 39
        3.3.1.8   Liquid Crystal Polymer (LCP) 39
        3.3.1.9   Carbon Nanotube (CNT) composites 39
        3.3.1.10 Polyimide 40
3.4   Recent advances in select technologies for implant fabrication 40
    3.4.1   Injectable implants 40
    3.4.2   On-demand implants 40
    3.4.3   Expandable implants 41
    3.4.4   3D printing 41
    3.4.5   Novel drug delivery system 41
    3.4.6   Polymers as a building block for DD system 41
    3.4.7   Polymer as drug carrier 42
    3.4.8   Chemically linked polymer matrix 42
    3.4.9   Physical entrapment of drug 42
    3.4.10 Liposomes 42
    3.4.11 Nanoparticles 42
    3.4.12 Microspheres 42

DOI: 10.1201/9781003319139-3

3.5   Mechanism of drug release from polymer device 43
       3.5.1   Diffusion-controlled system 43
       3.5.2   Matrix system 43
       3.5.3   Chemically control systems... 43
       3.5.4   Subcutaneous implant devices... 44
       3.5.5   Toxicological assessment... 44
3.6   Subcutaneous implantation and explant evaluation..................................... 45
       3.6.1   Preparation of single-cell suspension 45
       3.6.2   Polymeric implant toxicological assessment of extract for
                chromosomal aberration assays.. 46
       3.6.3   Preparation of extract for *Salmonella*/microsome and
                chromosome aberration assay... 46
       3.6.4   In vitro cytotoxicity analysis 46
                3.6.4.1   Proliferation assay.. 46
                3.6.4.2   The growth rate of fibroblasts....................................... 46
                3.6.4.3   Pharmacological evaluation 47
                3.6.4.4   Chromosome aberration assay 47
3.7   Conclusion 48
References.. 48

3.1   INTRODUCTION

With the advancement in the drug delivery system, implantable systems like drug pumps and depots emerged as new systems for better-sustained release at localized sites for better action. Implants include drug sizes ranging from microsphere to a few mm in size; hormones and cells can also be loaded in implants. Example includes are drug-loaded composites, stents, biosensors, catheters, scaffold for tissue engineering, heart valves, pacemakers, etc. (1, 2) Polymer used in implants can be biodegradable as well as non-biodegradable, which depends on compatibility with the drug. USFDA-approved polymeric implants are Atrigel, Atridox, Gliadel, etc. (3, 4). One of the major advantages of using implants is that they are free from preservatives making them more useful, and the property of a material to be implanted must-have thermal stability and biocompatibility, and it must enhance cell adhesion and their proliferation. On the basis of implants used, various types of polymer used, like injectable implants, contain low-viscous polymer solution. After getting injected, these polymers get solidified (5, 6).

With the advancement in technology for the production of new biomaterial, it is necessary for evaluating their biological parameter using experimental animals. For the selection of experimental animals, the researcher must follow a 3-hour condition that is reduction using the smallest possible number of animals refinement repeating use of the same animal for different experiments and replacement use of cell culture microorganism chemicals in silico model or another method (7, 8).

3.2   USE OF OLD POLYMERS BUT NEW COMPOSITES

The physical and chemical qualities of implant materials have a significant impact on the implant's usability and outcome. The effect of material and implant design, for example, has been demonstrated to affect the payload release profile in vitro and in vivo, as well as the implant biodegradation/integrity in vivo (9). Implant materials should have appropriate mechanical qualities, thermal stability, biocompatibility, and the ability to encourage cell adhesion and proliferation, depending on the application. Implant applications broaden the range of desirable material features and drive the development of novel materials and composites. Moving from the bench to the bedside necessitates scalable and cost-effective implant fabrication. As a result, research is focused on developing novel composites and sequence-specific polymers (10). The goal of developing new materials is to improve a variety of features held by polymers currently utilized for implant production, such as thermal and mechanical properties, as well as biocompatibility. When two or more polymers, such as chitosan and polypyrrole, are combined, a polymeric composite was developed with better hydrophilicity and durability to electrochemical erosion results compared to polypyrrole alone (11). Instead of being employed as a separate implant material, this novel composite was used as a coating on metal stents. Laminating numerous layers of polymers is another way to make novel composites. Biodegradable polymeric coatings on biodegradable implants have been proposed to allow for the sequential release of payloads while avoiding the high temperature exposure of pharmaceuticals that a hot-melt technique would cause. The lipophilic PLGA/polylactic acid (PLA) covering of the hydrophilic chitosan methotrexate implant, for example, provided for better control over the initial burst and release rate of methotrexate as well as implant swelling and disintegration (12–14). This is due to the fact that the bilayer coating was done by dipping the DL-lactide: L-lactide implant into a PLA solution containing the medication of choice (15). Similarly, 20–30 layers of the coating were achieved by dipping blank polycaprolactone (PCL) implants into a PCL polymer solution containing various anticancer drugs (16). This approach allows for the delivery of a mixture of agents with different physicochemical qualities or potentially incompatible substances. The dipping procedure can also assist in preventing the strong burst release of the payload that is prevalent with extrusion-prepared polymeric implants. This is achievable because laminating consecutive layers achieves a more homogeneous distribution of the payload across the layers, as opposed to the surface-rich layers found with the extrusion process. A novel composite made up of laminated chitin and PLA has recently been created to improve the mechanical and thermal properties of bone and dental implants (17). The composite was made by hot-pressing preprepared PLA and PLA-chitin films, and tensile strength, elongation at break, and E module all showed that the composite was stronger than either film alone. The created composite was recommended as a possible replacement for metallic and ceramic materials in bone implants; however, no direct comparison to such materials was provided. Particle filters are another method used to create novel polymeric materials from nanofibers. The formulation of a nanocomposite scaffold made of chitosan-graft-poly(acrylic acid-co-acrylamide)/hydroxyapatite in a multistep freeze-drying technique is an example of such an approach (18). Preprepared nanohydroxyapatite (NHAP) particles were used as a bioactive filler in this scaffold, resulting in a porous scaffold loaded with N-HAP, with the addition of HAP improving the scaffold's capacity to promote cell proliferation. The imparted porosity, which was associated with the amount of N-HAP employed in scaffold creation, was blamed for the observed impact. Chitosan was combined with PCL and magnesium oxide (MgO) particles to generate a nanofibrous composite because of its polysaccharide structure, which promotes cellular proliferation (19). As demonstrated in vitro employing fibroblasts, the nanofibrous scaffold had good mechanical properties, was low in cytotoxicity, and supported cell development. Electrospinning techniques were used to create the novel composite, eliminating the requirement for cross-linking chemicals, which have been demonstrated to have negative biocompatibility consequences (20). This contrasts with a nanofibrous scaffold made only of MgO particles and PCL (21). The inclusion of MgO nanoparticles as fillers increased the mechanical characteristics of the fibers (as determined by a tensile test). This is mostly owing to the fibers' homogeneous dispersion, which results in increased flexibility and strength. Despite the lack of bioactive fillers that have been considered to be important for mediating cell attachment in this composite, HAP developed on the surface of the composite scaffold but not on clean polymer sheets after incubation in simulated biological fluid. As a proof of concept, the composite was found to be biocompatible in vivo; however, no medicinal usage was investigated.

3.3   MATERIAL PREREQUISITES FOR DEVICES AND IMPLANTS

Designed for enduring usage in the human body, a device or implant must fulfill specified parameters. If conditions aren't met, the client may undergo negative side effects and otherwise possibly die. As a result, before being implanted into the human body, a gadget must be properly wrapped. In this research, the term "packaging" denotes to the interfacial material that exists amid the human environment and the device during the course of its operation within the body—the packaging functions as a barrier, averting waste products from moving between the device and the client. To allow a foreign object to be implanted into a human body, size is significant for not just throughout the implantation surgery but also for the period of the object's stay in the body. The object's survival and the client's ease are both governed by its size. As a result, the object must be packed in order to lessen trauma on the neighboring bones, muscles, and tissues wherever it has been implanted. The device's compact size also lets for negligibly intrusive installation practices. Even though smaller sizes compromise the structural integrity of robust devices, the need for ease frequently overrides structural integrity concerns (22). As a result, implant packaging and substrates must be comparable to a thin film covering the entire device.

Because the human body is always in motion, the packaging needs to handle pressures and jolts, as well as the rare abnormal and abrupt impulses arising from human activities and unexpected motions. Implants are utilized as an added infrastructure for the body's healing and redevelopment, for example, bone substitution. Furthermore, because the implants and gadgets are constantly exposed to the heat of the human body, the packaging needs to be efficient and functional at body temperature for a needed period of time. As a number of materials denatures when exposed to innumerable temperatures, and since edging can take place over time, the packaging and materials used need to work effectively and efficiently in over human body temperature range with, hampering its native function. As a result, electrical protection for packing films is essential to ensure that there is no excessive electrical interference under the influence of the external environment, such as muscles, bones, etc. The most popular pacemaker, for example, has polyurethane leads. Furthermore, certain implants and devices must be implanted in locations where electrical signals are present, such as the brain and spine. As a result of the insulation package, no electrical leaks to or from the device occur, which could damage the gadget or put the owner's health in danger.

3.3.1 MATERIALS

In biomedical device packaging and implants, a widespread series of polymers can be commissioned. It provides flexibility to tailor the conclusive qualities with regard to packaging material to meet specific needs. This topic is a hotspot in the market because of its applicability in various regions of the body. There are some polymer application methods in devices. Designers and medical implants have two options: Polymer can be used as an individual protecting covering or bonding agent to cap the gap amid two surfaces. Implantable sensors which oversee the gastrointestinal system pH level require biocompatibility to prevent oxidization from the acidic enzymes present in the stomach; hence, the sensor needs to use packaging that is both oxidization-resistant and allows for RF signal transmission. The Medtronic Bravo pH System device is one such commonly utilized device in the business, with patients reporting no discomfort after having it implanted (23). The device was packaged with an epoxy covering and nevertheless well-covered till the two-day assessment phase. Combinations of epoxy and glass, or silicone and glass, have been utilized as bonding agents in sealing devices used as implants to encapsulate structures and guard implants with the biological environment. Chang et al. competed for the two different methods to find out which would provide an extended lifespan within the body and established that the adhesion promoter and silicone amalgamation resulted in extensive lifespan; nonetheless, results did not show any significant confirmation of strain and stress effects on the packaging the aforementioned (24). Aside from epoxy, a variety of industrially accessible synthetic polymers are employed, with brief depictions of each provided beneath.

3.3.1.1 Polyethylene (PE)

Currently, there are two types of polyethylene first one is high-density polyethylene, and the second one is low-density polyethylene which is categorized on the basis of their molecular weight. With the increase in molecular weight, the material strength improves, but there is a decrease in elasticity (25). The techniques and characterization for ultra-high-molecular weight polyethylene are specified in depth. Ceramic polystyrene couplings showed less fracture rates and audible component-related noise when associated with typical ceramic to ceramic couplings, the ineffectiveness of PE for complete hip arthroplasty (25). Furthermore, the ceramic–polystyrene combination did not show reduced osteolysis. Hence, there were by no means substantial statistical variations. Polyethylene components, contrariwise, can be taken care of to minimize osteolysis (26, 27).

3.3.1.2 Polypropylene (PP)

It is a thermoplastic polymer that can be adjusted matching to density and classified into copolymer and homopolymer elements, with the main distinction being the material's strength. It is typically utilized in urogynecology to take care of stress, urine incontinence, and pelvic organ prolapse as a surgical mesh to reinforce weakening tissues as well as working as a scaffold for fibro-collagenous tissues to form on the mesh itself (28). Several researches have considered its application in further regions of the body, for instance, implant-based breast reconstruction (29). On the other hand, a certain dispute is about the usage of polypropylene materials in this application (30). An inflammatory reaction is caused by the usage of such implants, which leads to a slower recovery process. In disparity, Moalli et al. discovered that these inflammatory reactions are inevitable events of the body's recovery process, and therefore, PP meshes should be employed in the future (31). In fact, the usage of PP meshes should be encouraged because they have a low risk of causing cancer in humans. Because of the controversies surrounding the application of polypropylene hernia meshes, it is still unclear if PP is completely biocompatible (32). In the past, PP was utilized as a blood-oxygenator membrane; however, the body's immune system had responded in a number of ways. To increase blood compatibility, a variety of approaches have been used to surface-treat the PP membrane (33). Other materials have been discovered to perform better than PP membranes (34). As a result, it is thought that polypropylene is an excellent material with biocompatibility concerns that limit its usage as a biomedical implant. Surface treatments on the material surface should be researched further to increase biocompatibility before application in the human body. Graft polymerization with PEG is one such surface modification procedure that has been applied to the PP membrane surface (35, 36).

3.3.1.3   Polyurethane (PU)

PU may be easily changed to match diverse biomedical purposes in a broad array of implants. Chemical attacks on PU, on the other hand, might cause the breakdown of the material in vivo. When treated properly, this breakdown can aid in the formation of new tissues (37). PU has a decreased water permeability, which can be decreased even more with the help of small quantities of isopropyl myristate.

3.3.1.4   Polytetrafluoroethylene (PTFE)

Teflon is another prominent brand name for PTFE, created by DuPont. Zhang and colleagues were the first to use PTFE as a substrate for a high-frequency surface coil for MRI and spectroscopy (38). However, later discovered that PTFE did not attach fit to metals and had poor strength after being exposed to gamma radiation, making it unsuitable for some operations like gamma sterilization (39, 40). A silicone-covered stent and PU-covered stent were compared to an expanded polytetrafluoroethylene (e-PTFE)-covered biliary metal stent created to oppress tumor in-growth and cure benign biliary structures; as the stents were frequently subjected to bile during the six-month testing period, it was discovered that the e-PTFE was less biodurable.

3.3.1.5   Silicone, e.g., Parylene, PDMS

These are passive substances that come in a range of shapes as well as sizes. These implants have been earlier utilized in laryngeal procedures for tackling problems such as unilateral vocal fold paralysis, which leads to vocal dysfunction and partial glottis closure. Silicon materials have been frequently employed in surgeries to improve human looks and have been determined to be secure with minimal infection rates (41–43). As its smoother topography and lower surface energy, silicone was found to be trustworthy for enduring encapsulation in the body when associated with PU coatings and epoxy resin (44). These properties also prevent the polymer from absorbing cells and molecules. On the silicon surface, there were also fewer flaws, indicating improved protective functions.

3.3.1.6   Polymethylmethacrylate (PMMA)

PMMA is employed in a range of medical implants, comprising rhinoplasty, intra-ocular lenses, cranioplasty, as well as bone cement incomplete joint substitutions (45–49). Still, PMMA does not allow for osseointegration of the structure with other structures with which it comes into touch, limiting its use. To improve osseointegration, Goncalves et al. created two distinct formulations to induce calcium phosphate layer development on the surface of the cement disks (50).

3.3.1.7   Polyamide (PA)

Polyamides are macromolecules having amide bonds connecting repeating units. Polyamides can be natural as well as synthetic. Nonetheless, nylon is the utmost common type of polyamides utilized in biomedical devices and implants, and it is frequently used as a material for fiber's in composites to amplify the composite's mechanical strength; nevertheless, it is hardly ever used as a packaging film material (51, 52). Polyamides composites, on the other hand, are shown to be safe for use in bone formation scaffolds and typically used as nanofillers to improve the mechanical properties of composite materials (53, 54).

3.3.1.8   Liquid Crystal Polymer (LCP)

They have one of the greatest impact strengths and Young's modulus. The application of LCPs in microwave frequency electronics is also highly appealing. Recent research has revealed that LCPs can be used as biomaterials for a variety of devices and implants, including retinal and neurological prosthetic implants. The devices' RF properties were likewise unaltered with the thin film (55). It was discovered by employing LCP as both an encapsulating film and a substrate that a multilayered planar coil capable of supplying power and data to devices could be established.

3.3.1.9   Carbon Nanotube (CNT) composites

They are frequently recommended for usage as biomedical packaging films because of their unique mechanical, electrical, and surface qualities, which can help get better device operation. Carbon nanotube composites, with their tremendous tensile strength and elastic modulus, are undoubtedly the robust materials in this class. However, due to their hollow nature, they tend to be particularly feeble against shearing amid adjacent shells and are simply crushed. Compressive, bending, and torsional stresses are all-cause buckling. When CNTs are mixed with zeolite as a composite, they exhibit superconductivity along their unique axis (56, 57). A degradation monitoring device was also developed using a composite of poly (lactic acid) in addition to carbon nanotubes to analyze the deterioration of biodegradable polymers. It was also discovered that CNT coatings enable an electrically conductive fibrous surface layer at the interfaces. A PMMA/CNT/high-load HA cement coating composite was designed and refined, and it was discovered to cause calcium phosphate layer development on the surface of cement disks with higher cell survival and minimal apoptosis.

3.3.1.10   Polyimide

Polyimides are divided into several classes depending on their polymer chains, hydrocarbon residue types, and functional groups in the polymer chain. Their physical qualities and possible applications are determined by these properties.

3.4   RECENT ADVANCES IN SELECT TECHNOLOGIES FOR IMPLANT FABRICATION

3.4.1   INJECTABLE IMPLANTS

Implants are frequently associated with the disadvantage of requiring surgical implantation, which can negatively impact patient compliance. Recent studies have broadened their goals in developing medication delivery implants to include the ease of implant administration by developing injectable implants that can be administered noninvasively (58, 59). Injectable implants can be preformulated solid implants, such as the recently described anticancer fluorouracil (5FU)-loaded pellets that were extruded to an injectable diameter, allowing for a noninvasive way of implant administration and removing the need for surgical implantation. Most injectable implants, on the other hand, develop in situ. Low-viscosity polymeric implants that solidify or become semisolid when administered are known as in situ forming polymeric implants (60, 61). As an FDA-approved polymer, PLGA was used as a building block in several studies for a variety of applications, including allergies, ophthalmic usage, and analgesia (62, 63).

Many injectable implants for medication delivery and other medical uses have used hydrogels as the substrate (64–66). A novel application of hydrogels has been developed for cancer radiation (36). The manufactured hydrogel was presented as a biodegradable alternative to titanium seeds used in brachytherapy (a therapeutic technique for treating solid tumors that involves inserting titanium seeds enclosing radioactive material). Self-healing hydrogels are a newer type of hydrogel. Self-healing hydrogels, unlike standard hydrogels, can endure external impacts that can degrade gel mechanical characteristics and self-heal to regain function. Several evaluations (67–71) have focused on their self-repair mechanism, efficiency testing methodologies, and advancements in their formulations. This technique is increasingly being used for drug delivery as a stand-alone agent or in combination with a stimulus-responsive component, with cargos ranging from proteins to growth factors to antibiotics to chemotherapeutics (72–75).

3.4.2   ON-DEMAND IMPLANTS

Controlled drug delivery research goes beyond creating regulated and, in most cases, continuous and prolonged medication release characteristics. The capacity to release the payload from a medication delivery system when and where it is needed has become more important, especially in targeted and precision medicine. One method of reaching this goal is on-demand implants. On-demand implants make use of a stimulus-responsive drug carrier that allows a provider/clinician to cause the release of a precise dose of a certain payload as needed (76, 77).

3.4.3 Expandable implants

The word "expandable implant" refers to stents that are used to keep a channel open, such as a blood artery or the urethra. Although metallic stents are the most often utilized, there has been an increasing interest in using polymers in-stent production to improve drug-holding capacity and biocompatibility. As a result, polymer-coated stents arose, with the metal backbone providing the necessary mechanical support and the polymer coat providing a biocompatible and, if necessary, drug-laden layer (78–82).

3.4.4 3D printing

After the FDA approved the 3D printed tablet Spritam® in 2015, three-dimensional (3D) printing for drug delivery systems has gotten a lot of interest and is being used more in pharmaceutical formulations and research. Three-dimensional printing is the process of creating a medication delivery system layer by layer from a computer design (83–86). The technology allows for precision low-dose distribution, sophisticated dosage form composition, and spatial control of dosage form geometry, providing for the flexibility and luxury of building individualized and on-demand pharmaceutical solutions (87–88).

Implants come under a novel drug delivery system compared to the traditional drug delivery system.

3.4.5 Novel drug delivery system

Natural and synthetic polymer was used for new drug delivery systems over traditional dosage forms, including controlling the release of drugs from the implant at the target site. The released rate is nearly independent of environmental conditions such as pH, enzyme degradation, and drug metabolism in the body, excretions of drug moiety. Such systems are used for a longer duration of time. Controlled release preparation has many advantages, unlike conventional dosage forms like avoiding first-pass metabolism, improving patient's compliance, ensuring maximum stability of the drug, and masking unpleasant tastes or odors of the drug.

3.4.6 Polymers as a building block for DD system

According to the use of polymer and designed delivery system in order to attain maximum stability and biocompatible, polymers are selected with special features like non-toxic and which act as an additive, stabilizer, catalyst residue, and emulsifiers and they also do not undergo any chemical change and free from impurities. Mostly polymeric materials contain functional groups like CONH, ester, or anhydride bonds in their main chain. Properties of polymer like molecular weight, glass transition temperature, crystallinity, and solubility which come under physiochemical ones are the important consideration while designing a drug delivery system; other properties are like appropriate diffusion and solubility with the active pharmaceutical ingredient which must be stable (89).

3.4.7   POLYMER AS DRUG CARRIER

Bioactive agents can be incorporated into a copolymer matrix by either chemical bonding or physical entrapment.

3.4.8   CHEMICALLY LINKED POLYMER MATRIX

Cross-link between drug matrix and polymer leads to the formation of temporary hydrolyzable bonds such as anhydride, ester, acetyl, or thioester.

3.4.9   PHYSICAL ENTRAPMENT OF DRUG

If we add drugs in vehicles like microspheres, microcapsules, nanospheres, liposomes, and micelles are an example of physical entrapment of drugs, such as carriers are categorized into colloidal drug delivery system, particle size having range about 0.001–2000 µm.

3.4.10   LIPOSOMES

Liposomes are vesicular systems consisting of an alternating bilayer of lipid, separated by an aqueous compartment whose composition is influenced by the type of solution in which the structure is formed. Liposomes are mainly used in drugs, vaccines, and gene delivery systems. Drug molecules can be either encapsulated in the aqueous layer or intercalated into the lipid bilayer; the exact location of a drug in the liposome will depend upon its physicochemical characteristics and the composition of lipids (90). In particular, liposomes have appreciable value as drug carriers in the therapy of cancer and infections. Due to their high degree of biocompatibility, liposomes were initially conceived as a delivery system for intravenous delivery. Currently available liposomal formulations include doxorubicin and daunorubicin for the treatment of sarcoma (90).

3.4.11   NANOPARTICLES

Nanoparticles and nanospheres are colloidal polymer particles of size about nano in range and have been used as carriers for certain peptides: vaccine and anti-cancer agents. The drug may be entrapped in the polymer matrix in the particulate form, or it can be bound to the particle surface by adsorption (90).

3.4.12   MICROSPHERES

There are spherical particles having a size ranging from 1 µm to 500 µm. There are free-flowing powders prepared by standard techniques like solvent evaporation, emulsion, and various methods. Polymers of both natural origin and synthetic origin are used like bovine serum albumin, gelatin, chitosan, sodium alginate, starch, and polylactic acid. Some of them are degradable, while others are non-degradable polymers (91).

3.5 MECHANISM OF DRUG RELEASE FROM POLYMER DEVICE

There are two types of diffusion-controlled systems—reservoir and matrices.

Chemical control is accomplished by the polymer degradation & chemical cleavage of drug from the polymer. Solvent activation involves either swelling of the polymer or osmotic swelling effects.

3.5.1 DIFFUSION-CONTROLLED SYSTEM

Diffusion is a process in which no energy is used for the movement of molecules along their concentration gradients; here, a drug molecule is moved through a reservoir to surroundings fluids, and the drug is entrapped in the polymer system. It follows Fick's law. Usually, it follows zero-order kinetics, the movement of molecule varies by changing polymer coatings, but this process is ineffective for the drug having high molecular weight. This system offered a high cost. Drug-containing polymer in contact with the biological environment has a reservoir system that modulates the release of the drug; the rate-limiting step of this process is diffusion across the polymer to the ambient fluid. The advantage of this system is that there is no need to remove the implanted polymer since it degrades after releasing the active drugs (92).

3.5.2 MATRIX SYSTEM

Matrix system containing drug is evenly dispersed throughout solid, and polymer used in this system may be degradable and non-degradable type polymer. Drug diffusion through the polymer matrix is the rate-limiting stage in the reservoir system; this system offers advantages like it can deliver high-molecular weight compounds. It does not require a reservoir system, but it does not follow zero-order kinetics. The active drug becomes less soluble in the polymer matrix in a non-bioerodible matrix system, and the drug is discharged via a solution diffusion process. If the medication is insoluble in the polymer, it can be released through the intergranular opening by leaching. In matrix system, waxes are used like beeswax, carnauba wax, hydrogenated castor oil, and others to regulate medication dissolution by changing the porosity of the tablet, lowering its wettability, or slowing down its own disintegration. In such matrices, drug release is frequently first order. The medication is dispersed in molten wax, then solidified, and granulated. The major drawback of this non-degradable matrix system is that there is no biodegradability. As time passes, elevated levels of the active chemical extracted may lead to the erratic release of the drug (92).

3.5.3 CHEMICALLY CONTROL SYSTEMS

In this system, there is a modification in the chemical structure of polymer when it gets exposed to surrounding fluids. The polymer can be either a bioerodible or non-bioerodible system. In bioerodible polymer systems, which had distinct mechanisms first, they get hydrolysis degradation into a smaller unit, which is biologically safe. Degradation of polymer is of either two types, that is, bulk erosion and surface erosion. Bioerodible matrix system contains an active chemical that is disseminated in a polymer having bit by bit biologically wrinkled in a controlled manner. In nonerodible type, drug is uniformly scattered right through the polymer and depends on solution diffusion-type mechanism for controlled release, bioerodible systems release according to the rate of polymer bioerosion (93–95).

The major advantage of a bioerodible system is that the polymer is eventually absorbed by the body (126), and its release is controlled via three major mechanisms (127 sg). first one is water-soluble polymer insolubilized by degradable cross-links, second is water-insoluble polymer solubilized by hydrolysis, protonation of pendant side group, and example of such polymer is diethyl amino acetate, and third is water-insoluble polymer solubilized by backbone chain cleavage to small water-soluble molecule, for example, polylactic acids. A major class of drug-containing implantable devices includes three types. First, it consists of polymeric material, which exploits diverse types of polymer and its membranes in order to control the release of the drug into the natural system. Next, it consists of a matrix delivery system like rods and a microsphere (93–95). Third, it consists of a motorized pump that controls medication release using an infusion pump-like mechanism.

3.5.4 Subcutaneous Implant Devices

Currently, one of the most popular routes used to investigate the potential of controlled drug delivery in a particular implant is the surgical procedure involved in implantation removal and favorable absorption site as compared to oral or percutaneous routes.

3.5.5 Toxicological Assessment

For the assessment of polymeric material to be implanted there, the toxicological study includes experiments on animals so that we get a proper result at a lower caste cost. For this task, the researcher must use a minimal number of animals, following all protocols that minimize animals and give all comfort before, during, and after research. If a researcher had to sacrifice an animal, they must follow with initial euthanasia principles depending upon polymer nature and the site to be implanted. The selection of experimental animals must be precise with the material to be used (96). Animal testing cannot be performed if alternative methods for conducting analysis that achieves like software.

Biocompatibility before it refers to the introduction of a polymeric substance into the living organism and they're in the body. In ideal term, the inserted material shows maximum contact with that living system and does not cause any adverse effect, but due to different chemical nature, functional group number of polymeric substance has different behavior in the same environment, so their assessment is necessary by both and in vivo (96).

Various tests and their assessment for biocompatibility are carcinogenicity, mutagenicity, teratogenicity, antigenicity, implantation reaction and skin irritation hemolysis, and cytotoxicity (96).

3.6 SUBCUTANEOUS IMPLANTATION AND EXPLANT EVALUATION

For successful implantation, polymeric implants were soaked in the hydro-alcoholic solution for 15–20 min; then it's rinsed with a sterile solution of PBS three times, and stored experimental animals were given general anesthesia by gaseous means, and then removed hair of particular area which is exposed and washed with ethanol and applied betadine. By performing surgery, the given implant was inserted into the tissue, and the incision was closed by autoclips. Then, the behavior of the rat was examined and kept on a heating pad at 37°C to minimize their discomfort for 20 min (97). Rat movements and their behavior were closely monitored for the next 24 hrs. For their toxicological study, the sample was retrieved after the 7th day of implantation. For histological analysis, the polymeric implant was removed by two consecutive methods to assess the assessment of the toxicological method. We took a cross-section of tissue by cryostat and stained it with hematoxylin and eosin dye, further stained with immune histochemistry staining with CD68 counterstained with hematoxylin, then washed, and observed the presence of macrophages (97).

Gel electrophoresis is applied as an assessment for an implant for their evaluation of content genotoxicity. As medical implants are greatly used for the treatment and diagnosis of disease, it is important to evaluate their potential toxicity, such as genotoxicity, which means an alteration in the abnormality in the cell. Gel electrophoresis is used to evaluate the genotoxicity in which we detect the site of contact of medical devices. GE is used to detect the migration of DNA at the site of implantation. Extractable chemicals from the implant must be evaluated to check genetic toxicology. This test is performed by Ames test, chromosome aberration assay, mouse lymphoma assay, or in vitro micronucleus assay. (96).

For conduction of test, the extract had been carried from the implant and kept into a vehicle at 70°C up to 72 hrs. During this procedure, the extract had been taken out by implant device, which is held at vehicle solution at 70 to 72 hrs, so that leaching chemical get solubilized in the entire volume of vehicles, and high leaching chemical may cause DNA damage. To evaluate this, we take 8- to 10-week-old Wistar rats and give standard laboratory conditions. Randomly divided this animal into various groups, implants were placed on the body system like a subcutaneous pocket (97). Then, implant was taken out at 4–5 days, stained with fluorescein diacetate and ethidium bromide, and observed with a fluorescent microscope; it produces green color, then it is still living; if the sample produces red-colored, then it is a cytotoxic cell. Cytotoxicity study was also assessed by histopathology of both implant sites and liver. If there was any necrosis, apoptosis, degeneration, or inflammation, then it is a sign of toxicity (97).

3.6.1 PREPARATION OF SINGLE-CELL SUSPENSION

A tissue sample was pulverized briefly with ice-cold physiological solution with 20 nm EDTA and 10% DMSO and permissible to locate for a few minutes and then centrifuged, and supernatant of this cell was used by GE. Then, cell suspension about 5–10 μl was mixed with 75 μl of 0.5% agarose at 37°C and extended on the slide; and tolerable to set on ice and kept on ice-cold lysis buffer overnight. After performing cell lysis, the DNA in the cells was allowed to unravel in horizontal electrophoresis tanks supplied with buffer for 20 min. After electrophoresis, the slides were neutralized, dried, and stained with ethidium bromide, which was seen using a fluorescence microscope.

3.6.2 POLYMERIC IMPLANT TOXICOLOGICAL ASSESSMENT OF EXTRACT FOR CHROMOSOMAL ABERRATION ASSAYS

Sample having area of about 3 cm^2 was taken and kept in purified water at 50°C for 72 hr, so that proper extraction had been carried out at the end. If there was no change in color observed, then the material is said to be non-toxic. If there is an increased DNA migration, then it causes DNA damage (98).

3.6.3 PREPARATION OF EXTRACT FOR *SALMONELLA*/MICROSOME AND CHROMOSOME ABERRATION ASSAY

At the site of the implant, we extract out polymeric implant by two solvent systems, that is, water and DMSO at 50°C for 72 hrs. Thus, we obtained a clear extract containing no particulate matter. All clear extracts were administered to the test system within 12 h of preparation. For the *Salmonella*/ microsome assay, we checked leaked chemicals present in an implant for the evaluation of whether performing mutation or not. For this, we took two strains of bacteria, that is, the auxotrophic strain of *Salmonella* and the normal strain of *Salmonella*. Then, we put our extract into their respective culture media containing normal and auxotrophic strains, respectively. They were left for incubation period and examined for any sign of toxicity, and revertant colonies were counted normally (98–100).

3.6.4 IN VITRO CYTOTOXICITY ANALYSIS

3.6.4.1 Proliferation assay

The reasonability of cells had been chosen for evaluating this parameter and determined by using an MTT assay in which we used 3-(4, 5- dimethylthiazol-2yl) -2, 5-diphenyl tetrazolium bromide (101). For this, we take fibroblast cells which were incubated in a DMEM containing 10% bovine serum with varying concentration of tested copolymer in DMSO and polymer-free DMSO as a control on a 96-well microplate for 72 hr under 5% CO_2 atmosphere at 37°C. After the completion of the incubation period, this cell was further incubated with MTT solution for 4 hr at 37°C. If any complex formed, then isopropanol was added to solubilize this, and then absorption was determined at 540 nm using a microplate reader (101).

3.6.4.2 The growth rate of fibroblasts

It was measured by counting cells using a hemocytometer. Trypan blue solution was used to stain the cell so that viable cells were easily counted. We started with 5,000 cells per well and estimated and displayed the rise in multiplication as the number of cells at different time intervals.

3.6.4.3 Pharmacological evaluation

3.6.4.3.1 In vitro release

The specific amount of drug-loaded microspheres was transferred to a dialysis tube, and both sides were closed by making knots. A dialysis bag was introduced into a medium containing 100 ml of phosphate-buffered saline with 20% ethanol taken in a 250 ml stoppered conical flask. Perfect sink conditions were created, and the pH of the medium was maintained at 7.4. Samples were withdrawn at a specific interval of time, and the amount of drug present was determined by a UV spectrophotometer. The duration of study for drug release is up to several months (102).

3.6.4.3.2 In vivo evaluation

For this, we take rabbits for their evaluation. Prepared implants were loaded into 5-ml plastic syringes immediately prior to injection with 1 ml of sterile suspension medium, and the formulation carrier was mixed by agitation and injected intra-dermally on the marked flank region of the rabbits using a 12-gauge needle. Each rabbit's hair above the lower dorsal site was trimmed, and the skin was cleansed with an alcohol swab for the investigation; after injecting the solution, the blood sample was withdrawn at 1, 2, 4, 7, 10, 14, 18, 22, 26, and 30 days of the amount of 5 ml from rabbit marginal veins (102).

A blood sample is stored at 4°c overnight for clotting of fibrin aggregates of blood cells and a marginal separation of serum; the clarified serum was decanted meticu-lously, using individual disposable micropipette tips into fresh, labeled secondary sample tubes, and the Eppendorf vials were centrifuged at 18,000 rpm at 4°C for 30 min to separate the serum. Aliquots of individual serum samples were stored at −20°C until further use. Then, serum was measured using HPLC analysis for resid-ual drug content to determine the extent of drug release (102).

3.6.4.4 Chromosome aberration assay

Chromosomal research has gotten a lot of attention lately, thanks to a rising interest in evaluating the genotoxicity of environmental toxicants and carcinogens. In light of the rapidly increasing agricultural uses of chemicals, fertilizers, and pesticides, determining their genotoxic potential is essential for conducting proper risk assess-ments and ensuring a safer and more sustainable aquatic environment.

Significant alterations in chromosome structure that often affect many genes are referred to as chromosomal aberration (loci). It can be caused by a cell division defect (chromosome and chromatid non-disjunction), maternal age, or the environment. Chromosomal abnormalities are of two types, that is, numerical abnormalities like aneuploidy and polyploidy, and structural abnormalities like deletion, duplication, inversion, and translocation (103).

For evaluation of chromosomal aberration, we took the culture of human lympho-cytes; then, device extract was put into 48 hr. Then, we add colchicines at least 3 hr before so that cell division is stopped at the phase of metaphase. Before harvesting the cells, 0.075 M KCL was added and the cell was fixed in the medium by add-ing methanol or glacial acetic acid (3:1 v/v). Then, we prepared a slide from these fixed cells, which were further stained with Giemsa. Then, cells were observed under the microscope and scored for inhibition of cell cycle division and aberration of the chromosome. Then, we compared cultures treated with all implant extracts, resulting in frequencies of cells with standard aberration comparable to the concurrent untreated negative controls (103).

3.7 CONCLUSION

Despite the rapid expansion of drug-eluting implants in both research and clinical application in recent years, there is still room for improvement. In the area of synthetic materials, recent investigations have concentrated on individual materials rather than composite materials in biomedical devices and implants. It might be difficult to tell which materials are suitable for specific purposes. The quest for new materials and polymers is continuous; nevertheless, in terms of clinical translatability, it is more practical and desirable, to begin with authorized materials for implant manufacturing. We went through the broad classification of medical implants and devices, as well as the various materials that have been utilized, as well as the most recent research and advancements in the field of materials and composites. Rather than reporting novel polymers, we see more studies evaluating the prospects for new composites. The three main concerns with implant materials are safety, biocompatibility, and bioabsorbability.

Given the widespread attention that synthetic polymeric materials are receiving as a result of the global focus on health care, their future in the medical business is bright. Apart from that, work on improving the functionality of devices and implants is currently ongoing. Given the large spectrum of materials that are compatible with one another, the possibilities for material combinations as composites are virtually limitless. New composites are continually being created around the world, including blends of synthetic and natural polymers with the prospective to perform power-driven tasks analogous to those of the human body. Fabrication technology that makes use of such polymeric materials is also advancing, allowing for the quick and inexpensive creation of one-of-a-kind parts, allowing a larger series of applications. In prospect, what was formerly thought to create constant malfunction is now acknowledged to cause temporary impairment. This is a big step forward for the biomedical industry. Due to the development of numerous technologies, it has been reduced to a restricted disability with increased comfort, medical implants, and gadgets.

REFERENCES

1. Wang L, Huang K, Zhong C, Wang L, Lu Y. Fabrication and modification of implantable optrode arrays for in vivo optogenetic applications. *Biophys Rep*. 2018;4(2):82–93. doi: 10.1007/s41048-018-0052-4, PMID 29756008.
2. Flexner C, Thomas DL, Swindells S. Creating demand for long-acting formulations for the treatment and prevention of HIV, tuberculosis, and viral hepatitis. *Curr Opin HIV AIDS*. 2019;14(1):13–20. doi: 10.1097/COH.0000000000000510, PMID 30394948.
3. Ravivarapu HB, Moyer KL, Dunn RL. Sustained activity and release of leuprolide acetate from an in situ forming polymeric implant. *AAPS PharmSciTech*. 2000;1(1):E1. doi: 10.1208/pt010101, PMID 14727850.

4. Southard GL, Dunn RL, Garrett S. The drug delivery and biomaterial attributes of the ATRIGEL technology in the treatment of periodontal disease. *Expert Opin Investig Drugs.* 1998;7(9):1483–1491. doi: 10.1517/13543784.7.9.1483, PMID 15992045.

5. Brem H, Piantadosi S, Burger PC, Walker M, Selker R, Vick NA, et al. Placebo-controlled trial of safety and efficacy of intraoperative controlled delivery by biodegradable polymers of chemotherapy for recurrent gliomas. *The Polymer-brain Tumor Treatment Group. Lancet.* 1995;345(8956):1008–1012. doi: 10.1016/s0140-6736(95) 90755-6, PMID 7723496.

6. Perry J, Chambers A, Spithoff K, Laperriere N. Gliadel wafers in the treatment of malignant glioma: a systematic review. *Curr Oncol.* 2007;14(5):189–194. doi: 10.3747/co.2007.147, PMID 17938702.

7. Ashby LS, Smith KA, Stea B. Gliadel wafer implantation combined with standard radiotherapy and concurrent followed by adjuvant temozolomide for treatment of newly diagnosed high-grade glioma: a systematic literature review. *World J Surg Oncol.* 2016;14(1):225. doi: 10.1186/s12957-016-0975-5, PMID 27557526.

8. Palla S, Biswas J, Nagesha CK. Efficacy of Ozurdex implant in treatment of non-infectious intermediate uveitis. *Indian J Ophthalmol.* 2015;63(10):767–770. doi: 10.4103/0301-4738.171505, PMID 26655000.

9. Lin S, Chao PY, Chien YW, Sayani S, Kuma S, Mason M, et al. In vitro and in vivo evaluations of biodegradable implants for hormone replacement therapy: effect of system design and PK-PD relationship. *AAPS PharmSciTech.* 2001;2(3):E16. doi: 10.1208/pt020316, PMID 14727875.

10. Zhang Z, Zeng TY, Xia L, Hong CY, Wu DC, You YZ. Synthesis of polymers with on-demand sequence structures via dually switchable and interconvertible polymerizations. *Nat Commun.* 2018;9(1):2577. doi: 10.1038/s41467-018-05000-2, PMID 29968716.

11. Kumar AM, Suresh B, Das S, Obot IB, Adesina AY, Ramakrishna S. Promising bio-composites of polypyrrole and chitosan: surface protective and in vitro biocompatibility performance on 316-L SS implants. *Carbohydr Polym.* 2017;173:121–130. doi: 10.1016/j.carbpol.2017.05.083, PMID 28732850.

12. Manna S, Donnell AM, Kaval N, Al-Rjoub MF, Augsburger JJ, Banerjee RK. Improved design and characterization of PLGA / PLA-coated chitosan based micro-implants for controlled release of hydrophilic drugs. *Int J Pharm.* 2018;547(1–2):122–132. doi: 10.1016/j.ijpharm.2018.05.066, PMID 29857096.

13. Manna S, Banerjee RK, Augsburger JJ, Al-Rjoub MF, Donnell A, Correa ZM. Biodegradable chitosan and polylactic acid-based intraocular micro-implant for sustained release of methotrexate into vitreous: analysis of pharmacokinetics and toxicity in rabbit eyes. *Graefes Arch Clin Exp Ophthalmol.* 2015;253(8):1297–1305. doi: 10.1007/s00417-015-3007-1, PMID 25896109.

14. Manna S, Augsburger JJ, Correa ZM, Landero JA, Banerjee RK. Development of chitosan and polylactic acid based methotrexate intravitreal micro-implants to treat primary intraocular lymphoma: an in vitro study. *J Biomech Eng.* 2014;136(2):021018. doi: 10.1115/1.4026176, PMID 24317155.

15. Argarate N, Olalde B, Atorrasagasti G, Valero J, Carolina Cifuentes S, Benavente R, et al. Biodegradable bi-layered coating on polymeric orthopaedic implants for controlled release of drugs. *Mater Lett.* 2014;132:193–195. doi: 10.1016/j.matlet.2014.06.070.

16. Aqil F, Jeyabalan J, Kausar H, Bansal SS, Sharma RJ, Singh IP, et al. Multi-layer polymeric implants for sustained release of chemopreventives. *Cancer Lett.* 2012;326(1): 33–40. doi: 10.1016/j.canlet.2012.07.017, PMID 22820161.

17. Nasrin R, Biswas S, Rashid TU, Afrin S, Jahan RA, Haque P, et al. Preparation of chitin-PLA laminated composite for implantable application. *Bioact Mater.* 2017;2(4): 199–207. doi: 10.1016/j.bioactmat.2017.09.003, PMID 29744430.

18. Saber-Samandari S, Saber-Samandari S. Biocompatible nanocomposite scaffolds based on copolymer-grafted chitosan for bone tissue engineering with drug delivery capability. *Mater Sci Eng C Mater Biol Appl*. 2017;75:721–732. doi: 10.1016/j.msec.2017.02.112, PMID 28415522.

19. Rijal NP, Adhikari U, Khanal S, Pai D, Sankar J, Bhattarai N. Magnesium oxide-poly (ε-caprolactone)-chitosan-based composite nanofiber for tissue engineering applications. *Mater Sci Eng B*. 2018;228:18–27. doi: 10.1016/j.mseb.2017.11.006.

20. Ma B, Wang X, Wu C, Chang J. Crosslinking strategies for preparation of extracellular matrix-derived cardiovascular scaffolds. *Regen Biomater*. 2014;1(1):81–89. doi: 10.1093/rb/rbu009, PMID 26816627.

21. Suryavanshi A, Khanna K, Sindhu KR, Bellare J, Srivastava R. Magnesium oxide nanoparticle-loaded PCL composite electrospun fiber scaffolds for bone-soft tissue engineering applications: in-vitro and in-vivo evaluation. *Biomed Mater*. 2017;12(5):055011. doi: 10.1088/1748-605X/aa792b, PMID 28944766.

22. Bazaka K, Jacob MV. Implantable devices: issues and challenges. *Electronics*. 2012;2(4):1–34. doi: 10.3390/electronics2010001.

23. Kammula RG, Morris JM. Considerations for the biocompatibility evaluation of medical devices. *Med Dev Diagn Ind*. 2001;23(5):82–92.

24. Sastri VR. *Plastics in Medical Devices: Properties, Requirements, and Applications*. William Andrew Publishing; 2013.

25. Chang JH-C, Liu Y, Tai Y-C. Long term glass-encapsulated packaging for implant electronics. In: *Micro Electro Mechanical Systems (MEMS) 27th International Conference on*. Vol. 2014. IEEE Publications; 2014. pp. 1127–1130.

26. Kurtz SM. *UHMWPE Biomaterials Handbook: Ultra High Molecular Weight Polyethylene in Total Joint Replacement and Medical Devices*. Elsevier Science; 2009.

27. Amanatullah DF, Landa J, Strauss EJ, Garino JP, Kim SH, Di Cesare PE. Comparison of surgical outcomes and implant wear between ceramic-ceramic and ceramic-polyethylene articulations in total hip arthroplasty. *J Arthroplasty*. 2011;26(6);Suppl: 72–77. doi: 10.1016/j.arth.2011.04.032, PMID 21680138.

28. Green JM, Hallab NJ, Liao Y-S, Narayan V, Schwarz EM, Xie C. Antioxidation treatment of ultra high molecular weight polyethylene components to decrease periprosthetic osteolysis: evaluation of osteolytic and osteogenic properties of wear debris particles in a murine calvaria model. *Curr Rheumatol Rep*. 2013;15(5):1–5.

29. Zhou J, Huang X, Zheng D, Li H, Herrler T, Li Q. Oriental nose elongation using an L-shaped polyethylene sheet implant for combined septal spreading and extension. *Aesthetic Plast Surg*. 2014;38(2):295–302. doi: 10.1007/s00266-014-0299-1, PMID 24627142.

30. Scheidbach H, Tamme C, Tannapfel A, Lippert H, Köckerling F. In vivo studies comparing the biocompatibility of various polypropylene meshes and their handling properties during endoscopic total extraperitoneal (TEP) patchplasty: an experimental study in pigs. *Surg Endosc*. 2004;18(2):211–220. doi: 10.1007/s00464-003-8113-1, PMID 14691711.

31. Li X, Kruger JA, Jor JWY, Wong V, Dietz HP, Nash MP, et al. Characterizing the ex vivo mechanical properties of synthetic polypropylene surgical mesh. *J Mech Behav Biomed Mater*. 2014;37(0):48–55. doi: 10.1016/j.jmbbm.2014.05.005, PMID 24942626.

32. Zheng F, Xu L, Verbiest L, Verbeken E, De Ridder D, Deprest J. Cytokine production following experimental implantation of xenogenic dermal collagen and polypropylene grafts in mice. *Neurourol Urodyn*. 2007;26(2):280–289. doi: 10.1002/nau.20317, PMID 17009249.

33. Moalli P, Brown B, Reitman MT, Nager CW. Polypropylene mesh: evidence for lack of carcinogenicity. *Int Urogynecol J*. 2014;25(5):573–576. doi: 10.1007/s00192-014-2343-8, PMID 24614956.

34. Bergmann PA, Becker B, Mauss KL, Liodaki ME, Knobloch J, Mailänder P, et al. Titanium-coated polypropylene mesh (TiLoop Bra®)—an effective prevention for capsular contracture? *Eur J Plast Surg.* 2014;37(6):339–346. doi: 10.1007/s00238-014-0947-3.

35. Abednejad AS, Amoabediny G, Ghaee A. Surface modification of polypropylene blood oxygenator membrane by poly ethylene glycol grafting. *Adv Mater Res.* 2013; 816–817:459–463. doi: 10.4028/www.scientific.net/AMR.816-817.459.

36. Hinz J, Molder JM, Hanekop GG, Weyland A, Popov AF, Bauer M, et al. Reduced sevoflurane loss during cardiopulmonary bypass when using a polymethylpentane versus a polypropylene oxygenator. *Int J Artif Organs.* 2013;36(4):233–239. doi: 10.5301/ ijao.5000208, PMID 23504814.

37. Abednejad AS, Amoabediny G, Ghaee A. Surface modification of polypropylene membrane by polyethylene glycol graft polymerization. *Mater Sci Eng C Mater Biol Appl.* 2014;42(0):443–450. doi: 10.1016/j.msec.2014.05.060, PMID 25063140.

38. Rahimi A, Mashak A. Review on rubbers in medicine: natural, silicone and polyurethane rubbers. *Plast Rubber Compos.* 2013;42(6):223–230. doi: 10.1179/1743289811Y.0000000063.

39. Zhang X, Ugurbil K, Chen W. Microstrip RF surface coil design for extremely high-field MRI and spectroscopy. *Magn Reson Med.* 2001;46(3):443–450. doi: 10.1002/ mrm.1212, PMID 11550234.

40. Couty M, Woytasik M, Ginefri J-C, Rubin A, Martincic E, Poirier-Quinot M, et al. Fabrication and packaging of flexible polymeric microantennae for in vivo magnetic resonance imaging. *Polymers.* 2012;4(1):656–673. doi: 10.3390/polym4010656.

41. Niinomi M. *Metals for Biomedical Devices.* Elsevier Science; 2010.

42. Rupa S, Dutta B, Singh, SP, Rathor, A. Research article case report: Silicone implant in augmentation of saddle nose. *Int. J. Recent Sci. Res.* 2013;04, 1661–1662.

43. Elist JJ, Shirvanian V, Lemperle G. Surgical treatment of penile deformity due to curvature using a subcutaneous soft silicone implant: case report. *Open J Urol.* 2014;04(7):91–97. doi: 10.4236/oju.2014.47016.

44. Najafi M, Neishaboury M. Acute immunologic reaction to silicone breast implant after mastectomy and immediate reconstruction: case report and review of the literature. *Arch Breast Cancer.* 2014;1(2):33–36.

45. Kirsten S, Uhlemann J, Braunschweig M, Wolter KJ. Packaging of electronic devices for long-term implantation. In: *Electronics Technology (ISSE) 35th International Spring Seminar on.* Vol. 2012. IEEE Publications; 2012. pp. 123–127.

46. Pérez-Merino P, Dorronsoro C, Llorente L, Durán S, Jiménez-Alfaro I, Marcos S. In vivo chromatic aberration in eyes implanted with intraocular lenses. *Invest Ophthalmol Vis Sci.* 2013;54(4):2654–2661. doi: 10.1167/iovs.13-11912, PMID 23493299.

47. Terrada C, Julian K, Cassoux N, Prieur AM, Debre M, Quartier P, et al. Cataract surgery with primary intraocular lens implantation in children with uveitis: long-term outcomes. *J Cataract Refract Surg.* 2011;37(11):1977–1983. doi: 10.1016/j.jcrs.2011.05.037, PMID 21940141.

48. Kim BJ, Hong KS, Park KJ, Park DH, Chung YG, Kang SH. Customized cranioplasty implants using three-dimensional printers and polymethyl- methacrylate casting. *J Korean Neurosurg Soc.* 2012;52(6):541–546. doi: 10.3340/jkns.2012.52.6.541, PMID 23346326.

49. Rivkin A. A prospective study of Non-surgical primary rhinoplasty using a polymethylmethacrylate injectable implant. *Dermatol Surg.* 2014;40(3):305–313. doi: 10.1111/ dsu.12415, PMID 24438233.

50. Parida P, Behera A, Chandra Mishra SC. Classification of biomaterials used in medicine [international journal]. *Int J Advances Appl Sci.* 2012;1(3). doi: 10.11591/ijaas.v1i3.882.

51. Yangzes S, Seth NG, Singh R, Gupta PC, Jinagal J, Pandav SS, Gupta V, Gupta A, Ram J. Long-term outcomes of cataract surgery in children with uveitis. *Indian J Ophthalmol.* 2019 Apr;67(4):490–495. doi: 10.4103/ijo.IJO_846_18, PMID 30900580.

52. Gonçalves G, Portolés MT, Ramírez-Santillán C, Vallet-Regí M, Serro AP, Grácio J, et al. Evaluation of the in vitro biocompatibility of PMMA/high-load HA/carbon nano-structures bone cement formulations. *J Mater Sci Mater Med.* 2013;24(12):2787–2796. doi: 10.1007/s10856-013-5030-2, PMID 23963685.

53. Nanni F, Lamastra FR, Pisa F, Gusmano G. Synthesis and characterization of poly (ε-caprolactone) reinforced with aligned hybrid electrospun PMMA/Nano-Al2O3 fibre mats by film stacking. *J Mater Sci.* 2011;46(18):6124–6130. doi: 10.1007/s10853-011-5577-6.

54. Kubyshkina G, Zupančič B, Štukelj M, Grošelj D, Marion L, Emri I. Sterilization effect on structure, thermal and time-dependent properties of polyamides. *Conference Proceedings of the Society for Experimental Mechanics Series.* 2011;3:11–19. doi: 10.1007/978-1-4614-0213-8_3.

55. McMahon RE, Wang L, Skoracki R, Mathur AB. Development of nanomaterials for bone repair and regeneration. *J Biomed Mater Res B Appl Biomater.* 2013;101(2): 387–397. doi: 10.1002/jbm.b.32823, PMID 23281143.

56. Gendre L, Njuguna J, Abhyankar H, Ermini V. Mechanical and impact performance of three-phase polyamide 6 nanocomposites. *Mater Des.* 2015;66:486–491. doi: 10.1016/j.matdes.2014.08.005.

57. Jeong J, Lee SW, Min KS, Kim SJ. A novel multilayered planar coil based on biocompatible liquid crystal polymer for chronic implantation. *Sens Actuators A.* 2013;197(0): 38–46. doi: 10.1016/j.sna.2013.04.001.

58. Tang ZK, Zhang L, Wang N, Zhang XX, Wen GH, Li GD, et al. Superconductivity in 4 angstrom single-walled carbon nanotubes. *Science.* 2001;292(5526):2462–2465. doi: 10.1126/science.1060470, PMID 11431560.

59. Lortz R, Zhang Q, Shi W, Ye JT, Qiu C, Wang Z, et al. Superconducting characteristics of 4-A carbon nanotube–zeolite composite. *Proc Natl Acad Sci USA.* 2009;106(18): 7299–7303. doi: 10.1073/pnas.0813162106, PMID 19369206.

60. Hassler C, Boretius T, Stieglitz T. Polymers for neural implants. *J Polym Sci B Polym Phys.* 2011;49(1):18–33. doi: 10.1002/polb.22169.

61. Seung Woo Lee, Kyou Sik Min, Joonsoo Jeong, Junghoon Kim, Sung June Kim. Monolithic encapsulation of implantable neuroprosthetic devices using liquid crystal polymers. *IEEE Trans Biomed Eng.* 2011;58(8):2255–2263. doi: 10.1109/TBME.2011.2136341.

62. Malcolm RK, Edwards KL, Kiser P, Romano J, Smith TJ. Advances in microbicide vaginal rings. *Antiviral Res.* 2010;88;Suppl 1:S30–S39. doi: 10.1016/j.antiviral.2010.09.003, PMID 21109066.

63. Kaur M, Gupta KM, Poursaid AE, Karra P, Mahalingam A, Aliyar HA, et al. Engineering a degradable polyurethane intravaginal ring for sustained delivery of dapivirine. *Drug Deliv Transl Res.* 2011;1(3):223–237. doi: 10.1007/s13346-011-0027-1, PMID 25788241.

64. Pal S. Biomaterials and its characterization. In: *Design of Artificial Human Joints & Organs.* Springer; 2014. pp. 51–73. doi: 10.1007/978-1-4614-6255-2_4.

65. Kuo A, Pu Z. *Polymer Data Handbook.* Polymer Data Handbook; 1999.

66. Matbase MB. The free and independent online materials properties resource. Available from: http://www.matbase.com/material-categories/natural-and-synthetic-polymers/ [cited 17/5/2022].

67. Kawai H. The piezoelectricity of poly (vinylidene fluoride). *Jpn J Appl Phys.* 1969;8(7):975–976. doi: 10.1143/JJAP.8.975.

68. Klinge U, Klosterhalfen B, Ottinger AP, Junge K, Schumpelick V. PVDF as a new polymer for the construction of surgical meshes. *Biomaterials.* 2002;23(16):3487–3493. doi: 10.1016/s0142-9612(02)00070-4, PMID 12099293.

69. Ul Ahad I, Bartnik A, Fiedorowicz H, Kostecki J, Korczyc B, Ciach T, et al. Surface modification of polymers for biocompatibility via exposure to extreme ultraviolet radiation. *J Biomed Mater Res*. 2014;102(9):3298–3310. doi: 10.1002/jbm.a.34958.

70. Hayes, D. G. (). Pyrethroid-laden textiles for protection from biting insects. In: N. Pan, G. Sun (eds.), *Functional Textiles for Improved Performance, Protection and Health*. Woodhead Publishing; 2011. pp. 404–433.

71. Pruitt L, Furmanski J. Polymeric biomaterials for load-bearing medical devices. *JOM*. 2009;61(9):14–20. doi: 10.1007/s11837-009-0126-3.

72. Hussey M, Bagg M. Principles of wound closure. *Oper Tech Sports Med*. 2011;19(4): 206–211. doi: 10.1053/j.otsm.2011.10.004.

73. Hofstetter WL, Vukasin P, Ortega AE, Anthone G, Beart Jr RW. New technique for mesh repair of paracolostomy hernias. *Dis Colon Rectum*. 1998;41(8):1054–1055. doi: 10.1007/BF02237400, PMID 9715164.

74. Nathanael AJ, Oh TH. Biopolymer coatings for biomedical applications. *Polymers* (Basel). 2020 Dec 21;12(12):3061. doi: 10.3390/polym12123061, PMID 33371349.

75. Hieu LC, Zlatov N, Vander Sloten J, Bohez E, Khanh L, Binh PH, et al. Medical rapid prototyping applications and methods. *Assembly Autom*. 2005;25(4):284–292. doi: 10. 1108/01445150510626415.

76. Millán MS, Vega F, Poyales F, Garzón N. Clinical assessment of chromatic aberration in phakic and pseudophakic eyes using a simple autorefractor. *Biomed Opt Express*. 2019 Jul 22;10(8):4168–4178. doi: 10.1364/BOE.10.004168, PMID 31453002.

77. Kulik U, Wiklund A, Kugelberg M, Lundvall A. Long-term results after primary intra-ocular lens implantation in children with juvenile idiopathic arthritis-associated uveitis. *Eur J Ophthalmol*. 2019 Sep;29(5):494–498. doi: 10.1177/1120672118799623, Epub 2018 Sep 12, PMID 30207174.

78. Pöppe JP, Spendel M, Schwartz C, Winkler PA, Wittig J. The "springform" technique in cranioplasty: custom made 3D-printed templates for intraoperative modelling of polymethylmethacrylate cranial implants. *Acta Neurochir (Wien)*. 2022 Mar;164(3): 679–688. doi: 10.1007/s00701-021-05077-7, Epub 2021 Dec 6, PMID 34873659.

79. Jasin ME. Nonsurgical rhinoplasty using dermal fillers. *Facial Plast Surg Clin North Am*. 2013 May;21(2):241–252. doi: 10.1016/j.fsc.2013.02.004, PMID 23731585.

80. Heini PF, Berlemann U. Bone substitutes in vertebroplasty. *Eur Spine J*. 2001;10(2);Suppl 2:S205–S213. doi: 10.1007/s005860100308, PMID 11716020.

81. Akashi R, Ninomiya M. Liquid crystal-polymer composite film, electro-optical element using the same, and process for producing electro-optical element. Google Patents; 1997.

82. Jeong J, Lee SW, Min KS, Shin S, Jun SB, Kim SJ. Liquid crystal polymer (LCP), an attractive substrate for retinal implant. *Sens Mater*. 2012;24(4):189–203.

83. Kim JH, Min KS, An SK, Jeong JS, Jun SB, Cho MH, et al. Magnetic resonance imaging compatibility of the polymer-based cochlear implant. *Clin Exp Otorhinolaryngol*. 2012;5;Suppl 1:S19–S23. doi: 10.3342/ceo.2012.5.S1.S19, PMID 22701769.

84. Li X, Liu X, Huang J, Fan Y, Cui F-Z. Biomedical investigation of CNT based coatings. *Surf Coatings Technol*. 2011;206(4):759–766. doi: 10.1016/j.surfcoat.2011.02.063.

85. Guo HF, Li ZS, Dong SW, Chen WJ, Deng L, Wang YF, et al. Piezoelectric PU/PVDF electrospun scaffolds for wound healing applications. *Colloids Surf B Biointerfaces*. 2012;96:29–36. doi: 10.1016/j.colsurfb.2012.03.014, PMID 22503631.

86. Marques SM, Manninen NK, Ferdov S, Lanceros-Mendez S, Carvalho S. Ti1−xAgx electrodes deposited on polymer based sensors. *Appl Surf Sci*. 2014;317:490–495. doi: 10.1016/j.apsusc.2014.08.142.

87. Sharma T, Je S-S, Gill B, Zhang JXJ. Patterning piezoelectric thin film PVDF– TrFE based pressure sensor for catheter application. *Sens Actuators A*. 2012;177(0):87–92. doi: 10.1016/j.sna.2011.08.019.

88. Sobieraj M, Marwin S. Ultra-high-molecular-weight polyethylene (UHMWPE) in total joint arthroplasty. *Bull Hosp Jt Dis* (2013). 2018 Mar;76(1):38–46. PMID 29537956.

89. Piskin, E. Biodegradable polymers as biomaterials. *J Biomater Sci Polym Ed.* 1995;6(9):775–95.

90. Djošić MS, Bibić N, Mitrić MN, Šiljegović M, Stojanović JN, Jokić B, et al. Electrodeposited hydroxyapatite thin films modified by ion beam irradiation. *J Optoelectron Adv M.* 2009;11:1848–1854.

91. Sharma N. Nanomaterials in plants, algae and microorganisms. In: Durgesh Kumar Tripathi, Parvaiz Ahmad, Nawal Kishore Dubey (eds.), *Chitosan and Its Nanocarriers.* Academic Press; 2019. pp. 267–286. doi: 10.1016/B978-0-12-811488-9.00013-5.

92. Đošić M, Eraković S, Janković A, Vukašinović-Sekulić M, Matić IZ, Stojanović J, et al. In vitro investigation of electrophoretically deposited bioactive hydroxyapatite/chitosan coatings reinforced by graphene. *J Ind Eng Chem.* 2017;47:336–347. doi: 10.1016/j.jiec.2016.12.004.

93. Dorsett-Martin WA, Wysocki AB. Rat models of skin wound healing. In: Wanda A. Dorsett-Martin DVM, Annette B. Wysocki (eds.), *Sourcebook of Models for Biomedical Research.* Humana Press; 2008. pp. 631–638.

94. Louhimies S. Directive 86/609/EEC on the protection of animals used for experimental and other scientific purposes. *Altern Lab Anim.* 2002;30(2):217–219.

95. Borie E, Calzzani R, Dias FJ, Fuentes R, Salamanca C. Morphometry of Rabbit anatomical regions used as experimental models in implantology and oral surgery. *Biomed Res.* 2017;28(12):5468–5472.

96. Khurana RN, Porco TC. Efficacy and safety of dexamethasone intravitreal implant for persistent uveitic cystoid macular edema. *Retina.* 2015;35(8):1640–1646. doi: 10.1097/IAE.0000000000000515, PMID 25741813.

97. Sella R, Oray M, Friling R, Umar L, Tugal-Tutkun I, Kramer M. Dexamethasone intravitreal implant (Ozurdex®) for pediatric uveitis. *Graefes Arch Clin Exp Ophthalmol.* 2015;253(10):1777–1782. doi: 10.1007/s00417-015-3124-x, PMID 26228441.

98. Barbucci R, editor. *Integrated Biomaterials Science.* Springer Science+Business Media; 2002.

99. Langer R, Vacanti JP. Tissue engineering. *Science.* 1993;260(5110):920–926. doi: 10.1126/science.8493529, PMID 8493529.

100. Vacanti JP, Langer R. Tissue engineering: the design and fabrication of living replacement devices for surgical reconstruction and transplantation. *Lancet.* 1999;354;Suppl 1:SI32–SI34. doi: 10.1016/s0140-6736(99)90247-7, PMID 10437854.

101. Kohane DS, Langer R. Polymeric biomaterials in tissue engineering. *Pediatr Res.* 2008;63(5):487–491. doi: 10.1203/01.pdr.0000305937.26105.e7, PMID 18427292.

102. Vert M. Aliphatic polyesters: great degradable polymers that cannot do everything. *Biomacromolecules.* 2005;6(2):538–546. doi: 10.1021/bm0494702, PMID 15762610.

103. Stefanini GG, Holmes Jr DR. Drug-eluting coronary-artery stents. *N Engl J Med.* 2013;368(3):254–265. doi: 10.1056/NEJMra1210816, PMID 23323902.

4 Molecularly imprinted polymer-based materials for biomedical applications

Necla Yucel and Pinar Cakir Hatir

CONTENTS

4.1 Molecular imprinting...55
    4.1.1 Covalent binding..56
    4.1.2 Non-covalent interactions 56
4.2 MIP-based biomaterials..57
    4.2.1 Tissue scaffolds..57
    4.2.2 Drug delivery systems 60
    4.2.3 Drug targeting..61
    4.2.4 Controlled drug release...61
    4.2.5 MIP-based medicine...63
        4.2.5.1 Cell imaging...64
    4.2.6 MIPs as biosensors 65
    4.2.7 Fighting antibiotic resistance...66
4.3 Conclusions and future perspectives 67
References..68

4.1 MOLECULAR IMPRINTING

The molecular recognition mechanism in biological systems is one of the most essential features of nature. Molecular recognition can be defined as the intermolecular interactions between two or more molecules. Distinguishing one molecule from another without any mistake is critical for biological processes. Molecular recognition is the basis of many biochemical reactions in biomolecules such as substrate–enzyme, ligand–receptor, and antibody–antigen (Piletsky, 2006). Thanks to their specific molecular recognition properties, biomolecules have been employed in various biomedical and analytical applications for years, such as affinity chromatography (Gómez-Arribas et al., 2019), biosensors (Crapnell et al., 2020), and drug delivery systems (Shevchenko et al., 2022). However, concerning technological applications, biomolecules have certain disadvantages. They are often expensive since they are

DOI: 10.1201/9781003319139-4

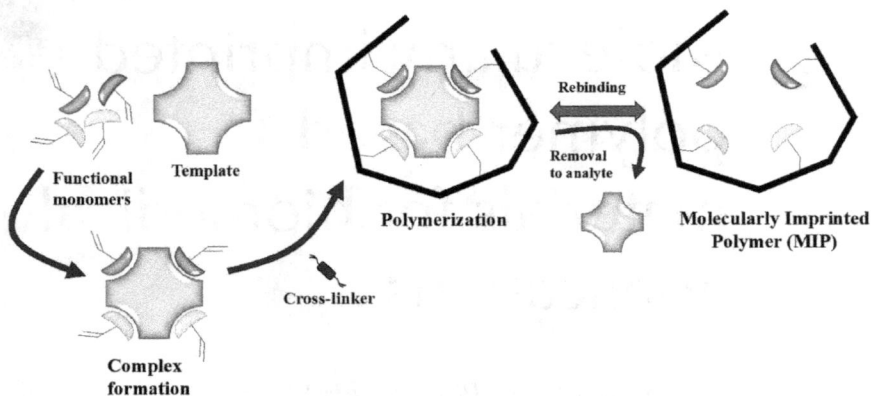

FIGURE 4.1   A schematic representation of molecular imprinting.

hard to obtain and to integrate into conventional industrial processes because they are unstable outside of their native environment (Haupt, 2012). Additionally, finding a natural bioreceptor for all kinds of target molecules is not easy. Thus, scientists have been working to build artificial recognition mechanisms inspired by nature for decades. One of the best ways to create custom-made receptors is the molecular imprinting technique.

Creating template-specific binding (recognition) sites in a polymer network is done using the molecular imprinting technique. In Figure 4.1, molecular imprinting is depicted schematically. The template molecule and functional monomers first form a self-assembled complex through covalent or non-covalent interactions. Following that, polymerization occurs in the presence of the crosslinker. After the polymer network formation, the template molecule is removed, leaving specific and selective binding sites that are complementary to the template in shape, size, and position of the functional groups. In the end, molecularly imprinted polymers (MIPs) are created with the molecular memory.

4.1.1 Covalent binding

The covalent approach involves the formation of covalent bonds between the functional monomers and the template molecule (Lee & Kunitake, 2012). The approach was developed initially by Wulff and Sarhan (1972). Upon forming the covalent bonds between the template and the monomer, the polymer is synthesized in the presence of the cross-linker. Then, the binding sites are created by the cleavage of these bonds. One of the most significant advantages of this approach is the creation of strong interactions, hence specific binding sites. However, at the same time, this strong binding may make it difficult for the template to remove from the polymer network.

4.1.2 Non-covalent interactions

One of the other approaches is the non-covalent approach involving non-covalent interactions between the template molecule and the functional monomers established originally by Mosbach (1981). This approach was inspired by nature, where there is a rich diversity of weak non-covalent interactions. Hydrophobic and ionic interactions, van der Waals forces, as well as hydrogen bonding, are examples of non-covalent interactions (Yilmaz et al., 2005). The most widely used non-covalent imprinting system contains methacrylic acid (MAA, a functional monomer) and ethylene glycol dimethacrylate (EGDMA, a cross-linker). Methacrylic acid is frequently preferred as the functional monomer since it can quickly form hydrogen bonding with numerous template molecules. The non-covalent approach's key benefits are its low cost and ease of use. On the other hand, template leakage and low selectivity may be the drawbacks of this approach (Sarpong et al., 2019).

4.2 MIP-BASED BIOMATERIALS

4.2.1 TISSUE SCAFFOLDS

Tissue scaffolds (TSs) are essential for tissue engineering because they must offer a proper mechanical and chemical environment for seeded cells to grow and operate normally, eventually forming completely functioning tissue. Any scaffold used in tissue engineering must first be biocompatible; cells must attach to the surface, operate correctly, move through the scaffold, initially multiply, then lay down a new matrix. Tissue engineering aims to gradually allow the body's cells to replace the implanted scaffold or tissue-engineered product. Also, scaffolds and structures are not meant to be permanent. Namely, the scaffold must be biodegradable so that cells may generate their extracellular matrix. The scaffold should have mechanical qualities that are compatible with the anatomical location into which it will be implanted. It should be robust enough to allow surgical manipulation during implantation. Scaffold design is crucial for tissue engineering. To allow cellular penetration and proper flow of nutrition to the extracellular matrix, these cells produce, high porosity and a networked pore structure is found to be ideal for scaffolds (O'brien, 2011). To sum up, when creating or establishing the appropriateness of a scaffold suitable for use in tissue engineering, several fundamental considerations are crucial, regardless of tissue types, such as biocompatibility, biodegradability, mechanical properties, scaffold architecture, and fabrication technology (Babensee et al., 1998; Hutmacher, 2000; O'brien, 2011).

Most tissue engineering techniques rely heavily on biomaterials. Biomimetic material design aims to create materials that can interact with surrounding tissues through specialized interactions, like how cells and extracellular matrix (ECM) proteins interact in natural tissues. Two critical design methodologies are used to establish biomolecular recognition of materials by cells. One method is to imbue biomaterials with bioactivity by incorporating soluble bioactive compounds into biomaterial carriers, such as growth factors and plasmid DNA. The bioactive molecule may be released and trigger or influence new tissue creation (Andreadis & Geer, 2006). The other strategy includes using ECM proteins and short peptide sequences produced from them to modify the surface and bulk of biomaterials via chemical or physical means, which can cause interactions with cell receptors (Hersel et al., 2003). Molecular imprinting (MI) technology is an approach to constructing enhanced artificial support structures that encourage cell adhesion and growth (Shea, 1994; Steinke

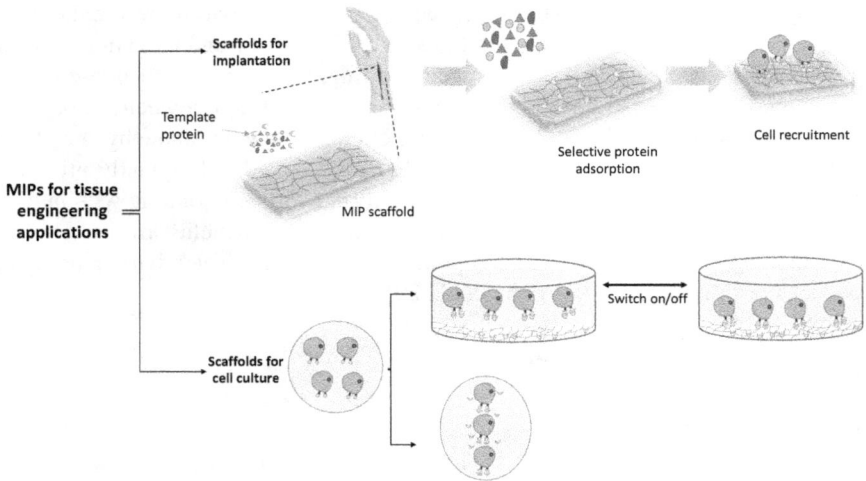

FIGURE 4.2   Tissue engineering applications of molecular imprinting.

et al., 1995; Mosbach & Ramström, 1996). MI technology is a viable replacement for biological molecular recognition systems. Indeed, macromolecular matrices created using this method may be stable even under extreme chemical and physical circumstances, have a long life span with no noticeable degradation in performance, and can be reused without losing memory (Svenson & Nicholls, 2001).

Molecular imprinting is a powerful method for creating scaffolds with high bioactivity and particular molecular recognition capability. Figure 4.2 displays tissue engineering (TE) applications of molecular imprinting. Protein molecular imprinting can help TE techniques, particularly scaffold-based bottom-up methodologies, for creating cellular scaffolds that can be used in cell culture or implantation.

Molecular imprinting can also be utilized to increase cell recruitment to the injury site, activate specific cell activities, and detect and adsorb a biomolecule that is present in situ or transported through the bloodstream (Neves et al., 2017).

Biomacromolecules are important in TE applications because they are involved in healing. Many research groups have developed protein-imprinted MIP systems in response to growing interest in macromolecule imprinting and its potential for therapeutic and pharmacological applications. Model macromolecules (template molecules) like lysozyme (Lyz), bovine serum albumin (BSA), and hemoglobin (Hb) are used in the bulk of protein MIP investigations. (Tabane, 2016; Suquila et al., 2018; Xu et al., 2018). However, biomolecules relevant to TE technologies, such as fibronectin (Fn), are only used in a few research (Zhu et al., 2015; Piletsky et al., 2020). The ECM contains the high-molecular-weight protein Fn, which plays a role in several biological processes, including tissue repair and wound healing (Valenick et al., 2005). Recent breakthroughs in protein imprinting demonstrate that molecularly imprinted smart scaffolds can have a significant impact on regenerative medicine technologies (Lee et al., 2007; Bergmann & Peppas, 2008; Sullivan et al., 2021).

MIPs made of synthetic materials with low degrees of cross-linking, likewise natural materials, have displayed promise for identifying, retaining, and even transporting macromolecules as MIPs have appeared in the biomedical sector (Clegg et al., 2017). Because of molecular imprinting's specificity and recognition capabilities, it has the potential to be used to design scaffolds with bioactivity and recognition capability for tissue engineering (TE) applications (Neves et al., 2017). Various MIP-based products are currently under development. For instance, Rosellini et al. (2010) described MIPs that recognize a pentapeptide fragment of an exposed fibronectin functional domain and their use as functionalization structures in constructing bioactive scaffolds. Because fibronectin was the principal ECM sticky glycoprotein and played a critical role in cell adhesion, migration, and repair, it was chosen as the molecule to be detected. The choice of fibronectin as the recognized molecule was supported by the fact that it is the primary ECM sticky glycoprotein and plays a critical role in cell adhesion, migration, and repair (Hersel et al., 2003). Rosellini and her team used precipitation polymerization to imprint a peptide sequence exposed by fibronectin onto MAA-based microgel spheres. In this work, researchers found that MI beads may preferentially bind to the entire fibronectin molecule as well as a single peptide sequence, promoting cell adhesion and proliferation when employed to functionalize the scaffold.

At many scale levels in natural systems, molecular identification is crucial. The immune system, for example, uses globular proteins (antibodies) that contain antigen-binding sites to identify foreign objects inside the body (using antigens). Fibrous and amorphous components of the ECM interact with cells via surface receptors (i.e., integrins). Cell–ECM interactions influence cell differentiation and proliferation, cell orientation, molecule secretion, and ECM remodeling (Li et al., 2017; Honig et al., 2020). Furthermore, growth factors (GFs) are attached to insoluble components of the ECM, which control their concentration and activity dynamically. Scaffolds must offer enough mechanical and structural support and actively guide and govern cell attachment, migration, proliferation, and differentiation in this respect. The scaffold's capabilities need to be expanded to include biological signals such as cues for interacting with cells and the capacity to administer GFs in a regulated manner (Biondi et al., 2008).

Pan and coworkers (2013) described a unique cell sheet harvesting product based on a PNIPAM-based MIP hydrogel layer with a thermoresponsive affinity for biomolecules. To show the proof-of-principle of their technique, the frequently utilized cell-adhesive peptide (RGDS) was selected as the target molecule. The MIPs' thermoresponsive recognition sites were utilized to create temperature-dependent interactions between RGDS molecules and the cell culture substrate throughout their development. A stable recognition of RGDS occurred at 37°C because of the thermoresponsive recognition sites on the MIP hydrogel layer. They triggered the release of RGDS when the temperature was lowered and the temperature-induced change in surface wettability. This is the first study that molecular imprinting has been used to biofunctionalized thermoresponsive cell culture substrates to harvest cell sheets for biomedical purposes.

Various aspects of MIP fabrication must be carefully considered when manufacturing material for TE applications. The selection of functional monomer(s) (and monomer ratios) is essential, especially after a suitable template molecule has been selected. Allowing for thermodynamically favorable and stable template–monomer complexes under reaction conditions, biocompatibility, and non-toxicity are important parameters for the chosen monomers (Kryscio & Peppas, 2012).

Biodegradability is particularly significant in bulk imprinted materials to allow for the exposure of new binding sites. The degree and kind of crosslinking employed in MIP can influence its biodegradability and flexibility. By decreasing mobility (e.g., swelling) and fixing binding sites, higher levels of cross-linking can induce better selectivity (Byrne et al., 2002). On the other hand, excessive cross-linking interactions might make template removal more difficult and diminish rebinding ability due to poor diffusion (Ou et al., 2004).

Biological uses of MIPs favor non-covalent approaches due to more gentle template removal procedures (Byrne et al., 2002), despite covalent and non-covalent cross-linking strategies for MIP formation.

4.2.2 DRUG DELIVERY SYSTEMS

Drug delivery systems (DDS) play a critical role in modern scientific medicine. DDS are engineered technologies that allow drug molecules to be delivered precisely and released in a regulated manner. DDS have two primary goals: to maximize the efficacy of the drug molecule and reduce its side effects (Puoci et al., 2010). Several significant improvements in developing novel technologies for optimizing drug delivery have been accomplished over the last decades. DDS should transport the drug molecule to the most appropriate location in the body, extending the drug molecule's action time while limiting side effects. Because of their strong affinity, MIP-based drug delivery systems may be attractive options for providing high loading capacity and prolonged release (Figure 4.3). MIPs act as a drug reservoir because they have cross-linked networks with complementary cavities for drug molecules. MIPs, on the other hand, may have a low cross-linking density, allowing the polymer network to alter conformation in response to external stimuli such as pH, temperature, solvent composition, electric fields, light wavelengths, and ionic strength (Zaidi, 2016). Not to mention that MIPs are very resistant to harsh environmental conditions,

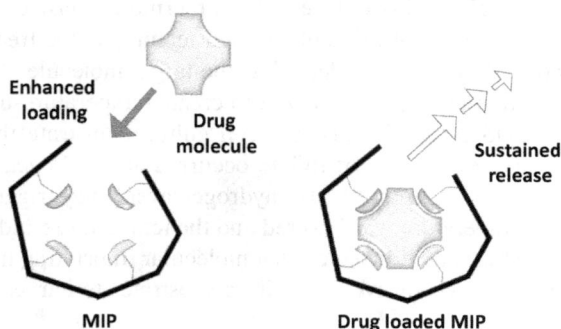

FIGURE 4.3   MIP-based drug delivery.

including highly basic and acidic pH, thermal and mechanical stresses. MIPs are ideal candidates for DDS because of all these properties.

Norell described one of the first potential MIP-based drug release systems (Norell et al., 1998).

They developed MIP to recognize the anti-asthmatic drug theophylline in the presence of its analog, caffeine, and showed that it could distinguish theophylline selectively. These studies demonstrated that MIP might be employed successfully in DDS due to its selective binding properties.

4.2.3 DRUG TARGETING

Active targeted drug delivery and passive targeted drug delivery are the two types of drug targeting approaches. Active targeting of drug molecules usually relies on biological ligands such as peptides, antibodies, and aptamers (Xu et al., 2021). Passive drug targeting is mainly based on the enhanced permeability and retention (EPR) effect, which causes nanoscale molecules to accumulate in tumor tissue much more than in healthy tissues (Matsumura & Maeda, 1986).

Biological ligands used in active targeting may have various unresolved challenges, including high-cost, time-consuming method, in vivo instability, and inherent immunogenicity. On the other hand, the MIP-based drug targeting approach provides specific recognition sites with a higher physical and chemical stability, better availability, and lower costs than biomolecules. The first successful example of a prospective active drug targeting application was published in 2000 (Allender et al., 2000). This study investigated histamine- and ephedrine-imprinted polymers as possible biological receptor mimics. The polymers were loaded with propranolol as a transdermal controlled release device. Tumor cells overexpress specific surface receptor proteins, making them perfect candidates for tumor cell identification. Therefore, all the protein-imprinted polymers are good candidates for active targeting strategy. For instance, cancer antigen 125 (CA125)-imprinted polymers were produced on the surface of graphene oxide for drug delivery, and the antitumor drug doxorubicin (DOX) was loaded into the composites (Han et al., 2019). The composites that bind to CA125 specifically could be used to target tumor cells and boost the efficacy of antitumor pharmaceuticals delivered into the tumor cells.

Takeuchi and colleagues revealed that human serum albumin (HSA)-imprinted nanogels allowed longer circulation (Takeuchi et al., 2017). The HSA-imprinted nanogels reacted with HSA in mice's blood after intravenous injection, forming an albumin-rich protein corona surrounding the nanogels and producing a prolonged circulation time in blood vessels with essentially minimal retention in liver tissue. According to this study, MIP nanogels have approximately sixfold higher accumulation in tumors than in healthy tissues, thanks to the EPR effect. This study is one of the best examples of MIPs targeting tumor tissues passively via the EPR effect.

4.2.4 CONTROLLED DRUG RELEASE

Controlling drug release, which relies on the stimuli-responsive systems, is critical for improving treatment efficacy. The development and application of functional nanomaterials are usually the basis for controlling drug release (Shevchenko et al., 2022). Most stimuli-responsive systems used in nano-based controlled drug release respond to environmental parameters, including temperature, pH, ion concentration, and external factors such as light and magnetic field (Hatır, 2020) (Figure 4.4). The adaptability of MIP-based drug delivery systems is critical for managing drug release, especially in cancer nanomedicine.

A MIP imprinted with a targeting moiety for the cellular biomarker and the imprinted medication for delivery may be seen in the left image. Different external and internal stimuli are shown in the right image to trigger MIP-mediated drug release that is responsive to those stimuli (lower part).

Because the tumor microenvironment is slightly acidic, drug delivery systems that are pH-sensitive play a significant role in cancer treatment. Non-covalent interactions created between the template molecule and the functional monomers, including hydrogen bonding and electrostatic interactions, can easily be affected by the pH of the medium. For instance, Wang and coworkers developed hollow microcapsules with doxorubicin (DOX)-imprinted shells to deliver the chemotherapy agent to the tumor cell (Wang et al., 2014). They demonstrated that the electrostatic interactions between DOX's amino group and MIP's carboxyl groups diminished at low pH, resulting in a pH-responsive release. At neutral pH, the hollow microcapsules released DOX slowly. However, they released the chemotherapy

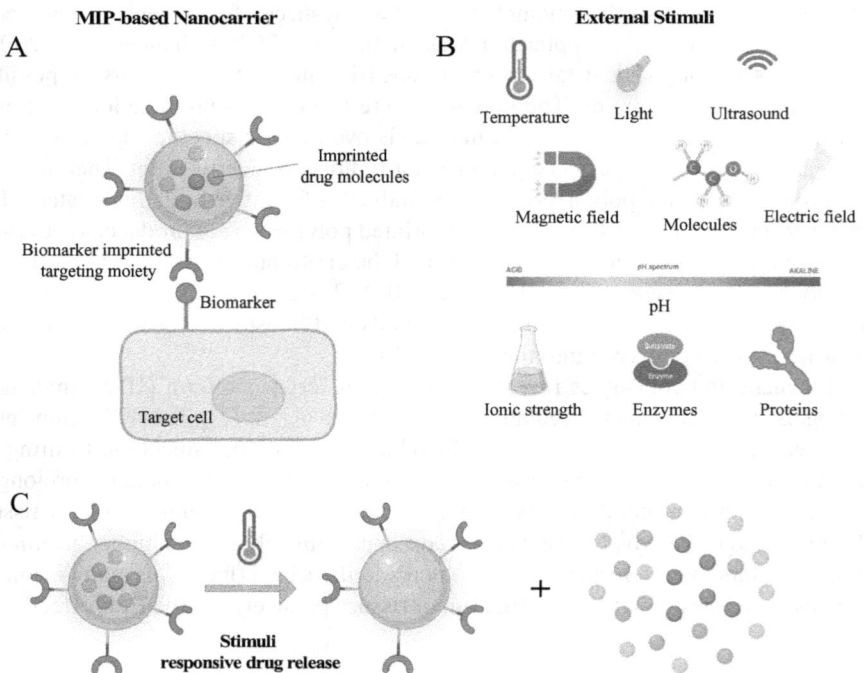

FIGURE 4.4 Drug delivery using molecularly imprinted polymers is shown schematically.

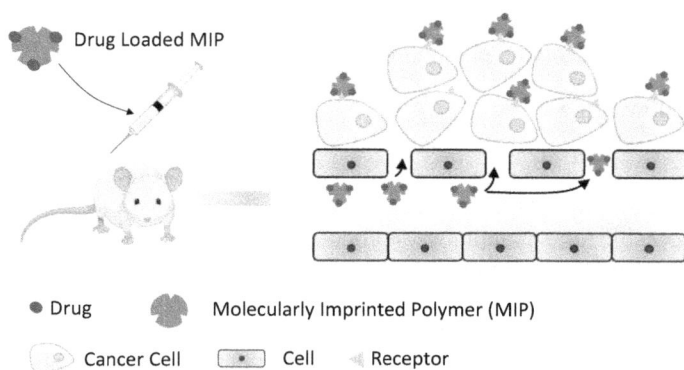

FIGURE 4.5 The MIP-based smart delivery system's schematic drug transport mechanism includes both active and passive targeting strategies.

agent quickly at acidic pH, which is advantageous in the acidic environment of tumor cells. Additionally, they articulated that DOX could trigger apoptosis of U373 malignant glioma cells and had better efficacy in terms of tumor inhibition within 144 hrs than free DOX.

Gu used the covalent approach to develop another pH-responsive MIP-based drug release system (Gu et al., 2021). Due to a strong covalent bond, the drug molecule could not be released from MIP at pH 7.4, while at pH 6.8, the covalent bond was disturbed, allowing the drug molecule to be gradually released. Sialic acid, a monosaccharide overexpressed in tumor cells, targeted the tumors. They employed 5′-deoxy-5-fluorocytidine (DFCR) as the prodrug, which can be converted to 5-fluorouracil (FU) in the tumor by thymidine phosphorylase. FU can inhibit DNA synthesis in cells via the inhibition of thymidylate synthase. The inhibition of thymidylate synthase by FU can prevent DNA synthesis in cells. The schematic representation of the drug transport mechanism in the MIP-based smart prodrug delivery system is shown in Figure 4.5, which illustrates both passive and active targeting. Through the EPR effect, drug-loaded MIP nanoparticles enter the cancerous tissue where they are bound to the cancer cell surface via receptors.

4.2.5 MIP-BASED MEDICINE

Apart from drug delivery systems, MIP itself can be used as medicine. For instance, the template peptides, the toxin melittin, have been recognized, neutralized, and cleared in the circulation in vivo utilizing molecularly imprinted polymeric nanoparticles with binding affinity and selectivity equivalent to natural antibodies (Hoshino et al., 2010). They demonstrated that they could obtain nanoparticles only slightly larger than proteins, with a high affinity and selectivity for the bee toxin melittin. They developed for the first time a plastic antibody that can be used to capture a toxin and neutralize it in the bloodstream of living animals. An exciting application was reported by Cutivet et al. (2009). They exhibited that MIP nanogels can be utilized to inhibit specific enzymes, which is the first example of a water-compatible molecularly imprinted microgel with biological activity.

4.2.5.1 Cell imaging

Single targets are frequently the focus of traditional screening paradigms. Powerful cellular imaging tools have been created to aid drug discovery in a cell or organism's more complicated physiological milieu. The development of these detection technologies has enabled the quantitative study of cellular events and the display of key cellular phenotypes. Cellular imaging makes it easier to include intricate biology into the screening process while also meeting high-content and high-throughput requirements. The employment of a system or technology capable of viewing a cell population, single-cell, or subcellular features, in conjunction with image analysis tools, is called cellular imaging. From a specific biological event or cell type, these technologies retrieve a two-dimensional pixel array of information (Lang et al., 2006).

At the hand of their superior optical qualities, fluorescent materials have been extensively employed as fluorescent probes for detection of analytes and imaging cells (Deng et al., 2013; Yuan et al., 2013). Furthermore, MIP-based fluorescent probes have been successfully used to image cells and detect analytes when combined with the excellent selectivity of MIPs. For example, in 2013, Deng's group designed a nanosensor based on fluorescent MIP created by covering multi-wall carbon nanotubes with imprinted polymer and treating them with fluorescein isothiocyanate (FITC) after the imprinting process. This developed material can be used in cell imaging studies. In another study, Song and coworkers (2014) designed lysozyme detection using an ultrasensitive carboxymethyl chitosan-quantum dot-based fluorescent "turn on–off" nanosensor. In recent research, Fang's team developed a fluorescent probe (CDs/SiO$_2$/MIP) to detect lysozyme, and cell imaging was created by combining the selectivity of MIP with the optical characteristics of carbon dots (CDs), using slightly cytotoxic CDs/SiO$_2$ and N-isopropylacrylamide (NIPAM). This study's significance is that CDs/SiO$_2$/MIP had low cytotoxicity, and HepG-2 cells displayed a high intracellular green fluorescence after being cultured with CDs/SiO$_2$/MIP for 48 hrs, showing that CDs/SiO$_2$/MIP could enter HepG-2 cells.

MIPs could be constructed with a specific binding affinity toward certain cell membrane molecules (e.g., proteins, lipids, etc.) or the ensemble of the cell membrane to detect a cell-in-cell imaging (Figure 4.6). Currently proposed approaches for MIP-mediated cell identification may be split into two groups based on this approach: cell membrane molecular imprinting and whole-cell imprinting (Pan et al., 2018).

Kunath and his colleagues (2015) used MIP antibody mimics to locate and quantify target molecules on the cell surface using molecular imaging of cells and tissue. Because molecular imprinting of complete biomacromolecules such as proteins or oligosaccharides is complex, the Kunath team used a technique inspired by nature dubbed the "epitope approach" (Rachkov & Minoura, 2001; Nishino et al., 2006). In this work, dye-labeled nanoparticles of produced MIP (the template molecule is glucuronic acid) were manufactured and utilized to photograph hyaluronan on human keratinocytes and adult skin specimens using epifluorescence confocal fluorescence microscopy (Kunath et al., 2015).

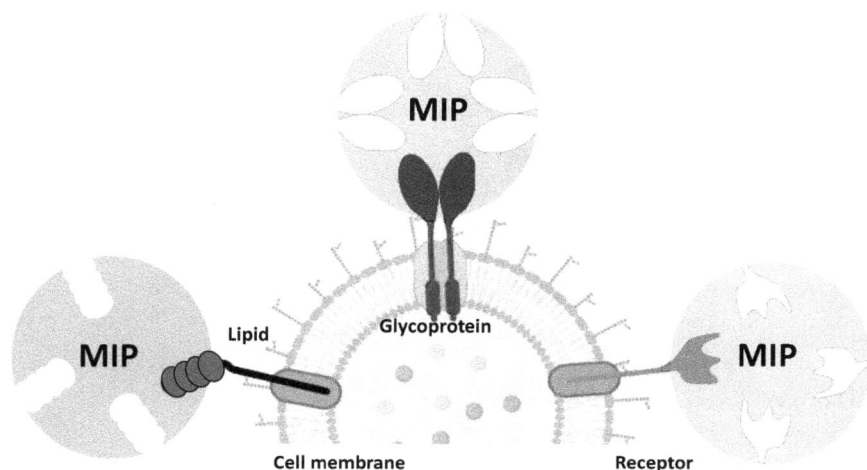

FIGURE 4.6 MIPs with cell recognition properties.

These results show that cell imaging with molecularly imprinted fluorescent probes using fluorescent materials and techniques such as cell imprinting with molecular imprinting is promising in diagnosing and treating diseases, especially drug applications.

4.2.6 MIPs AS BIOSENSORS

Biosensing relies heavily on molecular recognition. A biosensor is a "compact analytical instrument or unit combining a biological or biologically derived sensitive recognition element integrated or coupled with a physiochemical transducer" (Figure 4.7) (Turner, 2013; Jayanthi et al., 2017; Chen et al., 2019). A biosensor is defined as an electronic device that converts biological impulses into electrical signals (Wang et al., 2020). Many biosensors have been investigated and developed since Updike and Hicks established the first biosensor.

Biosensors are provided biochemical specificity and are in intimate association or integration within a physicochemical transducer, electrochemical, optical, mass sensitive, plasmonic nanosensor, etc. This detection approach performs well because it is simple, affordable, highly specific, and sensitive (Wang et al., 2020).

Electrochemical sensors that convert the interactions of an analyte with a receptor on the electrode surface into a proper analytical signal are widely used in many branches of industry, traffic, and environmental and medical monitoring for the study of metabolism and the control of biological processes. Electrochemical sensors are well-known and powerful methods for acquiring real-time information for process control using in situ chemical composition measurements rather than sampling (Guth et al., 2009). MIPs are used in electrochemical biosensors (Figure 4.7) thanks to their structure predictability, excellent sensitivity, and identification capabilities with the desired selectivity. Mosbach and Haupt were the first to integrate an electrochemical

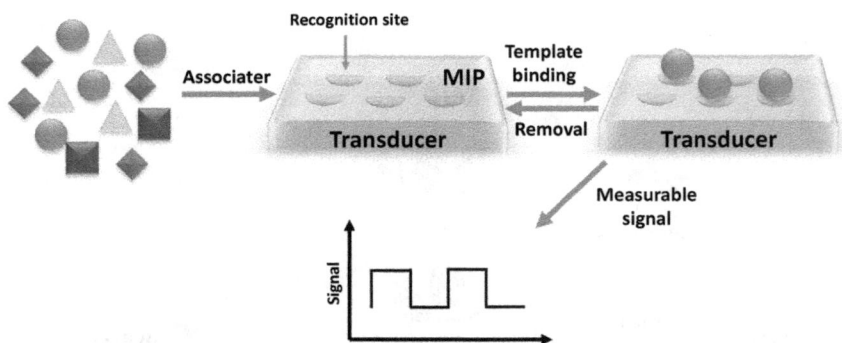

FIGURE 4.7   Schematic diagram of a MIP-based biosensor.

sensor with MIPs to create a MIPs-coated electrode, dubbed a molecularly imprinted electrochemical sensor in 1999 (Kröger et al., 1999). The MIP on the electrochemical sensor has recognition and transduction capabilities, meaning that it can precisely bind target analytes and provide a chemical or physical signal as a recognition element. For detection, a transducer converts the signal to a measurable output signal like potential, current, conductivity, or impedance change (Duan et al., 2018). Many applications of MIP-based electrochemical biosensors are reported in the literature (Xue et al., 2013; Russell et al., 2019; Crapnell et al., 2020). For example, Xue and coworkers' (2013) gold nanoparticles doped MIPs were used to create a highly sensitive and selective biomimetic electrochemical sensor to detect dopamine in human serums. Another study related MIP-based electrochemical biosensor design by Duan and coworkers (2018). The designed biosensor is as follows, 3D porous electrocatalytic framework materials and graphene-modified glassy carbon electrode, an electrochemical sensor for ultra-trace detection of biomacromolecule, which is bovine serum albumin (BSA).

Careful tuning of the synthesis, template removal, and detection parameters is essential to reach the levels of detection and reliability required for a successful bio-marker sensor. On the other hand, MIP-based biomimetic sensors are still inferior to biosensors in terms of sensitivity since MIPs and transducers must be further optimized. Considering the numerous benefits MIPs provide to sensor systems, it is expected that future research interest in this area and the development of more sensi-tive MIP-based sensors are expected.

4.2.7   FIGHTING ANTIBIOTIC RESISTANCE

Alexander Fleming discovered penicillin, the first antibiotic in history, in 1928. Since then, antibiotics have revolutionized medicine and extended life. Every person requires effective antibiotics since infections are a reality of life. Furthermore, effec-tive antibiotics are essential for patients who require organ transplantation, have sur-gery, or are undergoing cancer treatments. However, in recent years, microorganisms have become more resistant to traditional antibiotics due to multi-drug resistance (MDR) (Tse Sum Bui et al., 2022).

MIP-based strategies may be effective ways to combat resistant microorganisms. MIPs can capture ß-lactamase, quorum-sensing messengers, and extracellular polymeric substance (EPS) matrix components that support biofilm development. The most often prescribed conventional antibiotics are ß-lactam antibiotics, to which bacteria have slowly developed resistance through the expression of drug-deactivating enzymes, for instance, ß-lactamases. A MIP-based hydrogel was synthesized to recognize and inhibit the enzyme, ß-lactamase (Li et al., 2016). To assess the MIP's effectiveness in antibacterial applications, MIP was introduced to methicillin-resistant bacteria in the presence of penicillin G, one of the ß-lactam antibiotics. As a result, the bacterial viability dropped by 80%, the MIP was able to capture the ß-lactamase that the bacteria were excreting, thus reducing the bacterial resistance. Bacteria communicate with one another through a process called quorum sensing (QS) (Miller & Bassler, 2001). Small signaling molecules known as autoinducers are responsible for mediating QS. Bacteria can detect the density of their local population thanks to autoinducers. The concentration of autoinducers increases along with the bacteria population and biofilm formation is then triggered. MIPs can be designed to capture the signaling molecules. Piletska et al. demonstrated the first example of MIP to prevent the growth of biofilms to specifically capture signal molecules (Piletska et al., 2011). When MIP was present, as opposed to the control polymer, the growth of the biofilm was seen to be reduced by 80%.

4.3   CONCLUSIONS AND FUTURE PERSPECTIVES

In conclusion, this chapter explains significant progress in the application of MIPs, which has been documented repeatedly in the literature in recent years. MIPs are the most promising synthetic materials for molecular identification in several scientific domains because of their low cost, good stability, and continually improving performance (Vasapollo et al., 2011).

This part of the book reviews current breakthroughs in MIPs for biomedical applications, such as tissue scaffolds, biosensors, drug delivery, cell imaging, and drug targeting. MIPs have unique qualities such as high physicochemical stability, extended shelf life, ease of modification and functionalization, and superior biocompatibility, making them a viable alternative to natural antibodies in various medicinal applications (Choi et al., 2019).

The sensitivity of MIPs can be improved by adopting proportional fluorescence measurements (Geng et al., 2018). A lot of work is still needed to construct optimum recognition systems for each analyte chosen as the template molecule. Materials with a higher degree of accessibility and flexibility are required to facilitate the imprinting of larger biological molecules (Uzun & Turner, 2016).

The following stages in MIP-based drug delivery applications should involve research into MIP biosafety problems and clinical trials of innovative MIP-based devices (Choi et al., 2019). For all reasons above, more research on MIPs dedicated to biological applications is expected to be conducted in the near future, given the numerous potential problems.

REFERENCES

Allender, C. J., Richardson, C., Woodhouse, B., Heard, C. M., & Brain, K. R. (2000). Pharmaceutical applications for molecularly imprinted polymers. *International Journal of Pharmaceutics*, 195(1–2), 39–43.

Andreadis, S. T., & Geer, D. J. (2006). Biomimetic approaches to protein and gene delivery for tissue regeneration. *Trends in Biotechnology*, 24(7), 331–337.

Babensee, J. E., Anderson, J. M., McIntire, L. V., & Mikos, A. G. (1998). Host response to tissue engineered devices. *Advanced Drug Delivery Reviews*, 33(1–2), 111–139.

Bergmann, N. M., & Peppas, N. A. (2008). Molecularly imprinted polymers with specific recognition for macromolecules and proteins. *Progress in Polymer Science*, 33(3), 271–288.

Biondi, M., Ungaro, F., Quaglia, F., & Netti, P. A. (2008). Controlled drug delivery in tissue engineering. *Advanced Drug Delivery Reviews*, 60(2), 229–242.

Byrne, M. E., Park, K., & Peppas, N. A. (2002). Molecular imprinting within hydrogels. *Advanced Drug Delivery Reviews*, 54(1), 149–161.

Chen, Y., Liu, J., Yang, Z., Wilkinson, J. S., & Zhou, X. (2019). Optical biosensors based on refractometric sensing schemes: A review. *Biosensors and Bioelectronics*, 144, 111693.

Choi, J. R., Yong, K. W., Choi, J. Y., & Cowie, A. C. (2019). Progress in molecularly imprinted polymers for biomedical applications. *Combinatorial Chemistry & High Throughput Screening*, 22(2), 78–88.

Clegg, J. R., Wechsler, M. E., & Peppas, N. A. (2017). Vision for functionally decorated and molecularly imprinted polymers in regenerative engineering. *Regenerative Engineering and Translational Medicine*, 3(3), 166–175.

Crapnell, R. D., Dempsey-Hibbert, N. C., Peeters, M., Tridente, A., & Banks, C. E. (2020). Molecularly imprinted polymer based electrochemical biosensors: Overcoming the challenges of detecting vital biomarkers and speeding up diagnosis. *Talanta Open*, 2, 100018.

Cutivet, A., Schembri, C., Kovensky, J., & Haupt, K. (2009). Molecularly imprinted microgels as enzyme inhibitors. *Journal of the American Chemical Society*, 131(41), 14699–14702.

Deng, Q., Wu, J., Zhai, X., Fang, G., & Wang, S. (2013). Highly selective fluorescent sensing of proteins based on a fluorescent molecularly imprinted nanosensor. *Sensors*, 13(10), 12994–13004.

Duan, D., Yang, H., Ding, Y., Ye, D., Li, L., & Ma, G. (2018). Three-dimensional molecularly imprinted electrochemical sensor based on Au NPs@ Ti-based metal-organic frameworks for ultra-trace detection of bovine serum albumin. *Electrochimica Acta*, 261, 160–166.

El-Schich, Z., Zhang, Y., Feith, M., Beyer, S., Sternbæk, L., Ohlsson, L., & Wingren, A. G. (2020). Molecularly imprinted polymers in biological applications. *BioTechniques*, 69(6), 406–419.

Geng, Y., Guo, M., Tan, J., Huang, S., Tang, Y., Tan, L., & Liang, Y. (2018). A fluorescent molecularly imprinted polymer using aptamer as a functional monomer for sensing of kanamycin. *Sensors and Actuators B: Chemical*, 268, 47–54.

Gómez-Arribas, L. N., Urraca, J. L., Benito-Peña, E., & Moreno-Bondi, M. C. (2019). Tag-specific affinity purification of recombinant proteins by using molecularly imprinted polymers. *Analytical Chemistry*, 91(6), 4100–4106.

Gu, Z., Dong, Y., Xu, S., Wang, L., & Liu, Z. (2021). Molecularly imprinted polymer-based smart prodrug delivery system for specific targeting, prolonged retention, and tumor microenvironment-triggered release. *Angewandte Chemie*, 133(5), 2695–2699.

Guth, U., Vonau, W., & Zosel, J. (2009). Recent developments in electrochemical sensor application and technology—a review. *Measurement Science and Technology*, 20(4), 042002.

Han, S., Su, L., Zhai, M., Ma, L., Liu, S., & Teng, Y. (2019). A molecularly imprinted composite based on graphene oxide for targeted drug delivery to tumor cells. *Journal of Materials Science*, 54(4), 3331–3341.

Hatır, P. Ç. (2020). Biomedical Nanotechnology: Why "Nano"? In Pınar Çakır Hatır (Ed.), *Biomedical and Clinical Engineering for Healthcare Advancement* (pp. 30–65). IGI Global.

Haupt, K. (Ed.). (2012). *Molecular Imprinting* (Vol. 325). Springer Science & Business Media.

Hersel, U., Dahmen, C., & Kessler, H. (2003). RGD modified polymers: biomaterials for stimulated cell adhesion and beyond. *Biomaterials*, 24(24), 4385–4415.

Honig, F., Vermeulen, S., Zadpoor, A. A., De Boer, J., & Fratila-Apachitei, L. E. (2020). Natural architectures for tissue engineering and regenerative medicine. *Journal of Functional Biomaterials*, 11(3), 47.

Hoshino, Y., Koide, H., Urakami, T., Kanazawa, H., Kodama, T., Oku, N., & Shea, K. J. (2010). Recognition, neutralization, and clearance of target peptides in the bloodstream of living mice by molecularly imprinted polymer nanoparticles: a plastic antibody. *Journal of the American Chemical Society*, 132(19), 6644–6645.

Hutmacher, D. W. (2000). Scaffolds in tissue engineering bone and cartilage. *Biomaterials*, 21(24), 2529–2543.

Jayanthi, V. S. A., Das, A. B., & Saxena, U. (2017). Recent advances in biosensor development for the detection of cancer biomarkers. *Biosensors and Bioelectronics*, 91, 15–23.

Kröger, S., Turner, A. P., Mosbach, K., & Haupt, K. (1999). Imprinted polymer-based sensor system for herbicides using differential-pulse voltammetry on screen-printed electrodes. *Analytical Chemistry*, 71(17), 3698–3702.

Kryscio, D. R., & Peppas, N. A. (2012). Critical review and perspective of macromolecularly imprinted polymers. *Acta Biomaterialia*, 8(2), 461–473.

Kunath, S., Panagiotopoulou, M., Maximilien, J., Marchyk, N., Sänger, J., & Haupt, K. (2015). Cell and tissue imaging with molecularly imprinted polymers as plastic antibody mimics. *Advanced Healthcare Materials*, 4(9), 1322–1326.

Lang, P., Yeow, K., Nichols, A., & Scheer, A. (2006). Cellular imaging in drug discovery. *Nature Reviews Drug Discovery*, 5(4), 343–356.

Lee, K., Itharaju, R. R., & Puleo, D. A. (2007). Protein-imprinted polysiloxane scaffolds. *Acta Biomaterialia*, 3(4), 515–522.

Lee, S. W., & Kunitake, T. (Eds.). (2012). *Handbook of Molecular Imprinting: Advanced Sensor Applications*. CRC Press.

Li, W., Dong, K., Ren, J., & Qu, X. (2016). A β-lactamase-imprinted responsive hydrogel for the treatment of antibiotic-resistant bacteria. *Angewandte Chemie*, 128(28), 8181–8185.

Li, Y., Xiao, Y., & Liu, C. (2017). The horizon of materiobiology: a perspective on material-guided cell behaviors and tissue engineering. *Chemical Reviews*, 117(5), 4376–4421.

Matsumura, Y., & Maeda, H. (1986). A new concept for macromolecular therapeutics in cancer chemotherapy: mechanism of tumoritropic accumulation of proteins and the antitumor agent smancs. *Cancer Research*, 46(12 Part 1), 6387–6392.

Miller, M. B., & Bassler, B. L. (2001). Quorum sensing in bacteria. *Annual Review of Microbiology*, 55(1), 165–199.

Mosbach, K., & Ramström, O. (1996). The emerging technique of molecular imprinting and its future impact on biotechnology. *Bio/Technology*, 14(2), 163–170.

Neves, M. I., Wechsler, M. E., Gomes, M. E., Reis, R. L., Granja, P. L., & Peppas, N. A. (2017). Molecularly imprinted intelligent scaffolds for tissue engineering applications. *Tissue Engineering Part B: Reviews*, 23(1), 27–43.

Nishino, H., Huang, C. S., & Shea, K. J. (2006). Selective protein capture by epitope imprinting. *Angewandte Chemie*, 118(15), 2452–2456.

Norell, M. C., Andersson, H. S., & Nicholls, I. A. (1998). Theophylline molecularly imprinted polymer dissociation kinetics: a novel sustained release drug dosage mechanism. *Journal of Molecular Recognition: An Interdisciplinary Journal*, 11(1–6), 98–102.

O'brien, F. J. (2011). Biomaterials & scaffolds for tissue engineering. *Materials Today*, 14(3), 88–95.

Ou, S. H., Wu, M. C., Chou, T. C., & Liu, C. C. (2004). Polyacrylamide gels with electrostatic functional groups for the molecular imprinting of lysozyme. *Analytica Chimica Acta*, 504(1), 163–166.

Pan, G., Guo, Q., Ma, Y., Yang, H., & Li, B. (2013). Thermo-responsive hydrogel layers imprinted with RGDS peptide: a system for harvesting cell sheets. *Angewandte Chemie International Edition*, 52(27), 6907–6911.

Pan, J., Chen, W., Ma, Y., & Pan, G. (2018). Molecularly imprinted polymers as receptor mimics for selective cell recognition. *Chemical Society Reviews*, 47(15), 5574–5587.

Piletska, E. V., Stavroulakis, G., Larcombe, L. D., Whitcombe, M. J., Sharma, A., Primrose, S., & Piletsky, S. A. (2011). Passive control of quorum sensing: prevention of Pseudomonas aeruginosa biofilm formation by imprinted polymers. *Biomacromolecules*, 12(4), 1067–1071.

Piletsky, S. (2006). *Molecular Imprinting of Polymers*. CRC Press.

Piletsky, S., Canfarotta, F., Poma, A., Bossi, A. M., & Piletsky, S. (2020). Molecularly imprinted polymers for cell recognition. *Trends in Biotechnology*, 38(4), 368–387.

Puoci, F., Cirillo, G., Curcio, M., Iemma, F., Parisi, O. I., Spizzirri, U. G., & Picci, N. (2010). Molecularly imprinted polymers (PIMs) in biomedical applications. In *Biopolymers*. IntechOpen.

Rachkov, A., & Minoura, N. (2001). Towards molecularly imprinted polymers selective to peptides and proteins. The epitope approach. *Biochimica et Biophysica Acta (BBA)-Protein Structure and Molecular Enzymology*, 1544(1–2), 255–266.

Rosellini, E., Barbani, N., Giusti, P., Ciardelli, G., & Cristallini, C. (2010). Novel bioactive scaffolds with fibronectin recognition nanosites based on molecular imprinting technology. *Journal of Applied Polymer Science*, 118(6), 3236–3244.

Russell, C., Ward, A. C., Vezza, V., Hoskisson, P., Alcorn, D., Steenson, D. P., & Corrigan, D. K. (2019). Development of a needle shaped microelectrode for electrochemical detection of the sepsis biomarker interleukin-6 (IL-6) in real time. *Biosensors and Bioelectronics*, 126, 806–814.

Sarpong, K. A., Xu, W., Huang, W., & Yang, W. (2019). The development of molecularly imprinted polymers in the clean-up of water pollutants: a review. *American Journal of Analytical Chemistry*, 10(5), 202–226.

Shea, K. J. (1994). Molecular imprinting of synthetic network polymers: the de novo synthesis of macromolecular binding and catalytic sites. *Trends in Polymer Science*, 2, 166–173.

Shevchenko, K. G., Garkushina, I. S., Canfarotta, F., Piletsky, S. A., & Barlev, N. A. (2022). Nano-molecularly imprinted polymers (nanoMIPs) as a novel approach to targeted drug delivery in nanomedicine. *RSC Advances*, 12(7), 3957–3968.

Song, Y., Li, Y., Liu, Z., Liu, L., Wang, X., Su, X., & Ma, Q. (2014). A novel ultrasensitive carboxymethyl chitosan-quantum dot-based fluorescence "turn on–off" nanosensor for lysozyme detection. *Biosensors and Bioelectronics*, 61, 9–13.

Steinke, J., Sherrington, D. C., & Dunkin, I. R. (1995). Imprinting of synthetic polymers using molecular templates. *Synthesis and Photosynthesis*, 123, 81–125.

Sullivan, M. V., Clay, O., Moazami, M. P., Watts, J. K., & Turner, N. W. (2021). Hybrid Aptamer-Molecularly Imprinted Polymer (aptaMIP) nanoparticles from protein recognition—a trypsin model. *Macromolecular Bioscience*, 21(5), 2100002.

Suquila, F. A., de Oliveira, L. L., & Tarley, C. R. (2018). Restricted access copper imprinted poly (allylthiourea): the role of hydroxyethyl methacrylate (HEMA) and bovine serum albumin (BSA) on the sorptive performance of imprinted polymer. *Chemical Engineering Journal*, 350, 714–728.

Svenson, J., & Nicholls, I. A. (2001). On the thermal and chemical stability of molecularly imprinted polymers. *Analytica Chimica Acta*, 435(1), 19–24.

Tabane, T. H. (2016). A novel molecularly imprinted polymer for the selective removal of interfering hemoglobin prior to whole blood analysis (Doctoral dissertation, Botswana International University of Science & Technology (BIUST)).

Takeuchi, T., Kitayama, Y., Sasao, R., Yamada, T., Toh, K., Matsumoto, Y., & Kataoka, K. (2017). Molecularly imprinted nanogels acquire stealth in situ by cloaking themselves with native dysopsonic proteins. *Angewandte Chemie*, 129(25), 7194–7198.

Tse Sum Bui, B., Auroy, T., & Haupt, K. (2022). Fighting antibiotic-resistant bacteria: promising strategies orchestrated by molecularly imprinted polymers. *Angewandte Chemie*, 134(8), e202106493.

Turner, A. P. (2013). Biosensors: sense and sensibility. *Chemical Society Reviews*, 42(8), 3184–3196.

Uzun, L., & Turner, A. P. (2016). Molecularly-imprinted polymer sensors: realising their potential. *Biosensors and Bioelectronics*, 76, 131–144.

Valenick, L. V., Hsia, H. C., & Schwarzbauer, J. E. (2005). Fibronectin fragmentation promotes α4β1 integrin-mediated contraction of a fibrin–fibronectin provisional matrix. *Experimental Cell Research*, 309(1), 48–55.

Vasapollo, G., Sole, R. D., Mergola, L., Lazzoi, M. R., Scardino, A., Scorrano, S., & Mele, G. (2011). Molecularly imprinted polymers: present and future prospective. *International Journal of Molecular Sciences*, 12(9), 5908–5945.

Wang, P., Zhang, A., Jin, Y., Zhang, Q., Zhang, L., Peng, Y., & Du, S. (2014). Molecularly imprinted layer-coated hollow polysaccharide microcapsules toward gate-controlled release of water-soluble drugs. *RSC Advances*, 4(50), 26063–26073.

Wang, Q., Yang, Q., & Wu, W. (2020). Progress on structured biosensors for monitoring aflatoxin B1 from biofilms: a review. *Frontiers in Microbiology*, 11, 408.

Wulff, G., & Sarhan, A. (1972) The use of polymers with enzyme-analogous structures for the resolution of racemates. *Angewandte Chemie International Edition*, 11, 341–344.

Xu, K., Wang, Y., Wei, X., Chen, J., Xu, P., & Zhou, Y. (2018). Preparation of magnetic molecularly imprinted polymers based on a deep eutectic solvent as the functional monomer for specific recognition of lysozyme. *Microchimica Acta*, 185(2), 1–8.

Xu, S., Wang, L., & Liu, Z. (2021). Molecularly imprinted polymer nanoparticles: an emerging versatile platform for cancer therapy. *Angewandte Chemie International Edition*, 60(8), 3858–3869.

Xue, C., Han, Q., Wang, Y., Wu, J., Wen, T., Wang, R., ... & Jiang, H. (2013). Amperometric detection of dopamine in human serum by electrochemical sensor based on gold nanoparticles doped molecularly imprinted polymers. *Biosensors and Bioelectronics*, 49, 199–203.

Yilmaz, E., Schmidt, R. H., & Mosbach, K. (2005). The non-covalent approach in Molecularly Imprinted Materials: Science.

Yuan, L., Lin, W., Zheng, K., He, L., & Huang, W. (2013). Far-red to near infrared analyte-responsive fluorescent probes based on organic fluorophore platforms for fluorescence imaging. Chemical *Society Reviews*, 42(2), 622–661.

Zaidi, S. A. (2016). Molecular imprinted polymers as drug delivery vehicles. *Drug Delivery*, 23(7), 2262–2271.

Zhu, D. W., Chen, Z., Zhao, K. Y., Kan, B. H., Liu, L. X., Dong, X., ... & Zhang, L. H. (2015). Polypropylene non-woven supported fibronectin molecular imprinted calcium alginate/polyacrylamide hydrogel film for cell adhesion. *Chinese Chemical Letters*, 26(6), 807–810.

5 Polymeric materials for drug delivery systems

Aszad Alam

CONTENTS

5.1 Introduction and importance of drug delivery systems 73
    5.1.1 Familiarization with terminologies utilized in drug delivery 74
    5.1.2 Routes for delivering the drugs 76
5.2 Polymers in drug delivery systems 77
5.3 Various aspects for polymers in drug delivery: applications
and mechanism 78
    5.3.1 As fillers/excipients 78
    5.3.2 As encapsulation/coating 79
    5.3.3 For increasing the bioavailability of drugs 79
    5.3.4 For controlling the kinetics of drug release 80
        5.3.4.1 Mechanism of degradation and erosion of polymers for
release of drugs 81
5.4 Polymer-based novel materials having potential drug delivery applications 82
    5.4.1 Stimuli-sensitive polymers 82
        5.4.1.1 pH-responsive polymers and their mechanism 83
        5.4.1.2 Thermo-responsive polymers and their mechanism 83
        5.4.1.3 Redox-responsive polymers and their mechanism 84
    5.4.2 Conjugation of the therapeutic to the polymer: achieving the
need of the time 84
        5.4.2.1 Polymer–drug conjugate 86
        5.4.2.2 Polymer–protein conjugate 86
        5.4.2.3 Polymeric micelles 86
    5.4.3 Molecularly imprinted polymers 87
5.5 Challenges and way ahead 88
References 88

5.1 INTRODUCTION AND IMPORTANCE OF DRUG DELIVERY SYSTEMS

Drug delivery systems evolved to solve the issues that arise in administering and delivering a wide variety of therapeutic agents those are ranging from small molecules to nucleic acids, peptides, proteins, and antibodies as well as in maintaining their required dose for the therapeutic action at those intended sites. The primary

DOI: 10.1201/9781003319139-5

goal of a delivery system is to deliver treatments to the intended anatomical region while keeping the drug concentration within an effective range for the desired time. Countless medicinal treatments have been developed as a result of drug delivery methods, which enhance the health of the diseased person by improving therapeutic delivery to the intended site for a required period of time, decreasing the buildup of drugs other than the targeted sites, and increasing patient satisfaction and compliance [1–3].

The relevance and scope of the drug delivery system can be envisioned from a new report named "Drug Delivery Systems Market Report, 2022–2029" by Fortune Business Insights. According to the study, the worldwide drug delivery systems' market was valued at USD 34.70 billion in 2021 and USD 39.33 billion in 2022, respectively, and is expected to reach USD 71.75 billion by 2029. The increased frequency of chronic illnesses, along with patients' increasing preference for sophisticated medication delivery methods, are the main factors responsible to drive the research and market for drug delivery systems.

Polymers have been shown to have a significant share of this growing drug delivery market, as polymer-based drug delivery systems are gaining popularity due to the fascinating physicochemical and biocompatible properties of polymers, which provide a favorable research scenario for exploitation of their potential in the field of nanomedicines [4]. Polymer-based drug delivery systems may be classified according to polymeric materials, their drug release mechanism, production process, and distribution route, and therefore, the market can be classified as well. Polymer-type-based categorization, for example, classifies cellulose as a natural polymer and its derivatives as semi-synthetic polymers. Polymer-based drug delivery systems can also be categorized according to their release mechanisms, such as diffusion-controlled systems, solvent-activated systems, stimuli-sensitive systems, and biodegradable systems [5, 6]. Because of this, a brief explanation of all pertinent terms and fundamental mechanisms is required to comprehend the flow of this chapter, and they are all addressed in subsequent sections.

The present chapter opens with an introduction to the fundamental terminologies, concepts, and mechanisms of existing drug delivery methods based on polymeric materials, as well as their features. This chapter also discusses the relevant characteristics of polymers for various drug delivery modalities, as well as some of the critical aspects that govern drug delivery. Glimpses of the historical evolution of polymer-based drug delivery systems are also presented, as are newly created polymer-based innovative materials with potential use in drug delivery. Finally, this chapter attempts to investigate the breadth of polymer-based drug delivery systems in meeting current needs by addressing areas for improvement and hurdles to overcome in polymer-based drug delivery systems.

5.1.1 Familiarization with Terminologies Utilized in Drug Delivery

There are various terminologies used in drug deliveries. Some important types of terminologies are represented in Table 5.1

TABLE 5.1
Frequently used terminologies in the drug delivery

Sl. no.	Terminologies	Meaning	Ref
1.	Controlled drug release	Controlling the release of medications in order to maintain a steady amount in blood and tissue. The therapeutic agents are released in a predictable pattern through this mechanism.	[7]
2.	Sustained drug release	Intended to deliver therapeutics over a long period of time with minimal negative effects.	[8]
3.	Site-specific drug release	A site-specific delivery system targets a few specified tissues. Specifically in the context of cytotoxic medications.	[9]
4.	Active targeting	Active targeting uses a targeting moiety in the drug delivery system such as a ligand or an antibody is introduced to target and identify particular changes in diseased cells from surrounding healthy cells and tissues.	[10]
5.	Passive targeting	Passive targeting is the preferred accumulation of medications at diseased sites. Made possible by the specific alterations in diseased cells, and it may be targeted depending on the size of drug delivery system.	[10]
6.	Zero-order drug release	Zero-order kinetics releases therapeutics at a constant rate that is independent of their initial amount present in the system as well as time. Extend the therapeutic benefit while avoiding pharmacological adverse effects.	[11]
7.	Pharmacokinetics	Pharmacokinetics is the study of drug movement into, throughout, and then out of the body, all of them together involve the phenomena of absorption, distribution, metabolism, and excretion. It is determined by the drug's physicochemical qualities, intrinsic clearance, and interactions with diverse tissue types.	[12]
8.	Pharmacodynamics	Pharmacodynamics is the analysis of the link between the amount of therapeutics at the intended/diseased site and physiological or toxicological responses.	[13]
9.	Therapeutic window/range	The therapeutic window is the ideal dosage range that is effective for patients at acceptable levels. The crucial range between the lowest effective dose and the lowest harmful dose.	[14]
10.	Bioavailability	The percentage of the given therapeutic dosage that enters the systemic circulation is referred to as drug bioavailability.	[15]
11.	GI tract	Comprises mouth, esophagus, small intestine, and large intestine. Entrance route for the therapeutics into the body, which is taken orally.	[16]
12.	Half-life of drug	The half-life of any therapeutics is the time necessary for their concentration in plasma to be lowered to exactly half of its original concentration.	[17]

5.1.2 Routes for Delivering the Drugs

Oral formulations, such as tablets and capsules, are the most frequent medication delivery platform, with active pharmacological ingredients delivered via the gastrointestinal (GI) tract. This occurs as a result of passive absorption down a concentration gradient on the intestinal surfaces and is principally determined by the drug's amount of ionization, molecular weight, and oil/water partition coefficient.

Another frequently used drug delivery method is the parenteral route, which avoids the GI tract by direct injection, typically intravenously or interstitially. This method is much more straightforward and typically faster than oral delivery. This is used for therapeutic substances or proteins that lack the stability or characteristics required for their absorption in the GI tract. The delivery of pharmaceuticals with extremely limited therapeutic windows and when immediate drug availability is required can also be accomplished when using this route. The main drawbacks of this route are overdoses that are nearly impossible to prevent and shorter drug circulation due to rapid access to excretory mechanisms. Polymer materials must typically be soluble in aqueous environments in order to be used as carriers for the intravenous delivery of drugs.

Therapeutics can also be administered through mucous membranes, such as the sublingual, sublabial, buccal, rectal, and vaginal routes, which is known as transmucosal drug administration. These non-invasive techniques also allow for self-administration. Furthermore, their quick response time with decreased first-pass effect makes them appropriate for use in hospice and end-of-life care. Despite the many benefits, these transmucosal routes confront problems such as a relatively limited surface for optimal drug uptake, a tiny amount of fluid for drug disintegration, and the mucus barrier as an additional obstacle.

Table 5.2 summarizes the drug delivery routes, as well as examples of medications that may be administered via those routes and the relevance of these systems.

TABLE 5.2
Routes for drug delivery and their significance

Sl. no.	Drug delivery routes	Description	Examples	Significance
1.	Oral	Administered from the mouth and then via GI tract.	Tablets, syrups, pills, capsules.	Most common platform for drug delivery.
2.	Intradermal	Injection into the epidermis layer of the skin.	Allergy testing.	Enhances the availability of limited antigens.
3.	Intravenous	Injection into the vein	Chemotherapeutics.	Almost 100 percent bioavailability.
4.	Intramuscular	Injection into the muscle.	Vaccines.	Avoids gastric enzymes and first-pass effect.
5.	Subcutaneous	Injection into subcutaneous fat under the skin.	Insulin delivery.	Sustained absorption. A low dose is required.

(Continued)

TABLE 5.2
(Continued)

Sl. no.	Drug delivery routes	Description	Examples	Significance
6.	Transdermal	A drug-loaded patch is kept/ adhered to the skin.	Wound healing patch.	Avoid the first-pass effect. Painless approach.
7.	Nasal	Spray/inhalation of therapeutic agents via the nose.	Migraine drugs.	Self-administration. Higher bioavailability.
8.	Ocular	Drug solution/suspension or emulsion given to eye.	Eye drops.	More ocular bioavailability. For reduction of irritation.
9.	Otic	Drops in ear.	Ear drops.	Locally treat the infection.
10.	Sublingual	By keeping drugs beneath the tongue.	Nitroglycerin. Vitamin B12.	The rapid absorption of the drug through the
11.	Sublabial	By keeping the drugs between lips and gum.	Lozenges. Chewing gum.	mucous membrane into the systemic
12.	Buccal	By keeping the drugs between cheeks and gum.	Orally dis- integrable tablets.	circulation. Avoids stomach's harsh enzymatic environment.
13.	Rectal	Insertion of drug delivery system into the rectum.	Suppositories. Foam/sponges.	More amount of drug into the systemic
14.	Vaginal	Insertion of drug delivery system into the vagina.	Tables/gels. Enemas.	circulation. Less pain/irritation. No vomiting/nausea.
15.	Topical	Application of therapeutics onto the skin.	Lotions/gel. Spray/creams.	Minimal side effects. Easy to administer.

5.2 POLYMERS IN DRUG DELIVERY SYSTEMS

Not only polymeric materials are an important part of traditional drug delivery formulations and made a significant contribution to the treatment of various diseases, but the development of potent and targeted biological therapeutics has increased the demand for intelligent delivery systems, where polymers are paving the way [18].

As we know that the bioavailability of the drug in the bloodstream enables distribution to almost all bodily tissues whether it was given as an oral dose, through the parenteral route, or other methods, like inhalation or transdermal patches. Drugs then spread to all or the majority of tissues after entering the blood by overcoming endothelial barriers or by draining through endothelial holes in tissues with "leaky" vasculature. Additionally, a drug can be delivered to selective and specific targeted sites either by itself or with the help of suitable conjugation.

In these circumstances, polymeric materials have demonstrated their extraordinary utility as drug carriers and as polymer–drug conjugates that can disproportionally partition into the target tissue. Some of the recent advancements are made possible by polymers that can direct the drug within the cells or recognize molecules and receptors. The use of polymeric carriers and reservoirs as well as tuning the release kinetics accordingly is the first step in the hierarchical advancement of modern drug delivery.

We can say that advances in drug delivery are taking place as a result of the diverse properties of polymers and their easy tunability to perform specific biological functions, and are tailored for a specific cargo. Pharmaceuticals can now travel safely through hostile physiological regions, thanks to the development of hydrogels and other polymer-based carriers.

Additionally, the biodegradable properties of various polymers have been shown to be helpful in enhancing the release kinetics of drug delivery systems and preventing their buildup in the body. By altering the transport or circulation half-life properties of the pharmaceutical agents attached to them, polymeric materials enable both passive and active targeting of these therapeutic agents. Polymers can also be bioactive, and when they are combined with therapeutics, they offer their own therapeutic benefit. The most recently fabricated polymeric drug delivery has created polymeric carriers that make it easier to deliver novel therapeutics directly into the cells.

5.3 VARIOUS ASPECTS FOR POLYMERS IN DRUG DELIVERY: APPLICATIONS AND MECHANISM

We have seen quite a bit about the drug delivery systems and their routes in previous sections. Based on that, we can state that the dosage form, the form in which a drug is administered to the body, varies depending on the route of administration. These dosage forms can be solid, liquid, or semisolid. These include tablets, capsules, syrups, pills, lozenges, drops, creams, gels, lotions, ointments, implant systems, micro-/nano-particle-based systems, injectable systems, as well as patches.

If we discuss the function of polymers in drug delivery, we should also discuss their function in the creation of these therapeutic formulations, which includes the use of polymers as binders in drug formulations, matrices, and reservoirs for regulating drug release, and materials for coatings and patches. Additionally, polymeric materials may be used to stabilize or thicken therapeutic formulations. Polymers may also be used to speed up the process of a drug's absorption into the body and subsequent solubilization. Polymeric materials are also used in liquid dosage forms to emulsify or suspend the drug in the appropriate solvent. On the other hand, polymeric materials, particularly in semisolid dosage form, can function as bioadhesives or gelling agents [19].

5.3.1 As FILLERS/EXCIPIENTS

The use of polymeric materials as excipients in drug delivery systems is well known for enhancing both drug delivery and manufacturing process. These polymeric materials work in tandem with the drug to perform specific tasks, and in some cases, they have a direct or indirect impact on the amount or rate of drug release and absorption [20].

Excipients should ideally be non-toxic, stable, and readily available. Polysaccharides meet all of these criteria, and they do so at a reasonably low price. Even though these polymeric materials have varying physicochemical characteristics and a gelation nature that is sensitive to the environment, all of these characteristics are helpful in regulating the drug release in accordance with particular therapeutic needs [21].

For use as excipients, natural as well as synthetic polymers have both been thoroughly studied. Natural polymers, however, are more advantageous than synthetic ones for these applications because they outperform the later one on all of the aforementioned criteria, including renewability and sustainability [22]. However, there are a few potential issues with natural polymeric materials, such as their low yield due to a lengthy purification process and rigidity when mixing with other components, which are currently being resolved by altering such material.

5.3.2 As encapsulation/coating

The therapeutic agent is frequently coated with polymers, which are used for site-specific drug delivery systems for targeted delivery as well as to protect the therapeutic agent in hostile environments [23].

Due to the physiological circumstances in the body, this type of delivery can be carried out in certain areas of the body. Therapeutic agents are coated with polymeric materials that are either indigestible or have pH-dependent solubilities. Since they resist the GI enzymes and keep themselves intact in the upper part of the GI tract before being degraded by bacterial enzymes in the colon, these typically non-starch polymers, like linear polysaccharides, are well suited for colon targeted delivery. Consequently, these polymeric materials result in drug delivery systems that are undamaged in certain parts of the GI tract but are broken down by bacterial enzymes upon reaching the colon [24, 25, 5].

5.3.3 For increasing the bioavailability of drugs

Any drug's usefulness in its delivery system depends not only on its potency but also on how readily it is absorbed by the body. This ultimately determines whether frequent dosing is necessary and how well the patient will take the medication. Therefore, a major barrier to the development of drug delivery systems is the poor bioavailability of drugs, which results in insufficient clinical utility [26]. This situation occurs with 70–80% of newly discovered or developed drugs, so it is not that uncommon.

The difficulty of creating an ocular drug delivery system is one such example, as the drug's accessibility to the aimed ocular tissues is constrained by barriers like the outer lipid layer, pre-corneal layer, dynamic barriers, and static barriers. Due to the rapid removal of the drug and the resulting reduced bioavailability of eye drops, which ranges from 1 to 5%, high doses of the drug are necessary to produce a therapeutic effect and may result in toxicity and poor patient compliance. Additionally, with those drugs that have limited solubility in water, the problem of poor bioavailability may occur.

Poly alcohols, hydroxyethyl cellulose, hydroxypropyl cellulose, and carboxymethyl cellulose are examples of such polymers that have been thoroughly investigated for better drug absorption and retention time when given as eye drops. Such problems are well solved by these mucoadhesive polymers in the form of polymeric gels because they adhere to biological tissues, lengthen the contact time, and increase bioavailability, all of which improve the effectiveness of ocular drug delivery systems. Even these polymeric gels, also referred to as in situ, alter their viscosity at the targeted site. Due to their hydrophilic nature and adaptable properties, cellulose-based polymers are well suited for such solubility enhancement techniques. Since polymer-based solubility enhancement of such drugs or such types of above-mentioned delivery demonstrates their importance once more, this method has been extensively researched [27].

5.3.4 FOR CONTROLLING THE KINETICS OF DRUG RELEASE

The controlled molecular architecture of polymers can be used or tuned accordingly to give a well-defined response to external conditions since polymers and their behavioral transition to the external conditions are well known. Polymeric materials have shown their potential in achieving different kinds of drug release rates and mechanisms, which might be utilized in various kinds of disease conditions [28]. Based on the behavior of polymeric materials in the microenvironment of the body, different kinds of formulations have been developed and those will be discussed hereafter. Since the formulation of drug delivery systems is based on the rate of drug release that is necessary to maintain the therapeutic level of the drug in the specific organ or to provide significant bioavailability in the bloodstream, drug release kinetics are crucial in all drug delivery systems. As with polymeric drug delivery systems, they are categorized according to their release kinetics. Diffusion-controlled, solvent-activated systems, like swelling-controlled or osmotically controlled, and also release-controlled by an external trigger system, are included in this classification [29–31].

A drug is dissolved in a non-swellable or fully swollen polymeric matrix in diffusion-controlled drug delivery systems, where the matrix remains intact throughout the therapeutic life of the drug. Or sometimes, if the concentration exceeds the polymer's solubility limit, the drug may be dispersed rather than completely dissolved. Diffusion-controlled carriers typically have a straightforward, monolithic design [32].

On the other hand, solvent-activated systems are based on the polymers in the absence of a plasticizing aqueous solvent, which typically operate well below their glass transition temperatures and have very low diffusivities. In such systems, dehydrated drug-loaded hydrophilic polymers or hydrogels swell when exposed to an aqueous environment and absorb water. Drug delivery systems that operate as swelling-controlled systems change from their glassy to rubbery state as a result of solvent swelling, which relaxes polymer chains and dissolves the drug deposits that were dispersed into them. The release behavior of polymers will vary depending on their nature after swelling or dissolution; for example, erosion of the polymer will be preferred and an erosion mechanism will also appear in the absence of crystallinity and cross-linking. The erosion mechanism, if present, and the diffusion and swelling mechanism of drug release are all created by this process and move simultaneously.

TABLE 5.3
Drug release systems, their mechanisms, and the polymers utilized

Sl. no.	Drug release systems	Components	Release mechanism/ models	Polymers utilized
1.	Dissolution controlled	Drug is encapsulated in polymeric membrane.	Dissolution is a rate-limiting step. Reservoir system.	Derivatives of natural polymers.
2.	Diffusion controlled	Insoluble polymeric membrane trapping the drugs.	Rate-limiting step is the diffusion of drug from the membrane.	Vinyl acetate copolymers.
3.	Osmotic controlled	A semi-permeable membrane that covers osmotic agents.	The osmotic pressure buildup is responsible for the drug release.	Cellulose acetate. Ethylcellulose.
4.	Swelling controlled	Hydrophilic polymers containing the drug.	Glassy-to-rubbery transition of polymeric matrix results in drug release.	Ethylene vinyl alcohol. Cellulose ether. Polyvinyl alcohol.
5.	Polymer–drug dispersion	The biodegradable polymer contains uniformly dispersed drugs.	Polymer's degradation leads to drug release either by bulk erosion or by surface erosion.	Chitosan. Dextran. Poly(aspartamides).
6.	Polymer–drug conjugate	Grafting or covalent binding of drug to the polymer.	Bond cleavage between polymer and drug.	Poly(ethylene glycol). Poly(lactide-co-glycolide).

Diverse classes of polymers are utilized to achieve different mechanisms of drug release, a summary of which is given in Table 5.3.

5.3.4.1 Mechanism of degradation and erosion of polymers for release of drugs

Degradation and erosion, the two phenomena that are primarily responsible for the release of drugs from polymeric carriers, can take place as surface or bulk processes. Biodegradable and bioerodible polymers are a crucial class of materials for drug delivery when considering the aforementioned release mechanisms; occasionally, these two terms are even used synonymously. In contrast to erosion, which does not chemically alter the substance and only dissolves chain fragments in polymeric systems without cross-links, degradation occurs when covalent bonds in cross-linked polymeric systems are broken by chemical reactions. For this to happen, the polymer should soak up the aqueous liquid present in its surroundings and interact with water either via charge interactions or through hydrogen bonding. Even though the volume fraction of polymers largely stays unchanged, surface degradation gradually removes the polymer matrix from the surface to make room for drug molecules to be released. Contrarily, with bulk degradation, the physical size of the polymer carrier does not change significantly until it has almost completely eroded or degraded, but as time passes, less and less polymer is present in the carrier, which causes the encapsulated drug to release. These two types of degradation processes compete with one another, and these processes end up dominating depending on variables like how quickly the solvent penetrates the polymer. Because biodegradable hydrogels are frequently polymerized in the presence of an aqueous solvent, these rate aspects are particularly crucial when designing biodegradable polymeric drug delivery systems.

A significant proportion of biodegradable synthetic polymers rely solely on chemical degradation in which polymers should have bonds in their backbone or cross-linker that can be easily broken by hydrolysis. Examples include the hydrolysis of ester bonds or the production of ester derivatives like poly(-caprolactone), poly(lactic/glycolic acid), etc. Derivatives of poly(anhydrides), poly(orthoesters), poly(phosphoesters), poly(phosphazenes), and poly(cyanoacrylate) are indeed affected by hydrolysis. Because the degradation process may generate an acid product that may catalyze additional degradation or promotes hydrophobic structure to absorb more water, one should be aware that the degradation and dissolution processes can auto-accelerate. In this way, drug release can be tuned accordingly [33].

However, the same mechanism could cause serious safety issues because of an unforeseen or unpredictable release. Additionally, toxicity brought on by the distribution of fragment sizes is also possible. To combat these kinds of issues, it is ideal to administer some medications parenterally along with their polymeric carriers, where these polymeric carriers break down into small, physiologic substances that are supposed to be nontoxic and can get clear from the clearance mechanisms.

5.4 POLYMER-BASED NOVEL MATERIALS HAVING POTENTIAL DRUG DELIVERY APPLICATIONS

5.4.1 STIMULI-SENSITIVE POLYMERS

An important class of materials is known as stimuli-responsive polymers, also referred to as smart polymers. The extraordinary quality of the responsive polymers is their capacity to undergo a significant physical or chemical change in response to an outside stimulus, which can be categorized as physical or chemical stimuli [34].

Physical stimuli, because they all regulate the energy level of the polymer–solvent system, cause a polymer response at a certain level of energy. Physical stimuli include electric field, magnetic field, temperature, electromagnetic radiation, and ultrasound. Chemical stimuli, such as chemical agents, pH changes, ionic strengths, and redox potential, are another type of stimulus. They elicit a response by changing the molecular interactions between the solvent and the polymer. They affect the polymer chain backbone, the cross-linking, hydrophobic affiliation, or repulsive forces between the chains to change the hydrophobicity or hydrophilicity of the polymer–solvent system. The coil–globule transition of polymer chains, swelling/deswelling of covalently cross-linked hydrogels, the sol–gel transition of physically cross-linked hydrogels, and self-assembly of amphiphilic polymers are just a few examples of how these changes emerge.

A variety of polymeric systems, such as hydrogels, micelles, polyplexes, or polymer–drug conjugates, respond to external stimuli, which is why they are frequently used in targeted and site-specific drug release. Because of their physical or covalent cross-links, hydrogels, which are hydrophilic networks of copolymers capable of absorbing large volumes of water or biological fluids, are typically insoluble in water. Hydrogels can be formed to react to different stimuli and are proven to be very useful in the healthcare and biopharmaceutical industries. PEG-grafted hydrogels of polymers like poly(methacrylic acid) have been tested for delivery of protein through the oral route and have demonstrated pH-responsive behavior. Interpolymer complexation is used to successfully entrap, safeguard, and facilitate the delivery of medications in acidic environments, such as insulin. Some polymers, like block copolymers of poly(ethylene oxide) and poly(propylene oxide) or copolymers of poly(N-isopropyl acrylamide) (PNIPAAm) combined with water-soluble PEG, have the ability to form micelles and exhibit temperature-responsive micellization, leading to extensive research in drug delivery [35]. Additionally, polyplexes are also being widely researched for drug delivery, particularly for gene delivery. A good example of one such is when DNA and polyethyleneimine (PEI) interact electrostatically. However, the molecular weight, branching, cross-linking, and biodegradability of these polymeric materials ultimately determine how fascinating features they exhibit.

5.4.1.1 pH-responsive polymers and their mechanism

The use of pH-responsive polymeric materials takes advantage of the body's regular pH change, especially along the GI tract, where the stomach's acidic pH and enzymatic activity (pH around 2) degrade these pH-responsive carriers and cause the release of medication as a result. In addition to being significantly more alkaline, with a pH range of 6.2 to 7.5, the small intestine, physiological pH profiles also change within individual cellular compartments. One such instance is that the pH of endosomes is 5–6.8, whereas the pH of lysosomes is 4.5–5.5. Since diseased or inflamed tissues have different pH profiles than normal tissue, pH can also be used as a marker to distinguish between these two. This has led to the exploration of systems that can deliver therapeutic agents to those specific locations only. Since tumors are frequently reported to produce acidic conditions (pH 6.5) in the extracellular region, this pH-based distinction can be easily seen in cases where tumors are present. Utilizing these pH variations to deliver valuable therapeutics to particular sites or intracellularly is an intriguing option made possible by the polymeric materials. pH-responsive polymer delivery systems that provide well-controlled pH response and drug discharge can be created by carefully choosing the materials to use as well as modifying their structure [36].

5.4.1.2 Thermo-responsive polymers and their mechanism

A different intriguing class of polymers, like PNIPAAm, is capable of undergoing a temperature-dependent phase transition that is inherently reversible, when their environment temperature rises above the lower critical solution temperature (LCST), causing the polymer chains abruptly collapse into a hydrophobic globule. These polymers have an LCST below which they exist as a hydrophilic coil. The establishment and disruption of intra- and intermolecular electrostatic and hydrophobic interactions, which lead to a hydrophilic/hydrophobic balance of polymer chains, is thought to be the cause of this type of reaction to temperature change. This is because the local environment of polymer chains below the LCST contains water molecules in an

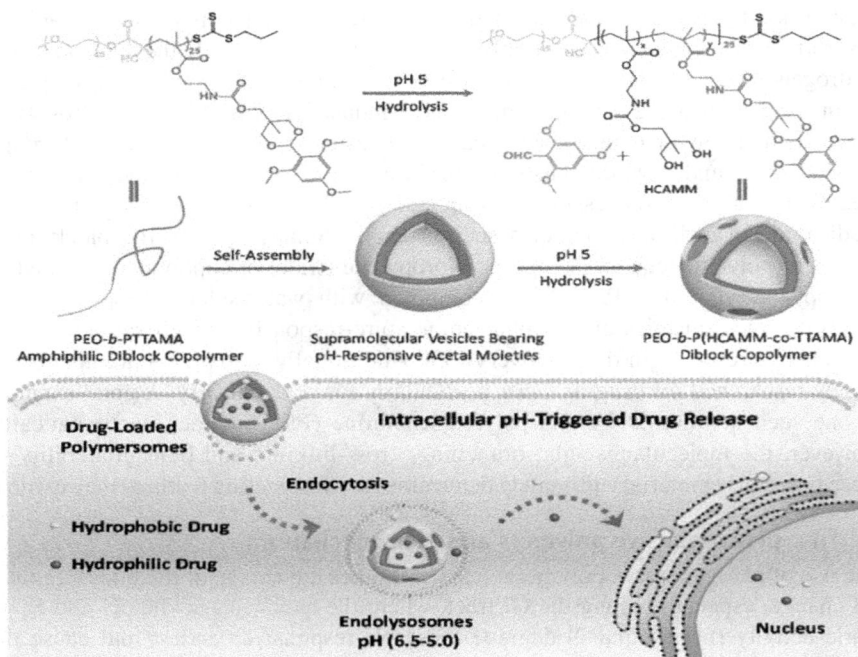

FIGURE 5.1 pH-sensitive polymeric materials and their role in drug delivery. Copyright 2022, *Chinese Chemical Letters*, Elsevier: Reproduced with permission [36].

ordered state, and raising the temperature above the LCST favors polymer–polymer hydrophobic interactions, which causes the polymer chain to collapse and cause drug release. As a result, the lower limit temperature for responsiveness will depend on how much of their hydrophobic hydration area is present, which causes them to collapse at lower temperatures. The LCST will rise, however, as the hydrophilic content of the polymer chain increases. These systems are now preferred for drug release because they allow for sustained release formulations from drug/polymer solution which is administered into a target site since the drug diffuses out of the solid gel as the solution warms to a relatively warm body temperature [37, 38].

5.4.1.3 Redox-responsive polymers and their mechanism

Redox fragile linkage polymers offer an alluring opportunity to create either biodegradable or erodible delivery systems [39].

5.4.2 CONJUGATION OF THE THERAPEUTIC TO THE POLYMER:
ACHIEVING THE NEED OF THE TIME

The term "polymer therapeutics" itself describes the significance of polymers in the pharmaceutics and drug delivery industries. This is because polymers have the ability to act as bioactive substances on their own or, more frequently, as an inert carriers

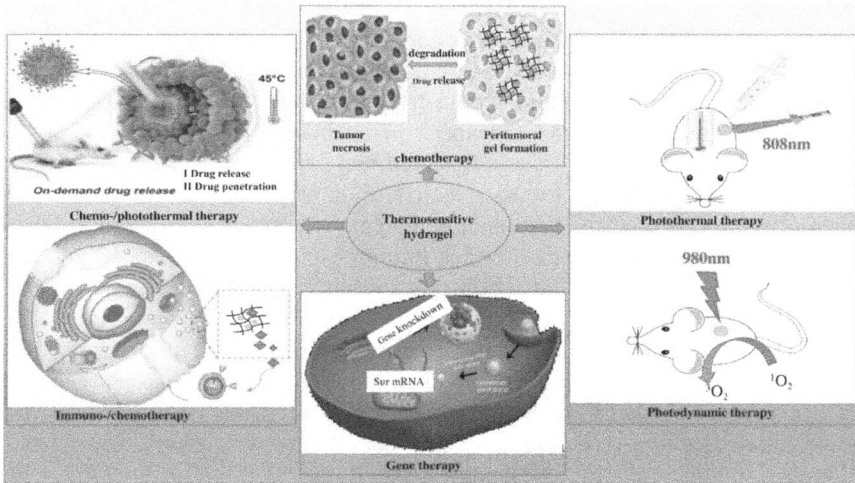

FIGURE 5.2 Application of thermo-responsive polymeric materials in cancer therapy. Copyright 2022, *Colloids and Surfaces B: Biointerfaces*, Elsevier: Reproduced with permission [37].

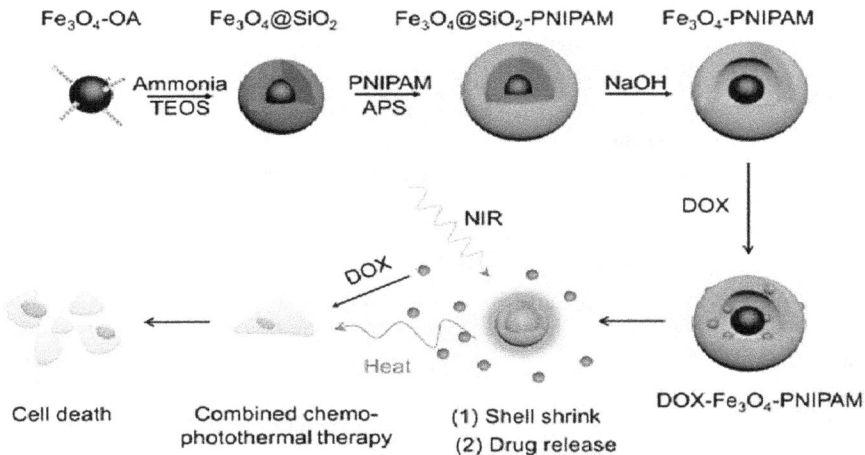

FIGURE 5.3 Drug release mechanism from thermo-sensitive polymers. Copyright 2022, *European Polymer Journal*, Elsevier: Reproduced with permission [38].

for the covalent bonding of drugs with themselves. The domain of polymer-based therapeutics has experienced tremendous growth since the development of controlled drug release polymer-based delivery systems, as attention has shifted to techniques that enable targeted release, particularly for anticancer drugs, which frequently have extremely harmful side effects if they are delivered by conventional routes and methods. Polymer–drug conjugates, polymer–protein conjugates, polymeric micelles, and multicomponent polyplexes are all products of this development happening in the field of drug delivery. These polymer conjugates play a variety of roles in the delivery of drugs, including those related to diabetes, rheumatoid arthritis, ischemia, hepatitis B and C, and anticancer therapeutics.

Because fewer doses must be administered more frequently, therapeutics can be conjugated with polymers to increase their plasma half-life, which will ultimately improve patient compliance. Additionally, polymeric conjugates shield those medications from proteolytic enzymes, lessen immunogenicity, and boost the solubility of medicines with low molecular weight. By altering the pharmacokinetic and pharmacodynamic properties in an aforementioned manner, these conjugated systems have increased efficiency in specifically delivering the drugs. Be it polymer–drug or polymer–protein conjugates, the typical polymer-based therapeutics typically have a polymer, drug, and linker between them. However, more advanced systems are now available that include extra components for targeted therapy delivery or combination therapies. Common polymers used as carriers in these systems include PEG, PEI, HPMA, poly(glutamic acid), dextran, chitosan, dextrin, and poly(L-lysine).

5.4.2.1 Polymer–drug conjugate

One of the most frequently researched subfields of polymer therapeutics is polymer–drug conjugates, which are primarily used for low-molecular-weight therapeutics or chemotherapeutic drugs [40]. The therapeutic's attachment to polymeric carriers limits the cellular uptake to endocytosis, prolongs circulation times, and aids in passive tumor targeting, which was difficult with free drugs because they typically disperse randomly throughout the body and cause harmful side effects [41]. The advancements in polymer chemistry to unique architectures like graft, branched, star polymers and fascinating features associated with them, so they are currently being investigated as conjugate carriers, like dendrimers are promising delivery systems for delivering poorly soluble drugs inside the cells [42].

5.4.2.2 Polymer–protein conjugate

Since the polymer–protein conjugate reduces toxicity as well as produces less antigenicity and immunogenicity, it is also preferred to be conjugated with the protein that is to be delivered inside the body [43]. These kinds of systems make it possible for specific conjugation to occur without the protein becoming cross-linked, allowing the therapeutic to be released [44]. PEGylation is an illustration of this, in which proteins and peptides are covalently joined to PEG.

5.4.2.3 Polymeric micelles

A promising area of polymer therapeutics is polymeric micelles, which are simple to conjugate for active targeting [45]. Besides that, the hydrophobic core of these particles has a high loading capacity, and the attributes of their nanosize favor quick cellular uptake. Unlike polymer–drug conjugates mostly used to passively target the sites, polymeric micelles enable active tumor targeting, and one such kind of micellar system manages to combine pH-induced anticarcinogenic therapeutic release with a conjugated ligand [46–48].

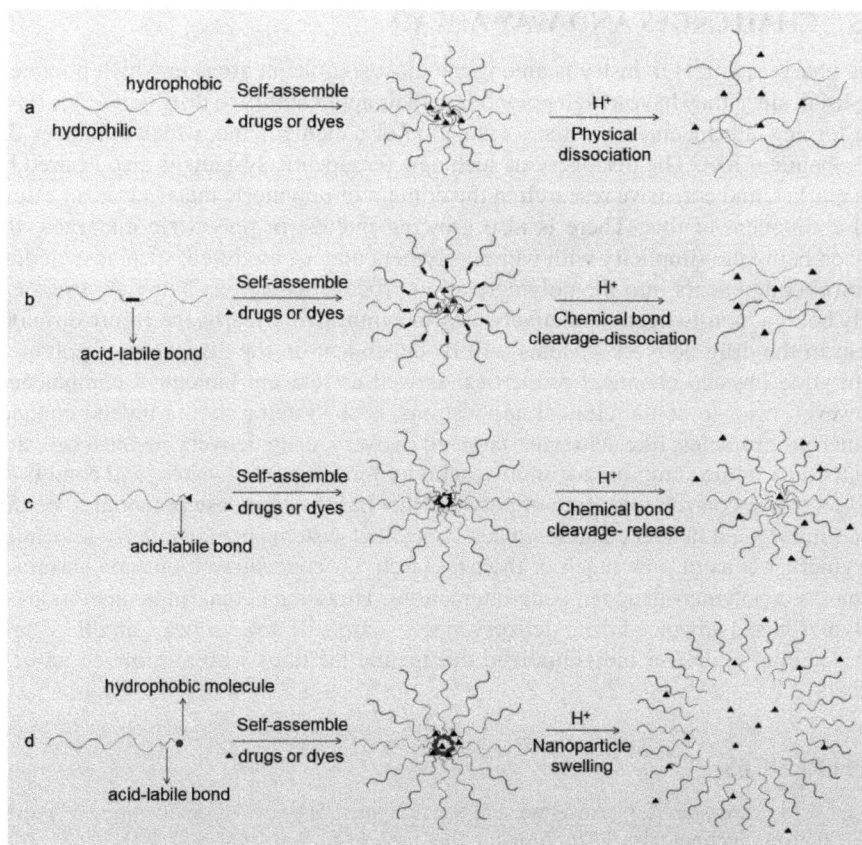

FIGURE 5.4 pH-sensitive release modes of polymeric micelles. Copyright 2022, *Open Nano*, Elsevier: Reproduced with permission [46].

5.4.3 MOLECULARLY IMPRINTED POLYMERS

Molecular imprinting of polymers, in which polymer networks function on a lock-and-key mechanism because they are formed with specific recognition for the desired template molecule, is a promising strategy that is currently being used in the field of drug delivery [49]. In this way, there would be a certain affinity between the polymer and the drug template, leading to their use in sophisticated drug delivery systems [50]. As a result, molecularly imprinted polymer-based drug delivery systems have the potential to produce zero-order drug release, and they can keep drug concentration in its therapeutic window for extended periods of time, so they do away with the need for regular highly concentrated doses [51]. These types of polymers are made from functional monomers that are polymerized in the involvement of the intended template and then exhibit a strong bias for the receptors that are unique to the template molecule [52].

5.5   CHALLENGES AND WAY AHEAD

The pharmaceutical industry is among the most significant areas in which polymers are used, since they have a high potential in their applicability to drug delivery, allowing for new advancements in the formulation of nanomedicine, which enhances the therapeutic effect. The discovery of such new therapeutic systems is also desired by the market, and extensive research in the domain of polymeric materials is an essential component of this. There is also growing interest in polymeric materials, the reason being the simplicity with which polymers may be modified, such as including natural components into the polymerization process, as well as being environmentally benign, non-toxic, and relatively easy to synthesize. Clearly, the future development in the drug delivery systems will be dependent on the discovery of polymers with good physico-chemical properties, as well as relevant biological competence. However, prior to actual clinical applications, such systems should indeed conquer numerous obstacles, like achieving targeted delivery, drug delivery inside a cell, and nontoxicity while combining stimuli sensitivity for different physiological conditions and feedback control. One kind of polymer that has the immense potential to be utilized in targeted delivery and feedback-controlled systems is molecularly imprinted polymers, but as of now much of their research has concentrated only on sustained release via polymer–drug template interactions. However, actual implementations of polymer-based advanced drug delivery systems are still a ways away, and they have the potential to deliver individualized therapeutic facilities with minimized adverse effects.

REFERENCES

1. A. M. Vargason, A. C. Anselmo, and S. Mitragotri, "The evolution of commercial drug delivery technologies," *Nat. Biomed. Eng.*, vol. 5, no. 9, pp. 951–967, 2021.
2. P. Davoodi *et al.*, "Drug delivery systems for programmed and on-demand release," *Adv. Drug Deliv. Rev.*, vol. 132, pp. 104–138, 2018.
3. P. Vega-vásquez, N. S. Mosier, and J. Irudayaraj, "Nanoscale drug delivery systems : From medicine to agriculture," *Front. Bioeng. Biotechnol.*, vol. 8, no. February, pp. 1–16, 2020.
4. N. Kamaly, B. Yameen, J. Wu, and O. C. Farokhzad, "Degradable controlled-release polymers and polymeric nanoparticles: Mechanisms of controlling drug release," *Chem. Rev.*, vol. 116, no. 4, pp. 2602–2663, February 2016.
5. J. Wang *et al.*, "4- Enzyme-responsive polymers for drug delivery and molecular imaging," in *Stimuli Responsive Polymeric Nanocarriers for Drug Delivery Applications, Volume 1*, A. S. H. Makhlouf and N. Y. Abu-Thabit, Eds. Cambridge: Woodhead Publishing, 2018, pp. 101–119.
6. S. Hajebi *et al.*, "Stimulus-responsive polymeric nanogels as smart drug delivery systems," *Acta Biomater.*, vol. 92, pp. 1–18, 2019.
7. P. W. S. Heng, "Controlled release drug delivery systems," *Pharm. Dev. Technol.*, vol. 23, no. 9, p. 833, 2018.
8. S. Jethara, M. Patel, and A. Patel, "Sustained release drug delivery systems: A patent overview," *Aperito J. Drug Des. Pharmacol.*, vol. 1, pp. 1–14, 2014.
9. T. Shukla, N. Upmanyu, S. P. Pandey, and M. S. Sudheesh, "Chapter 14- Site-specific drug delivery, targeting, and gene therapy," in *Nanoarchitectonics in Biomedicine*, A. M. Grumezescu, Ed. Norwich, NY: William Andrew Publishing, 2019, pp. 473–505.

10. T. D. Clemons, R. Singh, A. Sorolla, N. Chaudhari, A. Hubbard, and K. S. Iyer, "Distinction between active and passive targeting of nanoparticles dictate their overall therapeutic efficacy," *Langmuir*, vol. 34, no. 50, pp. 15343–15349, December 2018.
11. X. Li, Q. Li, and C. Zhao, "Zero-order controlled release of water-soluble drugs using a marker pen platform," *ACS Omega*, vol. 6, no. 21, pp. 13774–13778, June 2021.
12. S. C. Turfus, R. Delgoda, D. Picking, and B. J. Gurley, "Chapter 25- Pharmacokinetics," in *Pharmacognosy*, S. Badal and R. Delgoda, Eds. Boston: Academic Press, 2017, pp. 495–512.
13. M. Marian and W. Seghezzi, "Chapter 4- Novel biopharmaceuticals: Pharmacokinetics, pharmacodynamics, and bioanalytics," in *Nonclinical Development of Novel Biologics, Biosimilars, Vaccines and Specialty Biologics*, L. M. Plitnick and D. J. Herzyk, Eds. San Diego: Academic Press, 2013, pp. 97–137.
14. S. de Visser and H. Truebel, "Chapter 18- The pharmaceutical research and development productivity crisis: Can exploratory clinical studies be of any help?," in *Principles of Translational Science in Medicine (Third Edition)*, Third Edition, M. Wehling, Ed. Boston: Academic Press, 2021, pp. 239–245.
15. S. Chemtob, "Chapter 20- Basic pharmacologic principles," in *Fetal and Neonatal Physiology (Fourth Edition)*, Fourth Edition, R. A. Polin, W. W. Fox, and S. H. Abman, Eds. Philadelphia: W.B. Saunders, 2011, pp. 211–223.
16. C. A. Picut and G. D. Coleman, "Chapter 5- Gastrointestinal tract," in *Atlas of Histology of the Juvenile Rat*, G. A. Parker and C. A. Picut, Eds. Boston: Academic Press, 2016, pp. 127–171.
17. M. Schrag and K. Regal, "Chapter 3- Pharmacokinetics and toxicokinetics," in *A Comprehensive Guide to Toxicology in Preclinical Drug Development*, A. S. Faqi, Ed. Cambridge, MA: Academic Press, 2013, pp. 31–68.
18. K. Ulbrich, K. Holá, V. Šubr, A. Bakandritsos, J. Tuček, and R. Zbořil, "Targeted drug delivery with polymers and magnetic nanoparticles: Covalent and noncovalent approaches, release control, and clinical studies," *Chem. Rev.*, vol. 116, no. 9, pp. 5338–5431, May 2016.
19. H. A. Silva Favacho *et al.*, "Synergy between surfactants and mucoadhesive polymers enhances the transbuccal permeation of local anesthetics from freeze-dried tablets," *Mater. Sci. Eng. C*, vol. 108, p. 110373, 2020.
20. A. Bernkop-Schnürch, "Chitosan and its derivatives: Potential excipients for peroral peptide delivery systems," *Int. J. Pharm.*, vol. 194, no. 1, pp. 1–13, 2000.
21. N. Debotton and A. Dahan, "Applications of polymers as pharmaceutical excipients in solid oral dosage forms," *Med. Res. Rev.*, vol. 37, no. 1, pp. 52–97, 2017.
22. C. C. Kandar, M. S. Hasnain, and A. K. Nayak, "Chapter 1- Natural polymers as useful pharmaceutical excipients," in *Advances and Challenges in Pharmaceutical Technology*, A. K. Nayak, K. Pal, I. Banerjee, S. Maji, and U. Nanda, Eds. Cambridge, MA: Academic Press, 2021, pp. 1–44.
23. X. Tong, W. Pan, T. Su, M. Zhang, W. Dong, and X. Qi, "Recent advances in natural polymer-based drug delivery systems," *React. Funct. Polym.*, vol. 148, p. 104501, 2020.
24. A. Kumari, S. K. Yadav, and S. C. Yadav, "Biodegradable polymeric nanoparticles based drug delivery systems," *Colloids Surf. B: Biointerfaces*, vol. 75, no. 1, pp. 1–18, 2010.
25. R. Arévalo-Pérez, C. Maderuelo, and J. M. Lanao, "Recent advances in colon drug delivery systems," *J. Control. Release*, vol. 327, pp. 703–724, 2020.
26. P. Jana, M. Shyam, S. Singh, V. Jayaprakash, and A. Dev, "Biodegradable polymers in drug delivery and oral vaccination," *Eur. Polym. J.*, vol. 142, p. 110155, 2021.
27. B. Gupta, V. Mishra, S. Gharat, M. Momin, and A. Omri, "Cellulosic polymers for enhancing drug bioavailability in ocular drug delivery systems," *Pharmaceuticals*, vol. 14, no. 11, 2021.

28. R. Safdar, A. A. Omar, A. Arunagiri, I. Regupathi, and M. Thanabalan, "Potential of Chitosan and its derivatives for controlled drug release applications – A review," *J. Drug Deliv. Sci. Technol.*, vol. 49, pp. 642–659, 2019.

29. X. Yuan *et al.*, "Preparation of carboxylmethyl chitosan and alginate blend membrane for diffusion-controlled release of diclofenac diethylamine," *J. Mater. Sci. Technol.*, vol. 63, pp. 210–215, 2021.

30. S. Sur, A. Rathore, V. Dave, K. R. Reddy, R. S. Chouhan, and V. Sadhu, "Recent developments in functionalized polymer nanoparticles for efficient drug delivery system," *Nano-Structures & Nano-Objects*, vol. 20, p. 100397, 2019.

31. K. Kaur, R. Jindal, and D. Jindal, "RSM-CCD optimized microwave-assisted synthesis of chitosan and gelatin-based pH sensitive, inclusion complexes incorporated hydrogels and their use as controlled drug delivery systems," *J. Drug Deliv. Sci. Technol.*, vol. 48, pp. 161–173, 2018.

32. J. Siepmann and F. Siepmann, "Modeling of diffusion controlled drug delivery," *J. Control. Release*, vol. 161, no. 2, pp. 351–362, 2012.

33. K. Sevim and J. Pan, "A model for hydrolytic degradation and erosion of biodegradable polymers," *Acta Biomater.*, vol. 66, pp. 192–199, 2018.

34. A. Zhang, K. Jung, A. Li, J. Liu, and C. Boyer, "Recent advances in stimuli-responsive polymer systems for remotely controlled drug release," *Prog. Polym. Sci.*, vol. 99, p. 101164, 2019.

35. A. R. Kim, S. L. Lee, and S. N. Park, "Properties and in vitro drug release of pH- and temperature-sensitive double cross-linked interpenetrating polymer network hydrogels based on hyaluronic acid/poly (N-isopropylacrylamide) for transdermal delivery of luteolin," *Int. J. Biol. Macromol.*, vol. 118, pp. 731–740, 2018.

36. Z. Shi, Q. Li, and L. Mei, "pH-Sensitive nanoscale materials as robust drug delivery systems for cancer therapy," *Chinese Chem. Lett.*, vol. 31, no. 6, pp. 1345–1356, 2020.

37. Y. Xiao *et al.*, "Injectable thermosensitive hydrogel-based drug delivery system for local cancer therapy," *Colloids Surf. B: Biointerfaces*, vol. 200, no. January, p. 111581, 2021.

38. M. Jouyandeh, M. R. Ganjali, B. Shirkavand, M. Mozafari, and S. S. Sheiko, "Thermosensitive polymers in medicine: A review," *Eur. Polym. J.,* vol. 117, no. February, pp. 402–423, 2019.

39. X. Guo, Y. Cheng, X. Zhao, Y. Luo, J. Chen, and W.-E. Yuan, "Advances in redox-responsive drug delivery systems of tumor microenvironment," *J. Nanobiotechnology*, vol. 16, no. 1, p. 74, 2018.

40. S. Lee, A. Stubelius, N. Hamelmann, V. Tran, and A. Almutairi, "Inflammation-responsive drug-conjugated dextran nanoparticles enhance anti-inflammatory drug efficacy," *ACS Appl. Mater. Interfaces*, vol. 10, no. 47, pp. 40378–40387, November 2018.

41. I. Ekladious, Y. L. Colson, and M. W. Grinstaff, "Polymer–drug conjugate therapeutics: Advances, insights and prospects," *Nat. Rev. Drug Discov.*, vol. 18, no. 4, pp. 273–294, 2019.

42. C. Yu, L. Wang, Z. Xu, W. Teng, Z. Wu, and D. Xiong, "Smart micelles self-assembled from four-arm star polymers as potential drug carriers for pH-triggered DOX release," *J. Polym. Res.*, vol. 27, no. 5, p. 111, 2020.

43. J. H. Ko and H. D. Maynard, "A guide to maximizing the therapeutic potential of protein–polymer conjugates by rational design," *Chem. Soc. Rev.*, vol. 47, no. 24, pp. 8998–9014, 2018.

44. Y. Wang and C. Wu, "Site-specific conjugation of polymers to proteins," *Biomacromolecules*, vol. 19, no. 6, pp. 1804–1825, June 2018.

45. B. S. Makhmalzade and F. Chavoshy, "Polymeric micelles as cutaneous drug delivery system in normal skin and dermatological disorders," *J. Adv. Pharm. Technol. Res.*, vol. 9, no. 1, pp. 2–8, 2018.

46. Y. Mu, L. Gong, T. Peng, J. Yao, and Z. Lin, "Advances in pH-responsive drug delivery systems," *OpenNano*, vol. 5, no. August 2021, p. 100031, 2022.
47. Q. Zhou, L. Zhang, T. Yang, and H. Wu, "Stimuli-responsive polymeric micelles for drug delivery and cancer therapy," *Int. J. Nanomedicine*, vol. 13, pp. 2921–2942, 2018.
48. Y. Sun *et al.*, "Novel polymeric micelles as enzyme-sensitive nuclear-targeted dual-functional drug delivery vehicles for enhanced 9-nitro-20(S)-camptothecin delivery and antitumor efficacy," *Nanoscale*, vol. 12, no. 9, pp. 5380–5396, 2020.
49. S. He *et al.*, "Advances of molecularly imprinted polymers (MIP) and the application in drug delivery," *Eur. Polym. J.*, vol. 143, p. 110179, 2021.
50. A. E. Bodoki, B.-C. Iacob, and E. Bodoki, "Perspectives of molecularly imprinted polymer-based drug delivery systems in cancer therapy," *Polymers (Basel)*, vol. 11, no. 12, p. 2085, 2019.
51. N. Sanadgol and J. Wackerlig, "Developments of smart drug-delivery systems based on magnetic molecularly imprinted polymers for targeted cancer therapy: A short review," *Pharmaceutics*, vol. 12, no. 9, p. 831, 2020.
52. Y.-T. Qin, Y.-S. Feng, Y.-J. Ma, X.-W. He, W.-Y. Li, and Y.-K. Zhang, "Tumor-sensitive biodegradable nanoparticles of molecularly imprinted polymer-stabilized fluorescent zeolitic imidazolate framework-8 for targeted imaging and drug delivery," *ACS Appl. Mater. Interfaces*, vol. 12, no. 22, pp. 24585–24598, June 2020.

6 Analysis of polymeric composite material-based components using ANSYS workbench

Sajith T. A., Ajay Vasudeo Rane
and Krishnan Kanny

CONTENTS

6.1   Introduction 93
6.2   Composite Structures...94
6.3   Performance analysis of Composites...95
6.4   Conclusion 100
References... 100

6.1   INTRODUCTION

In response to an ever-increasing quantity and variety of applications, the variety and sophistication of polymer composite material systems and processing has risen dramatically. Understanding of polymer composite materials is far from complete due to the wide range of accessible materials as well as their ongoing development. As a result, the chapter's main objective is to disseminate to the general public knowledge regarding the links between properties of polymer composite materials and their processing, as well as their structural reaction. Analytical, experimental, and computational techniques that directly influence composite structure design are outlined in this chapter. Finite element analysis of composite materials made of polymers analysing structures built of composite materials is done using ANSYS®. This chapter's discussion of polymer composite materials covers both a microstructural and macrostructural investigation of the materials [1, 2].

This chapter provides a brief overview of the ideas involved in the in-depth analysis of composites, a thorough explanation of the mechanics required to convert those ideas into a mathematical representation of the physical world, and an explanation of how to calculate boundary values using finite element analysis software available commercially, such as ANSYS.

Nowadays, polymer composite materials are used extensively in a variety of industries, such as aerospace, automotive, civil infrastructure, sporting goods, and others. Composites are designed initially on the assumption that the laminate is

DOI: 10.1201/9781003319139-6

under plane stress. The geometry of the component, as well as the loading and support conditions, are also approximated in some way. In this approach, algebra may be used to do computations with relative ease and relatively easy analytical procedures. However, there are a number of drawbacks to preliminary analytical techniques that may be fixed with finite element analysis and advanced mechanics [3, 4].

6.2   COMPOSITE STRUCTURES

The majority of composite structures are constructed as shell and plate assemblies. This is so that the structure can carry membrane loads more effectively. The difficulty in manufacturing thick laminates is another significant factor. A hollow square tube with thin walls has a twice as much failure moment per unit area as a solid segment. Of course, the buckling of the thin walls restricts the failure moment. For polymer composites, buckling analysis is crucial because of this. Because the material is so strong and the thicknesses are so thin, the majority of composite structures are built with buckling limitations. As a result, structural failure like buckling is more common than material failure like yield stress in metallic structures. Plates are a specific type of shell since they don't have an initial curve. As a result, the sequel will solely address shells. Due to the fact that two dimensions (length and breadth) are substantially bigger than thickness, shells are treated as two-dimensional structures. The thickness coordinate is removed from the governing equations, which reduces the 3D issue to a 2D one. As a result, the thickness develops into a known parameter that is provided to the analysis model. Laminated composite modelling is distinct from modelling typical materials in three ways. First, each lamina's constitutive equations are orthotropic. Second, the kinematic presumptions of the shell theory applied and their incorporation into the element determine the constitutive equations of the element. Finally, when attempting to employ symmetry criteria in the models, material symmetry is just as crucial as geometric and load symmetry. Laminated composites may undergo deformation and stress analysis at many levels. The amount of post-processing wanted determines the level of detail required for the material description [1–4].

The strain and stress are calculated at the constituent level, that is, the reinforcement and matrix, when a high degree of detail is required. In this instance, it is important to explain the microstructure, in addition to the form and geometrical distribution of the reinforcement, as well as the material characteristics of the elements. Additionally, the composite should be studied as a solid, as indicated, when the composite material is a woven fabric, the laminate is extremely thick, or when researching localised phenomena like free edges effects. It should be highlighted, nonetheless, that the majority of laminated structures may be studied using the simplifications of plates and shells [1–2].

Most commonly, loads models are made using finite element analysis. It is sometimes also utilised to develop thorough stress models. The essence of finite element analysis may be summed up as follows: F = kX, where F is the applied force, k is the global stiffness matrix, commonly known as the stiffness of the entire structure, and X is the displacement (unknown). As we previously established, polymer composites are constructed from several tiny bits of discrete stiffness before being put together to form a single large stiffness matrix (which can be really big matrix depending on the model). Only using finite element analysis is feasible to numerically simulate the complicated stiffness of a complex structure made up of any number of pieces. The applied load F and the structure's stiffness k, which already have the requirements for static equilibrium built in, are the known quantities in the static finite element analysis. Therefore, the displacement and its derivative numbers are the only things that are unknown. Here is where the finite elemental solver's magic happens. The solver's role is basically as follows:

1. Gather all the models' numerical data.
2. Put the global stiffness matrix together.
3. Check the model's numerical definition, load distribution, and constraint balance.
4. Create all of the equilibrium equations by inverting this substantial stiffness matrix.
5. Next, resolve each of these equations to determine the undetermined displacements.
6. The solver then calculates all the derivative values, such as stresses and strains, etc., once the displacements have been solved for.

The majority of composite structures have thin walls. This is a logical outcome given the following circumstances:

6.3   PERFORMANCE ANALYSIS OF COMPOSITES

Composites outperform traditional materials in strength. Then, with a tiny area and hence a small thickness in most components, it is feasible to bear very large weights. In comparison to normal materials, composites are more costly. Therefore, there is a significant incentive to minimise the volume and, consequently, the thickness. With increasing rigidity, polymer composites become more expensive. The fibre-dominated rule of mixtures can be used to determine stiffness in the fibre direction. To enhance the moment of inertia of beams and stiffeners without increasing the cross sectional area, there is hence great motivation. The best course of action is to enhance the moment of inertia by lowering the thickness and extending the cross sectional area. The combination of the aforementioned characteristics frequently results in the design of composite structures with thicker walls and bigger cross sections, with buckling-prone failure modes. In contrast to material failure, buckling is a loss of stability brought on by geometrical factors. However, if the resulting deformations are not con-trolled, it may result in material failure and collapse. Most constructions can function within a range of linear elastic. In other words, when the load is removed, they revert to their original configuration. If the elastic range is surpassed, like when polymer matrix cracking happens in a composite, permanent deformations follow. Only in-plane stress is produced in the interior of symmetric laminates when they are loaded in-plane. Due to the imbalance of the in-plane stress components at the free edge, interlaminar stresses are generated close to the free edges [1–4]. The elastic modulus, shear modulus, Poisson's ratio, and other elastic characteristics of composite materi-als were believed to be accessible. Numerous material characteristics are required for heterogeneous materials, such as composites, and experimental evaluation of these numerous qualities is a time-consuming and expensive procedure. Additionally, the values of these characteristics vary depending on the volume proportion of reinforcement, among other factors. Utilising homogenisation techniques to forecast the elastic properties of the composite based on the elastic properties of the elements is an alternate method, or at the very least a supplement to testing (matrix and reinforcements). The approaches used to derive approximations of the characteristics of the composite are known as micromechanics methods or techniques because homogenisation models are based on more or less precise models of the microstructure [1–4]. Empirical, semiempirical, analytical, and numerical micromechanics models may all be divided into these categories. Numerical techniques, primarily the finite element method, are used to explore the nonlinear material behaviour of composites having periodic microstructure. The behaviour of the microstructure under a certain load history has been examined in nonlinear finite element analysis of metal matrix composites. The finite element approach has been used to determine bounds on composites' overall instantaneous elastoplastic characteristics. Materials' time-dependent responses can be divided into elastic, viscous, and viscoelastic categories. We are interested in viscoelasticity because viscoelasticity manifests itself in the creep behaviour of polymer composites. In composite materials, a variety of damage mechanisms, such as matrix fractures, fibre breakage, fibre-matrix debonding, and others, can be seen. Each of these damage mechanisms, their evolution with regard to load, strain, time, number of cycles, etc., and their impact on stiffness, remaining life, etc., have all been extensively studied. All of these failure types are represented by continuum damage mechanics (CDM) based on the impact they have on the material's mesoscale behaviour (lamina level). In other words, CDM uses continuum damage variables to determine the lamina and laminate's deteriorated moduli. Then, damage initiation is detected using either strength or fracture mechanics failure criteria [1–4].

It is acceptable to infer that the matrix only supports a small amount of the imposed load, and that no matrix damage is anticipated during loading if a lamina is subjected to tensile stress in the fibre direction. The strength of a bundle of fibres may then be calculated in order to precisely anticipate the eventual tensile strength of the composite lamina. The gauge length employed during fibre strength testing affects the fibre strength. The ineffective length is the range of lengths that influences how much of the fibre strength is really utilised in a composite. The ineffective length is the distance over which a fibre recovers a significant portion of its load, measured from the fibre break point [1–4].

When under load, matrix fractures expand perpendicular to the fibre orientation, showing that the lamina's cracks are aligned with the fibre direction. The rigidity of the fractured lamina is decreased by these parallel sets of cracks, which transfers some of the load to the uncracked laminas.

The fracture density, which is calculated as the inverse of the distance between two adjacent cracks, is used to illustrate the damage that this collection of parallel cracks causes in each lamina. As a result, the only state variable required to depict the degree of damage in the fractured lamina is the crack density. It should be noted that the theory, called discrete damage mechanics, models the real, discrete fractures (DDM) [1–4].

A prevalent mode of failure that affects the structural performance of composite laminates is delamination. Because the connection between two adjacent laminas depends only on the matrix parameters, the interface between laminas provides a low-resistance channel for crack formation. Delamination can be the result of manufacturing flaws, fatigue cracks, low velocity impact cracks, stress concentration around geometrical/material discontinuities such as joints and free edges, or high interlaminar stresses. Fracture mechanics and cohesive damage models can be used to investigate delamination [2].

The flow during vacuum infusion, sheet moulding compound (SMC), the autoclave process, and twin-screw extrusion have all been modelled using computational fluid dynamics (CFD). The study of three-dimensional geometries and the homogeneous treatment of multiphase flows and porous media has been done by various researchers. As an example, the porous media for the vacuum infusion process may be situated in a complicated mould with shifting borders and may have anisotropic, spatially, and temporally variable permeability. If shear-thinning effects are taken into consideration, it is possible to forecast the pressure inside the mould during compression moulding of SMC. A complete 3D flow in a thin, porous material with an anisotropic, spatially, and temporally dependent permeability defines vacuum infusion's impregnation. Additionally, the compliance of the fibre network may vary as it is wetted, and the form of the porous medium might change over time due to pressures from the difference in pressure between the atmosphere and the mould.

Utilising three distinct methods, compression moulding of SMC has been examined with CFD. This includes a study where various rheological models, including the shear-thinning effect, are compared, a methodology for surrogate-based optimisation applied to simulations with a straightforward rheology model, and a study where the layers of the compound closest to the surfaces of the mould are given much lower viscosities than the bulk layers [5].

CFD simulations of heat transport to a tool within an autoclave have been performed both with and without accounting for thermal radiation. The pressure within the autoclave is raised, and hot air is blasted over the tool. Particularly for simulations when thermal radiation was considered in the model, the anticipated temperature at a number of discrete points on the tool agrees with experimental observations provided in. A position with relatively easy flow is frequently where the points with strong agreement are found. However, there were certain locations where there was less agreement, and these spots were frequently found in places where the flow was more complicated. The mismatch may be attributed to problems with the mesh quality for a more complex flow and turbulence modelling. However, it can be said that thermal radiation should be taken into account when modelling heat transfer for such a situation and that CFD may be used to anticipate the heat transmission within an autoclave during the manufacture of composites. The study demonstrates the significance of using an appropriate input velocity profile [5].

Liquid-mediated melt compounding of nanocomposites in twin-screw extruders is a new technique that combines melt mixing with solution assistance to address the drawbacks of each technique alone. After the liquid has evaporated, the liquids utilised serve as plasticizers as well as temporary carriers of nanomaterials. It is difficult to model the flow of thermoplastic polymers in twin-screw extruders because of the mixing, variable solvent volume ratios, and non-spherical particle additions. In the current scenario, a two-phase flow technique is used, and it is expected that the particles would travel with the carrier fluid through the extruder's mixing section [5].

The content up above provides a very quick overview of ANSYS and its uses in relation to polymers and polymer composites. Below, we list a few studies that employ ANSYS as a workbench for the design and analysis of polymer composites.

A metal or ceramic femoral head is combined with an acetabular cup made of ultra-high-molecular-weight polyethylene (UHMWPE) to provide an enhanced model of wear in the spherical joint of a complete hip prosthesis. In line with all other research works that have been documented in the literature, the wear model is based on the traditional Archard–Lancaster equation. According to ISO 14242-1 specifications, the contact problem between the cup and the head was solved using finite elements while subject to loads and rotational rotations. When the wear factor is set to be a function of contact pressure, the polymer wear is first assessed in terms of cumulative linear wear and volume wear [6].

Following total hip replacement (THA), periprosthetic bone loss is a severe problem that can result in implant failure before it should. According to Wolff's law, a rigid prosthesis causes significant bone loss close to the implant. To create long-lasting prosthetics, flexible implants must be designed, and their impact on the process of bone remodelling must be thoroughly studied. In this work, the mechano-biochemical bone adaption model was used to compare bone remodelling around a relatively new biomimetic polymer composite-based (CF/PA12) hip implant to that in a metallic one (made of titanium) (irreversible thermodynamic-based model). The findings showed that compared to a titanium stem, a composite stem causes lower density changes (bone loss) [7].

The acetabular cup of an existing complete hip prosthesis made of UHMWPE in conjunction with a metal or ceramic femoral head and based on the conventional Archard equation is updated and enlarged. With the help of this model, investigations are carried out using finite element analysis to determine cumulative linear and volumetric wear for the ISO 14242-1 requirements as well as extra conditions for walking gait. Additionally, they are performed with a head diameter of 28 mm, both with a constant wear factor and with a variable wear factor, the latter of which is derived using a modified formula for the dependency on contact pressure [8].

In the prosthesis-bone system, the pressures placed on the prosthesis during human activity cause dynamic stresses that change over time and may lead to stress shielding, and decrease the stress buffering effect as a result. In order to determine which of these models performs best, this study used finite element analysis to examine how PEEK and carbon/PEEK composite coating materials on a titanium alloy hip implant stem could reduce the stress shielding effect associated with various human activities, including standing up, regular walking, and climbing stairs. For the purposes of finite element analysis, a 3D finite element model of the femur, hip implants, and coating layers using composite (carbon/PEEK) and polymeric (PEEK) coating materials was created. The prosthetic head was subjected to a time-dependent cycling load. In comparison to an uncoated prosthesis, the highest increase in load transmission to the bone was 207% for the prosthesis covered with carbon/PEEK configuration I (fibres oriented with 0, +45, −45, and 90 degrees). The carbon/PEEK composite material (configuration I) appears to be a good option to distribute the applied load and transmit it to the bone, reducing stress shielding issues and extending the lifespan of the prosthesis-bone system, according to numerical results. Aseptic loosening will be avoided, and the system's stability will be improved [9].

Medical waste made of single-use plastic that comes from petroleum-based sources is building up in landfills and leaking into the environment. Utilising biodegradable polymers can assist to solve the pressing environmental dilemma of managing plastics and medical waste. The project's goal is to lessen single-use plastics' harmful environmental consequences. The focus of the current work is on the creation and description of bioplastics based on banana peel starch and using glycerine as an adhesive or plasticizer. Three different samples of bioplastic made from banana peel starch were created using different ratios of corn starch, banana peel starch, vinegar, glycerine, and distilled water. The assessment tests for all three samples— moisture content, water absorption, water and alcohol solubility, soil degradation, tensile strength study, and FTIR analysis—show that the banana peel starch-based bioplastic sample II possesses the requisite physiochemical and mechanical qualities. Utilising ANSYS software, an intravenous tube was modelled, and its flow and velocity patterns were examined and tested. Future printing and moulding of the same design as an intravenous tube utilising the suggested bioplastic material for infusion and transfusion purposes is conceivable [10].

For the diagnosis and treatment of human illness, both engineering and medical disciplines are essential. One of the therapeutic sources for treating bone loss in the modern scientific world is the technology of alternative bone scaffolds. The design and study of a porous scaffold created using the additive manufacturing technology are the main topics of this research work. For this bone scaffold, a variety of biocompatible materials with various properties are employed. In this research, a material composition comprising biocompatible polyamide (PA) and hydroxyapatite (HA) is mixed to have a high load-bearing capability. Since HA has the property of enhanced tissue cell seeding proliferation, it is added to the formulation. With a pore size of 800 microns and a porosity range of 40% to 70%, the porous scaffold models with various configurations of cubical pore, spherical pore, shifted cubical pore, and shifted spherical pore are created using solid works software. ANSYS software is used to examine each and every CAD model. Based on the static structural study, the shifted cubical scaffold was chosen for manufacturing using a selective laser sintering machine because it has reduced stress concentration. The load-bearing strength of the specimens is determined experimentally after they are constructed in three distinct construction orientations. This study takes into account four distinct material compositions: 100% PA, 95% PA with 5% HA, 90% PA with 10% HA, and 85% PA with 15% HA [11].

A balloon-like protrusion in the blood artery wall known as an aneurysm can develop in the main arteries of the heart and brain. For wide-neck complicated aneurysms, biodegradable polymeric stent-assisted coiling is anticipated to be the best option. In order to treat aneurysms, this report describes the development of fabrication and design techniques for biodegradable polymeric stents. First, a system for fabricating coil and zigzag patterns of biodegradable polymeric stents was created using a dispensing-based rapid prototyping (DBRP) technique. The radial deformation of the stents made with the coil or zigzag construction was then evaluated using compression testing. The findings showed that the zigzag-shaped stent had more radial rigidity than the coil-shaped one. Based on this, the zigzag-structured stent was selected for the creation of a finite element model to simulate the actual compression testing. The outcome shows that the biodegradable polymeric stents finite element model is appropriate within a range of radial deformation, approximately 20%. Additionally, the zigzag structure was optimised using ANSYS DesignXplorer, and the findings showed that by adjusting the structure's characteristics, the total deformation could be reduced by 35.7%. This would be a considerable improvement in the radial stiffness of biodegradable polymeric stents [12].

6.4 CONCLUSION

The choice of material and its proportions are, as we all know, the primary requirements for practically all components. In order to get effective results utilising ANSYS quickly, numerous analyses are performed along with effective component design and selection of the right material.

REFERENCES

1. Dill, E.H., 2012. *The finite element method for mechanics of solids with ANSYS applications* (Vol. 6000). New York: CRC Press.
2. Barbero, E.J., 2013. *Finite element analysis of composite materials using ANSYS* (Vol. 2103). Boca Raton: CRC Press.
3. Blaabjerg, F. and Ionel, D.M. eds., 2017. *Renewable energy devices and systems with simulations in MATLAB® and ANSYS®*. Boca Raton: CRC Press.
4. Chen, X. and Liu, Y., 2018. *Finite element modeling and simulation with ANSYS Workbench*. Boca Raton: CRC Press.
5. Lundström, T.S., 2016. Computational fluid dynamics applied to composites manufacturing. In *Proceedings of 13th International Conference on Flow Processing in Composite Materials (FPCM13)*, Kyoto Institute of Technology, Japan.
6. Pakhaliuk, V., Polyakov, A., Kalinin, M. and Kramar, V., 2015. Improving the finite element simulation of wear of total hip prosthesis' spherical joint with the polymeric component. *Procedia Engineering, 100*, pp. 539–548.
7. Avval, P.T., Samiezadeh, S. and Bougherara, H., 2014. Bone remodeling in response to a new biomimetic polymer-composite hip stem: Computational study using mechano-biochemical model. In *ECCM16-16th European Conference on Composite Materials, Seville, Spain* (pp. 22–26).
8. Pakhaliuk, V., Poliakov, A., Kalinin, M., Pashkov, Y. and Gadkov, P., 2016. Modifying and expanding the simulation of wear in the spherical joint with a polymeric component of the total hip prosthesis. *Facta Universitatis. Series: Mechanical Engineering, 14*(3), pp. 301–312.
9. Darwich, A., Nazha, H. and Abbas, W., 2019. Numerical study of stress shielding evaluation of hip implant stems coated with composite (carbon/PEEK) and polymeric (PEEK) coating materials. *Biomedical Research, 30*(1), pp. 169–174.
10. Vijayalaksmi, M., Vigneshwari, N., Gokul, M., Govindaraj, V., Nithila, E.E., Bebin, M., Prasath, T.A., Kiran, V.G. and Varsha, A.K., Synthesis and Characterization of Banana Peel Starch-Based Bioplastic for Making Intra Venous Tubes.
11. Kumaresan, T., Gandhinathan, R., Ramu, M., Ananthasubramanian, M. and Pradheepa, K.B., 2016. Design, analysis and fabrication of polyamide/hydroxyapatite porous structured scaffold using selective laser sintering method for bio-medical applications. *Journal of Mechanical Science and Technology, 30*(11), pp. 5305–5312.
12. Han, X., Wu, X., Kelly, M. and Chen, X., 2017. Fabrication and optimal design of biodegradable polymeric stents for aneurysms treatments. *Journal of Functional Biomaterials, 8*(1), p. 8.

7 Anti-microbial activities of nano-polymers for biomedical applications

Sawna Roy

CONTENTS

7.1 Introduction 101
7.2 Types of anti-microbial polymers.. 101
7.3 Biocidal agents in anti-microbial nano-polymers... 102
7.4 Role of anti-microbial nano-polymers in various biomedical applications..... 106
7.5 Methods of generating anti-microbial polymer coatings.............................. 114
7.6 Conclusion 115
References.. 116

7.1 INTRODUCTION

Infections caused by pathogenic micro-organisms are a significant concern in the biomedical field, including surgical equipment, medical devices, tissue engineering, orthopedic implants, dental restoration, and healthcare products. Micro-organisms threaten humans every year, causing numerous infections and diseases. More than 1.2 million individuals – and probably a lot of millions – died in 2019 as an immediate result of antibiotic-resistant micro-organism infections, per the initial comprehensive estimate of the worldwide impact of anti-microbial resistance [1]. These omnipresent germs (bacteria, viruses, fungi, and protozoa) produce infections through touching, eating, consuming, or respiration, including germ containment [2]. Continuous overuse of anti-microbial agents, known to kill microbes, leads to resistance development in strains that evolve naturally by rapidly mutating genes on exposure to such agents.

7.2 TYPES OF ANTI-MICROBIAL POLYMERS

Anti-microbial polymers are classified into three types based on their polymeric system [3]:

i. **Biocidal polymers**: Biocidal polymers (Figure 7.1a) have an intrinsic anti-microbial activity. The biocidal polymers include natural polymers such as chitosan, poly(ε-lysine), and synthetic polymers, which contain cationic

DOI: 10.1201/9781003319139-7

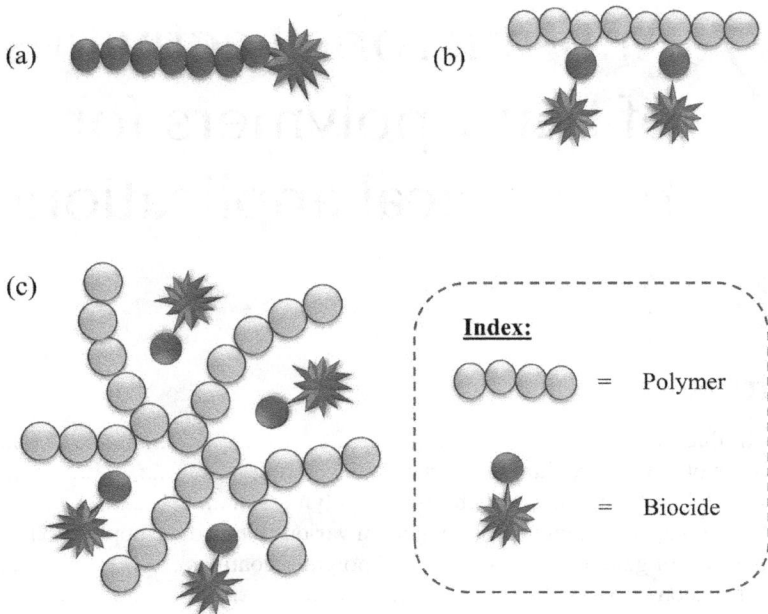

FIGURE 7.1   Types of anti-microbial polymers. (a) Biocidal polymers, (b) Polymeric biocides, (c) Polymer-releasing biocides.

salts such as quaternary phosphonium salts (QPS) or quaternary ammonium salts (QASs).

ii. **Polymeric biocides:** Polymeric biocides (Figure 7.1b) are polymers having backbones with attached biocidal molecules. Polymerization can either increase or decrease the anti-microbial activity of bioactive functional groups. Microbes typically have a negative charge at the cell's outer membrane. Cationic charges present in biocidal molecules, such as tertiary sulfonium, quaternary ammonium, benzimidazole, and halogen, cause cell surface destabilization leading to the induction of microbial death.

iii. **Polymer-releasing biocides**: Polymer-releasing biocides (Figure 7.1c) are polymers loaded with biocidal molecules [4]. Incorporating antibiotics or nanoparticles with anti-microbial properties in polymers under a controlled release system is helpful in biomedical applications.

7.3   BIOCIDAL AGENTS IN ANTI-MICROBIAL NANO-POLYMERS

1. **Antibiotics:** Antibiotics either encapsulate or conjugate with polymers to facilitate anti-microbial properties. Antibiotics inhibit growth or kill microbes by disrupting cell envelope or inhibiting protein and nucleic acid synthesis. Guadalupe et al.'s electrospun PCL nanofibers contained PNF1 (model angiogenic factor) and gentamicin and were used in wound dressing

[5]. Penicillin modifications to polytetrafluoroethylene (PTFE) were carried out to suppress *Staphylococcus aureus* development on PTFE material [6]. Gustafson et al. used photopolymerization to create charged hydrogels based on sodium methacrylate (OPF/SMA) and oligo(PEG-fumarate) as a vancomycin delivery method in surgical applications [7]. Combining biocidal polymers extends antibiotic efficacy, especially after depleting antibiotics, and the contact-active function can protect the surface against contamination [8].

2. **Nanoparticles:** Metallic nanoparticles are toxic to pathogens by various mechanisms, including generating massive oxidative stress, causing DNA damage, cell membrane disruption, or lipid peroxidation (Figure 7.2). Silver (Ag), cobalt (Co), copper (Cu), gold (Au), iron (Fe), nickel (Ni), mercury (Hg), manganese (Mn), bismuth (Bi), lead (Pb), tin (Sn), platinum (Pt), antimony (Sb), titanium (Ti), and zinc (Zn) are the heavy metals that are known to interact with microbes and show anti-microbial activity [9].

   i. **Silver Nanoparticles (AgNPs):** AgNPs adhere to the microbe's cell wall, form a pit by causing structural change, and enhance permeability, leading to cell death. AgNPs can be synthesized by easily using a chemical reduction method. Reducing agents such as tri-sodium citrate, sodium borohydride, chitosan, sodium alginate, etc., can be added,

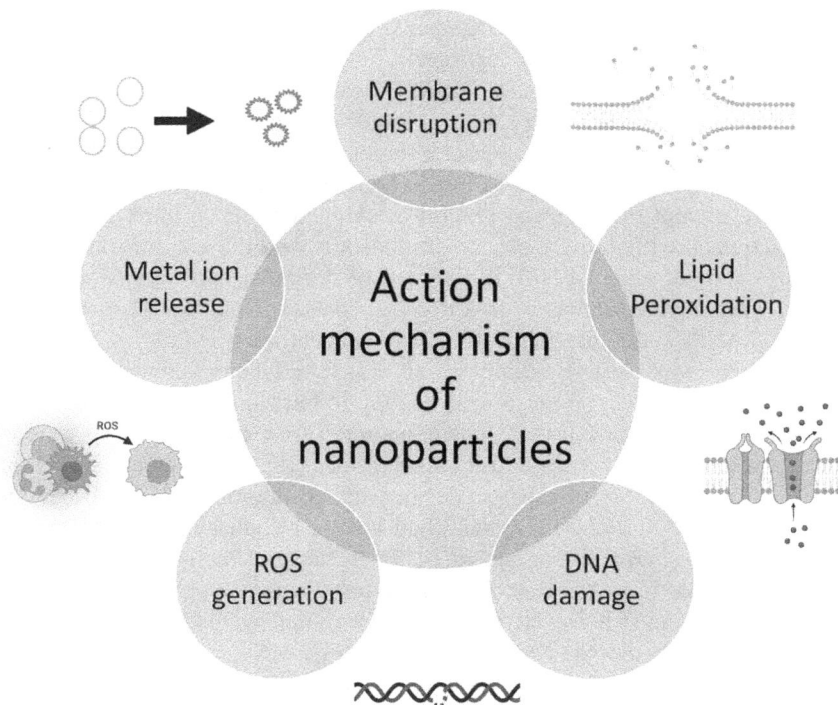

FIGURE 7.2   Action mechanism of nanoparticles in anti-microbial nano-polymers.

which can also act as stabilizing agents. Antiviral effects of AgO2 solutions (different concentrations varying from 0.025% to 0.1%) on vaccinia virus, herpes simplex type 1, papovavirus SV-40, adenovirus, and poliovirus were reported by Kadar et al. [10]. To suppress the growth of certain bacteria such as *Listeria monocytogenesis, S. aureus, Escherichia coli*, and *Pseudomonas fluorescens*, AgNPs are often used [11]. Wound dressing, drug delivery, tissue scaffolding, and protective coating applications can all benefit from AgNP-based nanosystems and nanomaterials.

ii. **Copper Nanoparticles (CuNPs):** Cu is a structural component of various enzymes in living organisms, and when it is in free ionic form, it can have hazardous consequences by creating reactive oxygen species (ROS) that damage DNA and amino acid synthesis at high concentrations [12]. The methods for synthesizing CuNPs include microemulsion and chemical reduction, electrochemical or hydrothermal. Size and surface charge influence the toxicity of CuNPs. Devi et al. investigated the antibacterial activity of bulk, as-prepared, and annealed CuO NPs against *E. coli, Proteus mirabilis,* and *Klebsiella spp.* and found that their effect was comparable to that of gentamycin on these strains [13, 14]. The antibacterial potential of CuNPs allows the development of a wide range of products, ranging from anti-microbial solutions used to disinfect surfaces and medical equipment to anti-microbial wound dressings, textiles, and coatings.

iii. **Gold:** Gold nanoparticles (AuNPs) can be synthesized using a variety of ways, including chemical routes such as solvothermal processes, physical means such as laser ablation, and green approaches such as bioaccumulation and biomineralization [15]. AuNPs were shown to disrupt the bacterial biofilm by Ahmed et al., *S. aureus* on being treated with AuNPs, spaced dramatically, and the biofilm was significantly eliminated [16]. In the case of drug-resistant fungi (for example, fluconazole-resistant *Candida albicans*), indolicidin-conjugated AuNPs – the minimum inhibitory concentration is only one-sixth of free indolicidin – exhibit strong anti-*C. albicans* activity, establishing a new way of antifungal therapy in burn infections [17]. Anionic AuNPs are harmless to cells in another investigation, whereas cations are moderately hazardous to all cell lines [18]. Zhang et al. discovered that coating the transparent device with 4,6-diamino-2-pyrimidinethiol (AuDAPT) and AuNPs modified having a high antibacterial impact on *Porphyromonas gingivalis* [19]. Because of their biocompatibility and ease of production, AuNPs are promising prospects for medicinal applications; however, whether intracellular agents can impact them remains explored [20].

iv. **Zinc nanoparticles:** Zinc is an active metal with excellent reduction characteristics and can oxidize quickly to generate zinc oxide [21]. The anti-microbial activity of ZnO NPs has piqued the interest of researchers worldwide, owing to the use of nanotechnology to create particles in the nanometer range [22]. ZnO NPs can be prepared via the physiochemical sol-gel method, the sol-gel combustion method, chemical synthesis at low temperatures, and the mechanical method [21]. The characteristics of ZnO NPs can also be altered by modifying with PEG or starch [23]. ZnO interactions with other antibiotics, metal oxides, metallic nanoparticles or metal doping, and some other biomaterials offer a broad-spectrum antibacterial activity that can be tailored for multi-therapeutic choices and used to improve their usefulness in clinical translation platforms [24].

v. **Iron nanoparticles:** Iron oxide magnetic nanoparticles or IONPs are chemically and physically stable, biocompatible, and ecologically friendly, making them ideal for clinical use [25]. Iron and its oxide-based nanoparticles can be synthesized using thermal decomposition, sol-gel, precipitation, etc. SPIONs (Superparamagnetic iron oxide nanoparticles) can employ a combination of targeting and imaging approaches and has the potential to improve infection treatment even further by increasing the uptake of nanoparticles by microbes [26]. Wang et al. described a hydrogel nanocomposite made by copolymerizing acrylamide (Am) and N-isopropyl acrylamide (NIPAm), which was then combined with vinyl-Fe3O4@SiO2 for photothermal therapy and drug targeting [27] (Table 7.1).

Various other metallic nanoparticles blending with polymers lead to the formation of nano-polymers which enhances the functionality in the biomedical application of polymers.

TABLE 7.1
List of methods for synthesizing nanoparticles [28]

Method for synthesizing nanoparticles

Physical method

(a) Chemical vapor deposition (CVD)	The substrate is exposed to volatile precursors, which break down on it and generate the desired deposit of nanoparticles
(b) Microwave irradiation	The metallic salt solution irradiates and synthesizes NPs
(c) Pulse laser method	The disc rotates on an aqueous solution of metallic salts. The laser beam generates hotspots where it reduces the salts and forms NPs

Chemical method

(a) Thermal decomposition method	At high temperatures, the chemical bond breaks, and the synthesis of NPs occurs
(b) Polyol method	Polyol, which is a non-aqueous liquid, is used as a reducing agent
(c) Microemulsion	Metallic nanoparticles in water-in-oil microemulsion are usually prepared by combining microemulsions containing a reducing agent and metal salt

7.4   ROLE OF ANTI-MICROBIAL NANO-POLYMERS IN VARIOUS BIOMEDICAL APPLICATIONS

1. **Surgical Implants:** Cardiovascular devices, vascular and urinary catheters, and cerebrospinal shunts are globally implanted every year. The implant's location determines the most likely colonizing pathogen for indwelling devices. For example, coagulase-negative *staphylococci* and *S. aureus* are more prone to colonize vascular implants, but *E. coli* and *Enterococcus sp.* are more likely to occupy urinary devices [29].

1.1 Surgical implants' polymer properties
i.   Malleability: Polymers used in medical implants should be malleable and flexible, i.e., they can be easily reshaped as per the need for implantation in a complex body system.
ii.   Biocompatible: Since surgical implants are in vivo, they are supposed to be biologically inert, non-allergic, and non-toxic for the recipient.
iii. Ease of fabrication: Implant polymers should have ease of fabrication to be fabricated easily in a short period.
iv.   Smart polymers:- They can respond to temperature, pH, light, or magnetic field to be helpful in specific medical applications.

1.2 Polymers in surgical implants
1.2.1 *Poly(methyl methacrylate) (PMMA)*
PMMA (Figure 7.3a) has been utilized in various medical implants, including intraocular lenses, rhinoplasty, cranioplasty, and bone cement in total joint replacement [30–32]. Porous PMMA space maintainers have also been designed for use in patients with craniofacial tissues and bones damaged or lost and cannot be repaired [33]. These space maintainers can also provide stability to the nearby tissues, potentially facilitating soft tissue recovery around the damaged structure [34]. On being examined, tissue growth for PMMA orbital implants showed that fibrovascular ingrowth of tissues from surrounding orbital tissues in the eyes was possible with no evidence of infection [35]. With the evolution of 3D printing, PMMA has become more widely used in patient-specific biomedical applications, such as the manufacture of porous-tailored freeform structures [36].

1.2.2 Polypropylene (PP)
PP (Figure 7.3b) has been widely utilized as a surgical mesh to fortify weakening tissues while also functioning as a scaffold for fibrocollagenous tissues to develop on the mesh itself [37]. It is mainly used in urogynecology to treat stress urinary incontinence and pelvic organ prolapse [37]. PP has also been blended with titanium to develop a mesh with a smaller capsular contracture, which is a crucial problem in implant-based breast reconstruction [5]. It is also a promising substance for strengthening soft tissue structure. PP has previously been utilized as a blood oxygenator membrane; nevertheless, the body has had numerous immune system reactions [38]. Surface

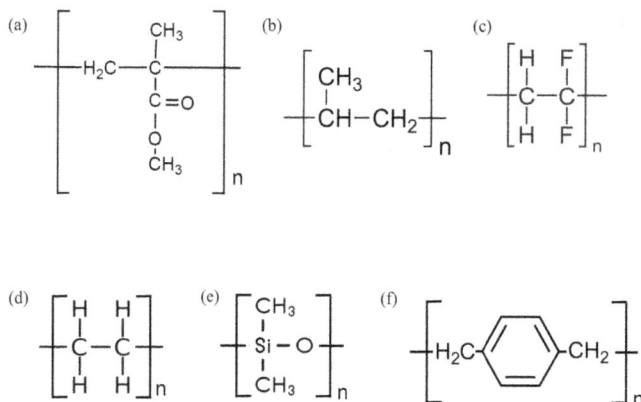

FIGURE 7.3 Structure of anti-microbial polymers. (a) Poly(methyl methacrylate) (PMMA), (b) Polypropylene (PP), (c) Polyvinylidene fluoride (PVDF), (d) Polyethylene (PE), (e) Polydimethylsiloxane (PDMS), (f) Parylene-C.

modification or surface coating with a bio-inert material can improve its biocompatibility.

1.2.3 Polyvinylidene Fluoride (PVDF)

PVDF is nonreactive, making it an excellent material (Figure 7.3c) for sutures and surgical meshes [39]. Its piezoelectric properties make it an ideal material for wound healing; it may also be used as a sensor substrate [40]. However, due to the inability to make smooth films and poor adherence to other materials, it is incredibly uncommon to obtain a pure PVDF film in biomedical devices used as packing films [34]. It has also been observed that energy may be gathered from the expansion and contraction of blood vessels in the human body by coupling PVDF nanofibers with graphene [34]. Given the complexity of thin film manufacturing, additional advances in PVDF fabrication techniques are important for future nanoscale device use, which would tremendously benefit the biomedical field [34].

1.2.4 Polyethylene (PE)

Porous high-density polyethylene (pHDPE) (Figure 7.3d) surgical implants have been used to repair a variety of bone abnormalities, including maxillofacial, cranial, and spinal surgery [34]. Material strength improves as molecular weight increases, but elasticity decreases. Ceramic–polystyrene couplings revealed lower fracture rates and less audible component-related noise than typical ceramic–ceramic couplings that employed PE for total hip arthroplasty [41]. Surface modification of PE-related materials has also been carried out in order to improve various qualities for diverse applications. One example is laser light modulating the surface roughness and wettability of ultrahigh molecular weight polyethylene [42].

1.2.5 Silicone-derived polymer

Silicone implants are inert substances utilized in laryngeal procedures to address difficulties such as unilateral vocal fold paralysis, which causes partial glottis closure and vocal dysfunction, and an encapsulant material in implants [34]. Polydimethylsiloxane (PDMS) (Figure 7.3d) and parylene (Figure 7.3e) are two silicone by-products that are extensively utilized in biomedical implants [34]. Shunts, esophageal replacements, mammary prostheses, cochlear implants, pacemakers, catheters, blood pumps, and implant packaging material electrical devices and sensors are made from PDMS [43]. PDMS can be synthesized from octamethylcyclotetrasiloxane (D4) monomers polymerized with hexamethyldisiloxane in a base state [44].

Parylene is the vernacular name for a group of vapor-deposited coatings that give chemical and moisture resistance to various items [45]. Due to its simplicity of application, low cost, and significant barrier qualities, parylene-C is the most widespread form of coating used in biomedical implants [46]. Altogether, silicone-derived polymers are widely utilized in implant materials and have been found to give structural support for various device applications; nevertheless, this material is relatively fragile when used in bulk. Its long-term consequences have not been studied [34].

2. **Dental restoration:** The most widespread oral disease is dental caries. The acidic environment is the primary causal agent in this disease which promotes the growth of microbes, such as *S. aureus*, *Lactobacillus* spp., *Actinomycetes,* and so on [47]. Polymeric resin and fillers are currently in demand for restoring dental cavities because of their anti-microbial and biocompatible nature. Resin type and filler type are two significant resin composites useful in dental restoration.

2.1 Anti-microbial polymer properties

Different anti-microbial agents target the microbes using various mechanisms, making them useful in dental restoration. The three essential properties of anti-microbial polymers are:

i.   *Drug release and effectiveness*: These antibacterial molecules can coat onto biomaterials via impregnation, physical adsorption, conjugation, or complexation. These functional coatings intend to serve as carriers of anti-microbial compounds released in higher concentrations in the surrounding media and are thus transported to the attached bacterial cells after implantation to limit initial invasion and avoid biofilm formation on implanted dental surfaces.

ii. *Biocompatibility*: Dental patients are exposed to anti-microbial monomers for treatment and polymers following dental restorations, which can cause local mucosal irritation or allergic reactions [48, 49]. It is critical to address the biocompatibility of anti-microbial polymers used in dental resin composites, resulting in unexpected issues when a new anti-microbial monomer is added [50].

iii. *Shelf life*: The polymer should be stable over long periods and have a long shelf life.

2.2 Anti-microbial polymer in dental restoration
2.2.1 *2-Methacryloyloxyethyl phosphorylcholine (MPC)*
The membrane of most pathogenic bacteria is bilipid in nature, where the inner layer is of negatively charged phospholipids like phosphatidylserine. In contrast, the outer layer is mainly composed of zwitterionic lipid phosphatidylcholine [51]. MPC (Figure 7.4a) could be synthesized by reacting 2-hydroxyethyl methacrylate with 2-chloro-2-oxo-1,3,2-dioxaphospholane, then ring-opening the intermediate alkoxyphospholane with trimethylamine [52]. The biocompatible MPC polymers mimic the biomembrane and reduce protein adsorption, bacterial adhesion, and cell attachment [53]. The addition of a methacryloyl group in MPC enabled polymerization reactions, and the PC headgroup is bioactive. Zhang et al. combined MPC and a quaternary ammonium dimethylaminohexadecyl methacrylate, DMAHDM, into a dental composite and inhibited biofilm growth and lactic acid production more effectively [50, 54]. Choi et al. documented that bonding synergetically increases with the addition of MPC and MBN (mesoporous bioactive glass nanoparticles) at appropriate ratios, with antibacterial, protein-repellent, and anti-demineralization effects [55].

2.2.2 *Quaternary Ammonium Methacrylates (QAMs)*
QASs are positively charged compounds containing four bonded heterocyclic, aryl, or alkyl groups to nitrogen [56]. Because QASs lack active functional groups in their chemical structures, they cannot chemically attach to dental resin networks, which may result in QAS burst release [50]. The addition of active functional moieties such as the methacryloyl group leads to converting QASs into QAMs. QAMs include quaternary ammonium methacrylate polymer (QAMP), quaternary ammonium dimethacrylate (QADM), 2-acryloxyethyltrimethylammonium chloride (ATA), quaternary ammonium polyethyleneimine (PEI), methacryloxyl ethyl-cetyl-dimethyl ammonium chloride (DMAE–CB), and dimethylaminododecyl methacrylate (DMADDM) (Figure 7.4b) [57]. The chemical synthesis of QAMs is

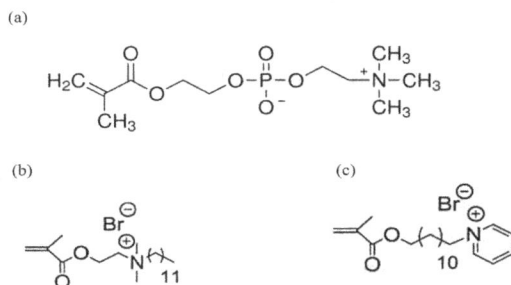

FIGURE 7.4 Structure of anti-microbial polymers used in dental restoration. (a) 2-Methacryloyloxyethyl phosphorylcholine (MPC), (b) Dimethylaminododecyl methacrylate (DMADDM), (c) Methacryloyloxydodecylpyridinium bromide (MDPB).

primarily on a radical polymerization basis, which is a challenge in gaining valuable control over macromolecular structures, configurations, and functions [50].

2.2.3 *Methacryloyloxydodecylpyridinium Bromide (MDPB)*

The development of anti-microbial dental resin, methacryloyloxydodecyl-pyridinium bromide (MDPB) monomer (Figure 7.4c), is based on an incorporating antibacterial agent, hydroxy-dodecyl pyridinium bromide [58]. MDPB imparts antibacterial and polymerizable characteristics by the addition of a methacryloyl group. MDPB is successfully copolymerizing with the typical methacrylates when formulated into a dental filling composite which is composed of 2,2-bis[4-(3-methacrylic-2-hydroxypropyl) phen-ylpropane (Bis-GMA), triethyleneglycoldimethacrylate (TEGDMA), and dimethylaminoethylmethacrylate (DMAEMA) at a weight percent between 0.1 and 0.2, respectively [50].

3. **Medical equipment and devices**: The widespread availability of high-quality, clean, sterile equipment at reasonable prices enabled the widespread expansion of smaller hospitals and clinics where the sick and injured could obtain medical care [59].

3.1 Polymer properties useful in medical devices and equipment

i. *Functionality*: Device components must be designed to utilize the resulting device or instrument without an issue. For example, multi-biomarkers can be detected by a single medical detection device.

ii. *Compatibility*: Not in terms of biocompatibility, but nano-polymers should be compatible in mixing with other materials for achieving desired properties.

iii. *Weightless*: In terms of transportation, polymeric material consumption and production cost can be reduced by using and designing medical devices that are less heavy and easier to use by the recipient.

iv. Eco-friendly: Most medical device manufacturers understand the importance of being environmentally responsible in designing their devices, manufacturing them, using them, and even how they can decompose after usage.

3.2 Polymers useful in equipment and medical devices
3.2.1 Biopolymers

a. *Chitosan*: Chitosan is a cationic polymer (Figure 7.5a), derived from chitin's deacetylation and synthesized by giving alkaline treatment at high temperatures [60]. Chitosan is primarily used in implants for bone, ligament, cartilage, tendon, liver, neural, stents, and skin regeneration. For improving mechanical qualities, Chen et al. created a polymeric stent consisting of chitosan-based sheets attached by genipin [61]. Chitosan is also grafted with heparin to improve its anti-coagulant and angiogenic characteristics and its affinity for growth factors [62]. These alterations provide the resulting products with distinct new features. For CNS regeneration, biomaterial scaffolds are designed with the needed

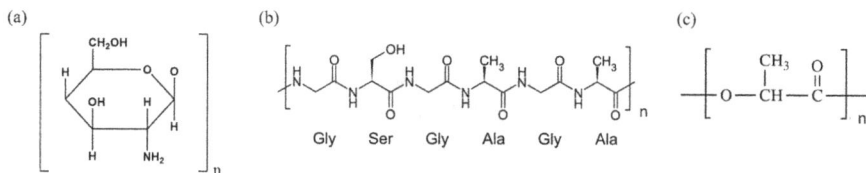

FIGURE 7.5   Structure of bio-polymers. (a) Chitosan, (b) Silk fibroin, (c) Poly-lactic acid (PLA).

structure and qualities for tissue restoration by doing modifications in chitosan. The layer of nanoparticles such as silicate [63], silver, iron [64], manganese dioxides, and cetyltrimethylammonium bromide modified rectorite (REC) matrices are used for the fabrication of anti-microbial packaging films [65].

b. *Silk:* Silk fibers are a sustainable protein biopolymer with high mechanical characteristics and biocompatibility. The silkworm's natural silk thread comprises two structural proteins – 72–81 wt% of fibroin (Figure 7.5b) and 19–28 wt% of sericin – and traces of 0.8–1% of fat/wax and 1–1.4% of color/ash [66]. However, because the sericin protein in silk can generate an immunological response, it is removed from the silk fibroin before scaffold processing [67]. The feasibility of gel-spun silk frameworks in bladder tissue engineering is evaluated by Franck et al., along with the impact of various extracellular matrix protein layers on the ability of silk matrices to facilitate cell responses [68]. They indicated that physical morphology and the existence of special tissue-specific protein coatings were significant determinants in the effectiveness of silk biomaterials [68]. Conducting polymers such as polypyrrole combined with silk fibroin creates viable neural tissue scaffolds [69]. Pancreatic islets enclosed in silk hydrogel containing laminin, collagen, and MSC (mesenchymal stromal cells) demonstrated improved graft survival [70]. Janani et al. employed a fusion of non-mulberry and mulberry silk fibroin to create a functional liver construct useful for an extracorporeal device [71]. Though there are still certain obstacles in the regulatory elements of many silk-based technologies and goods, the benefits of employing silk-based solutions outweigh the challenges in developing final valuable products for the future [72].

c. *Poly-lactic acid (PLA)*: PLA is a versatile biodegradable biopolymer with thermoplastic properties. Polymerization of lactide monomers results in the creation of PLA (Figure 7.5c). Enzymatic polymerization or azeotropic dehydration polycondensation is carried out for direct synthesis [73]. PLA has high bio-resorption properties, allowing it to interact with recipient cells and tissues helping in bone grafting. Tamai et al. created PLA-based biodegradable stents that showed promising outcomes in human models [74]. PLA-PGA (-polyglycolic acid) copolymer-based orthopedic devices have been employed for the treatment of fractures and to fill in bone deformities. Su et al. discovered that the embedding rate of hemoglobin was only 7.9% when PLA was utilized as the membrane material. The embedding rate was 90% when employing a PLA–PEG copolymer [75]. Fangueiro et al. have patented a technique for producing braided corrugated vascular prostheses composed of polyethylene terephthalate (PET) and PLA, which restores blood flow in compromised blood vessel segments and is especially valuable in vascular surgery [76]. The 3D-printed biodegradable scaffolds possess enhanced angiogenesis and osteogenesis properties and aid bone formation and regeneration [76]. According to certain studies, PLA scaffolds manufactured with 3D printing technology cause less inflammation, making them a viable material for healing bone injury [76].

3.2.2 Synthetic polymers

a. *Polyurethane (PU):* Elastomers, which resemble human proteins, are used to synthesize PU, making it a versatile polymer. The backbone, diisocyanate, and chain extender are PUs' three essential building components. Aromatic or aliphatic diisocyanates help make PUs (Figure 7.6a). Aromatic diisocyanates include benzene rings, resulting in more rigid, stronger, and less expensive PUs than aliphatics. PUs have mechanical and physical qualities equivalent to natural tissues, unlike many other synthetic and biopolymers. PU is useful in various biomedical applications with minimal in vitro protein adsorption and platelet adhesion. Jiang et al. developed an innovative amphiphilic poly(dimethylsiloxane)-based PU network coupled with carboxy betaine, showing 97.7% antibacterial efficiency with anti-adhesive capabilities indicating tremendous promise for biomedical devices and marine applications [77]. Zanini et al. used a multistep procedure that included a vapor-phase plasma-induced graft polymerization of acrylic acid to coat PU catheters with 3-(trimethoxysilyl)-propyldimethyloctadecylammonium chloride; the coated catheters had antibacterial action against *E. coli* [78]. To reduce tissue inflammation and obstruction, polyethyleneimine brushes effectively incorporate neural stem cells (NSC) into biodegradable PU gels using a 3D printing technology and further introduce them into zebrafish to restore a damaged nervous system [79]. In 2016, Duxbury and Harvey published a systematic evaluation that indicated that PU implants are a promising substitute for contoured silicone implants [80].

b. *Polytetrafluoroethylene*: Teflon® or PTFE (Figure 7.6b) is synthesized from four ingredients – fluorspar, chloroform, hydrofluoric acid, and water – in a reaction chamber, mixed, and heated to between 590°C and 900°C. PTFE is a widely used material for implants and medical devices because of its high biocompatibility and high biocompatibility inertness [81]. Its qualities can benefit the blood arteries, nose, eyes, heart, table jawbone, or abdominal wall in the event of sickness or injury [81]. The sterile packing of equipment and medication also has a PTFE coating to prevent the surfaces from sticking together throughout

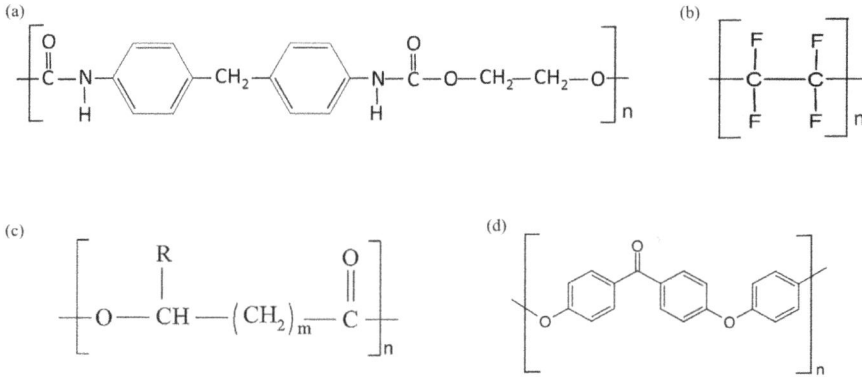

FIGURE 7.6 Structure of synthetic polymers. (a) Polyurethane, (b) Polytetrafluoroethylene, (c) Polyhydroxyalkanoates, (d) Polyether ether ketone.

the heating, transportation, and administration operations. To improve the PTFE's bonding strength at the bone contact, coatings containing the bone mineral hydroxyapatite were applied using radio frequency magnetron sputtering [82]. PTFE causes only minor inflammation in the body and causes some tissue ingrowth that can be reduced by surface modification.

c. *Polyhydroxyalkanoates (PHAs)*: PHAs (Figure 7.6c) are biocompatible and biodegradable polymers of R-hydroxy alkanoic acid polyesters. They are produced as distinct cytoplasmic inclusions in bacterial cells under nutrient-limiting conditions with excess carbon. PHAs on the market, in general, were not designed for use as biomedical implants, hence lacking the quality required for FDA approval. It is necessary to generate high-purity PHAs, test their biodegradation in vivo, fabricate scaffolds, and alter their surface [83]. In the 1960s, a polyhydroxybutyrate tube was utilized to repair ureter injury [84]. Because PHAs are piezoelectric, they can also use to heal injured nerves [85]. Also, PHA is more flexible than PLA and PGA, making it better suited for use as leaflets inside a tri-leaflet valve [86]. Articular cartilage repair, adhesion barriers, meniscus repair devices, cardiovascular patch grafting, orthopedic pins, staples, and screws, repair patch, rivets and tacks, stents, surgical mesh, sutured fasteners, and others are the most promising devices which can be designed after modifying PHAs [87].

d. *Polyaryletherketones and their derivatives*: Polyaryletherketones (PAEKs) are semi-crystalline high-performance engineering thermoplastic materials with a rare blend of chemical resistance, thermal stability, and outstanding chemical properties and mechanical qualities throughout a wide temperature range. The nucleophilic and electrophilic routes can both be used to make PAEKs (Figure 7.6d). Ether bonds are formed during the polymerization phase of the nucleophilic route, while

TABLE 7.2

List of common synthetic polymers used in biomedical devices

Common devices	Synthetic polymers used
Central venous access device	Polyethylene, polyamide, polytetrafluoroethylene
Pacemakers	Polyethylene, polypropylene, polyamide, polytetrafluoroethylene, polydimethylsiloxane, polyhydroxyalkanoates
Nasal reconstruction implants	Polydimethylsiloxane, parylene, silicone, liquid crystal polymer
Artificial urinary sphincter implant	Polyethylene, polyhydroxyalkanoates, silicone, polydimethylsiloxane, polypropylene, polyamide, polytetrafluoroethylene
Artificial intraocular lens	Polyamide, polymethyl methacrylate, polyethylene, polytetrafluoroethylene
Orthopedic implants	Polyethylene, polyhydroxyalkanoates, polyether ether ketones
Intra-uterine device (IUD)	Polyurethane, polypropylene, silicone

carbonyl bridges are formed during the electrophilic route. Pure PEEK (polyether ether ketone) has a limited bio-interfacial affinity between its surface and the surrounding tissue due to its hydrophobicity and bio-inertness [88]. Scotchford et al. investigated the in vitro biological reaction of human osteoblasts and murine macrophages to sliced carbon-fiber-reinforced (CFR)-PEEK polymer to develop a total hip replacement [89]. The amount of osteoblast adhesion was not significantly different between CFR-PEEK and titanium alloy (Ti_6Al_4V) discs (Table 7.2).

7.5 METHODS OF GENERATING ANTI-MICROBIAL POLYMER COATINGS

Medical implants or devices are surrounded by tissues or extracellular matrices, such as polysaccharides and proteins, which encourage bacterium colonization and biofilm development, increasing antibiotic tolerance of bacteria. Two main methods to generate anti-microbial polymer coating on the surface of medical devices and implants are:

a. Grafting: The term "grafting on" (Figure 7.7) refers to the chemical process of grafting a polymeric chain covalently onto the material surface of the device through its reactive functional groups. "Grafting from" refers to polymerizing target monomers using initiative groups created beforehand on the substrate's surface [90].

b. Layer-by-Layer (LbL): The LbL approach is a technique for fabricating thin films by alternatively applying layers of oppositely charged elements. Spray coating, spin coating, and dip coating (Figure 7.8) are a few methods used to create layers.

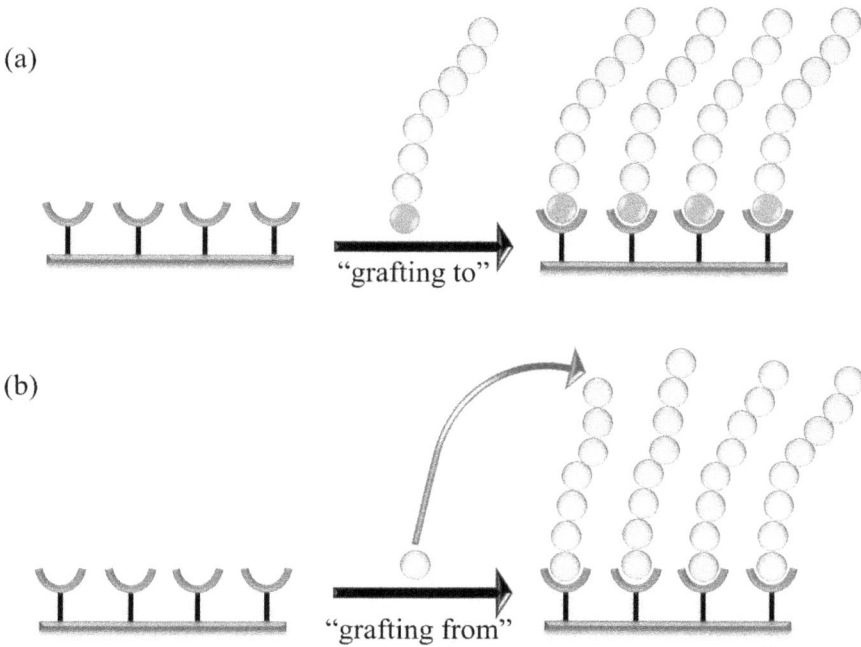

FIGURE 7.7 Strategies of polymer grafting. (a) "grafting to", (b) "grafting from".

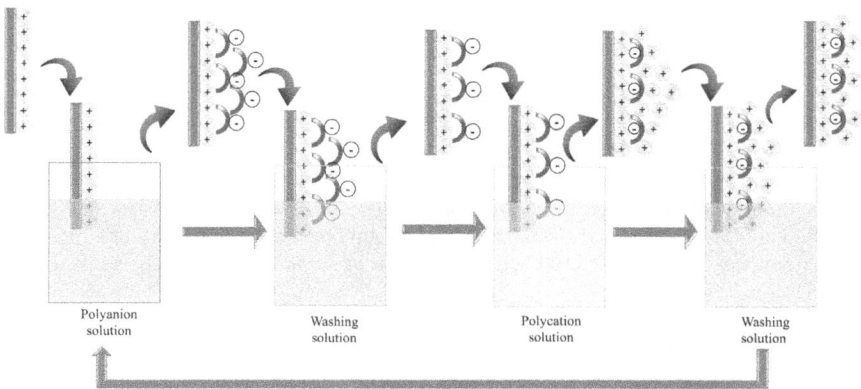

FIGURE 7.8 Layer-by-layer coating using dip method for polymer coatings.

7.6 CONCLUSION

The anti-microbial polymers arose as an up-and-coming method with excellent efficiency, a meager chance of resistance development, and the ability to remove a broad spectrum of bacteria. Significant advancements in this strategy should be expected, spurred by the inherent advantages over alternative approaches. Despite significant scientific advances in recent years, a massive amount of research remains to be done to address important challenges such as improving anti-microbial activity, broadening the range of micro-organisms that each material can effectively remove, raising the long-term stability of anti-microbial polymers, reducing the toxicity associated with some approaches, and developing cost-effective solutions.

REFERENCES

1. Sumathi, K., WD. Bencer, and C. Keerthana, Common infectious disease conditions and antibiotic resistance in pediatric population. *Journal of Medical Pharmaceutical and Allied Sciences*, 2022. 11(2): pp. 4503–4506.
2. Xue, Y., H. Xiao, and Y. Zhang, Anti-microbial polymeric materials with quaternary ammonium and phosphonium salts. *International Journal of Molecular Sciences*, 2015. **16**(2): pp. 3626–3655.
3. Huang, K.C., et al., Recent advances in antimicrobial polymers: A mini-review. *International Journal of Molecular Sciences*, 2016. **17**: p. 1578.
4. Barzic, A. and S. Ioan, *Concepts, Compounds and the Alternatives of Antibacterials*. 2015, InTech.
5. Guadalupe, E., et al., Bioactive polymeric nanofiber matrices for skin regeneration. *Journal of Applied Polymer Science*, 2015. **132**(16): pp. 1–10.
6. Kugel, A., et al., Anti-microbial polysiloxane polymers and coatings containing pendant levofloxacin. *Polymer Chemistry*, 2010. **1**(4): pp. 442–452.
7. Gustafson, C.T., et al., Controlled delivery of vancomycin via charged hydrogels. *PLoS One*, 2016. **11**(1): p. e0146401.
8. Chen, A., et al., Biocidal polymers: A mechanistic overview. *Polymer Reviews*, 2016. **57**: pp. 276–310.
9. Rakowska, P.D., et al., Antiviral surfaces and coatings and their mechanisms of action. *Communications Materials*, 2021. **2**(1): p. 53.
10. Kadar, M., et al., *Antiviral Effect of New Disinfectant Containing A Silver Complex and Hydrogenperoxide as Active Agents*. 1993: na.
11. Olmos, D. and J. González-Benito, Polymeric Materials with Antibacterial Activity: A Review. *Polymers*, 2021. **13**(4): p. 613.
12. Esteban-Tejeda, L., et al., The antibacterial and antifungal activity of a soda-lime glass containing silver nanoparticles. *Nanotechnology*, 2009. **20**(8): p. 085103.
13. Naika, H.R., et al., Green synthesis of CuO nanoparticles using Gloriosa superba L. extract and their antibacterial activity. *Journal of Taibah University for Science*, 2015. **9**(1): pp. 7–12.
14. Devi, A.B., et al., Novel synthesis and characterization of CuO nanomaterials: Biological applications. *Chinese Chemical Letters*, 2014. **25**(12): pp. 1615–1619.
15. Samanta, S., et al., Biomolecular assisted synthesis and mechanism of silver and gold nanoparticles. *Materials Research Express*, 2019. **6**(8): p. 082009.
16. Ahmed, F., et al., Beta galactosidase mediated bio-enzymatically synthesized nano-gold with aggrandized cytotoxic potential against pathogenic bacteria and cancer cells. *Journal of Photochemistry and Photobiology B: Biology*, 2020. **209**: p. 111923.
17. Rahimi, H., et al., Antifungal effects of indolicidin-conjugated gold nanoparticles against fluconazole-resistant strains of Candida albicans isolated from patients with burn infection. *International Journal of Nanomedicine*, 2019. **14**: p. 5323.
18. Yah, C.S., The toxicity of Gold Nanoparticles in relation to their physio-chemical properties. *Biomedical Research* (0970-938X), 2013. **24**(3).

19. Zhang, M., et al., Biological safe gold nanoparticle-modified dental aligner prevents the Porphyromonas gingivalis biofilm formation. *ACS Omega*, 2020. **5**(30): pp. 18685–18692.
20. Rabiee, N., et al., Silver and gold nanoparticles for antimicrobial purposes against multi-drug resistance bacteria. *Materials*, 2022. **15**: p. 1799.
21. Gudkov, S.V., et al., A mini review of antibacterial properties of ZnO nanoparticles. *Frontiers in Physics*, 2021. **9**: p. 641481.
22. Sirelkhatim, A., et al., Review on zinc oxide nanoparticles: Antibacterial activity and toxicity mechanism. *Nano-Micro Letters*, 2015. **7**(3): pp. 219–242.
23. Nair, S., et al., Role of size scale of ZnO nanoparticles and microparticles on toxicity toward bacteria and osteoblast cancer cells. *Journal of Materials Science: Materials in Medicine*, 2009. **20**(1): pp. 235–241.
24. Jin, S.E. and H.E. Jin, Antimicrobial activity of zinc oxide nano/microparticles and their combinations against pathogenic microorganisms for biomedical applications: From physicochemical characteristics to pharmacological aspects. *Nanomaterials (Basel)*, 2021. **11**(2): p. 263.
25. Lu, A.H., E.E.L. Salabas, and F. Schüth, Magnetic nanoparticles: synthesis, protection, functionalization, and application. *Angewandte Chemie International Edition*, 2007. **46**(8): pp. 1222–1244.
26. Suci, P.A., et al., High-density targeting of a viral multifunctional nanoplatform to a pathogenic, biofilm-forming bacterium. *Chemistry & Biology*, 2007. **14**(4): pp. 387–398.
27. Wang, Y.-H., et al., Chelerythrine loaded composite magnetic thermosensitive hydrogels as a novel anticancer drug-delivery system. *Journal of Drug Delivery Science and Technology*, 2019. **54**: p. 101293.
28. Cele, T., *Preparation of Nanoparticles. Engineered Nanomaterials-Health and Safety*. 2020: IntechOpen.
29. Zhang, Z. and V.E. Wagner, *Anti-Microbial Coatings and Modifications on Medical Devices*. 2017: Springer.
30. Pérez-Merino, P., et al., In vivo chromatic aberration in eyes implanted with intraocular lenses. *Investigative Ophthalmology & Visual Science*, 2013. **54**(4): pp. 2654–2661.
31. Kim, B.J., et al., Customized cranioplasty implants using three-dimensional printers and polymethyl-methacrylate casting. *Journal of Korean Neurosurgical Society*, 2012. **52**(6): pp. 541–546.
32. Rivkin, A., A prospective study of non-surgical primary rhinoplasty using a polymethylmethacrylate injectable implant. *Dermatologic Surgery*, 2014. **40**(3): pp. 305–313.
33. Actis, L., et al., Anti-microbial surfaces for craniofacial implants: State of the art. *Journal of the Korean Association of Oral and Maxillofacial Surgeons*, 2013. **39**(2): pp. 43–54.
34. Teo, A.J.T., et al., Polymeric biomaterials for medical pmplants and devices. *ACS Biomaterials Science & Engineering*, 2016. **2**(4): pp. 454–472.
35. Miyashita, D., et al., Tissue ingrowth into perforated polymethylmethacrylate orbital implants: an experimental study. *Ophthalmic Plastic & Reconstructive Surgery*, 2013. **29**(3): pp. 160–163.
36. Espalin, D., et al., Fused deposition modeling of patient-specific polymethylmethacrylate implants. *Rapid Prototyping Journal*, 2010. **16**(3): pp. 164–173.
37. Scheidbach, H., et al., In vivo studies comparing the biocompatibility of various polypropylene meshes and their handling properties during endoscopic total extraperitoneal (TEP) patchplasty: An experimental study in pigs. *Surgical Endoscopy*, 2004. **18**(2): pp. 211–220.
38. Abednejad, A.S., G. Amoabediny, and A. Ghaee, Surface modification of polypropylene membrane by polyethylene glycol graft polymerization. *Materials Science & Engineering. C, Materials for Biological Applications*, 2014. **42**: pp. 443–450.

39. Klinge, U., et al., PVDF as a new polymer for the construction of surgical meshes. *Biomaterials*, 2002. **23**(16): pp. 3487–3493.
40. Low, Y.K., et al., β-*Phase poly(vinylidene fluoride) films encouraged more homogeneous cell distribution and more significant deposition of fibronectin towards the cell-material interface compared to* α-*phase poly(vinylidene fluoride) films. Materials Science & Engineering C-Materials for Biological Applications*, 2014. **34**: pp. 345–353.
41. Amanatullah, D.F., et al., Comparison of surgical outcomes and implant wear between ceramic-ceramic and ceramic-polyethylene articulations in total hip arthroplasty. *Journal of Arthroplasty*, 2011. **26**(6 Suppl): pp. 72–77.
42. Riveiro, A., et al., Laser surface modification of ultra-high-molecular-weight polyethylene (UHMWPE) for biomedical applications. *Applied Surface Science*, 2014. **302**: pp. 236–242.
43. Rahimi, A. and A. Mashak, Review on rubbers in medicine: Natural, silicone and polyurethane rubbers. *Plastics, Rubber and Composites*, 2013. **42**(6): pp. 223–230.
44. Auliya, D.G., et al., Synthesis of low viscosity polydimethylsiloxane using low grade of octamethylcyclotetrasiloxane. *Materials Science Forum*, 2021. **1028**: pp. 365–370.
45. Kim, H., et al., Parylene-C coated microporous PDMS structure protecting from functional deconditioning of platelets exposed to cardiostimulants. *Lab Chip*, 2020. **20**(13): pp. 2284–2295.
46. Hassler, C., et al., Characterization of parylene C as an encapsulation material for implanted neural prostheses. *Journal of Biomedical Materials Research Part B: Applied Biomaterials*, 2010. **93**(1): pp. 266–274.
47. Zhang, Y., et al., Quaternary ammonium compounds in dental restorative materials. *Dental Materials Journal*, 2018. **37**(2): pp. 183–191.
48. Shahi, S., et al., A review on potential toxicity of dental material and screening their biocompatibility. *Toxicology Mechanisms and Methods*, 2019. **29**(5): pp. 368–377.
49. Leggat, P.A. and U. Kedjarune, Toxicity of methyl methacrylate in dentistry. *International Dental Journal*, 2003. **53**(3): pp. 126–131.
50. Xue, J., et al., Application of antimicrobial polymers in the development of dental resin composite. *Molecules*, 2020. **25**(20): p. 4738.
51. Seydel, U., G. Schröder, and K. Brandenburg, Reconstitution of the lipid matrix of the outer membrane of Gram-negative bacteria as asymmetric planar bilayer. *The Journal of Membrane Biology*, 1989. **109**(2): pp. 95–103.
52. Ma, J., et al., Synthesis and applications of 2-methacryloyloxyethyl phosphorylcholine monomer and its polymers. *Progress in Chemistry*, 2008. **20**(0708): p. 1151.
53. Fujiwara, N., et al., 2-Methacryloyloxyethyl phosphorylcholine (MPC)-polymer suppresses an increase of oral bacteria: A single-blind, crossover clinical trial. *Clinical Oral Investigations*, 2019. **23**(2): pp. 739–746.
54. Zhang, N., et al., Protein-repellent and antibacterial dental composite to inhibit biofilms and caries. *Journal of Dentistry*, 2015. **43**(2): pp. 225–234.
55. Choi, A., et al., Enhanced anti-microbial and remineralizing properties of self-adhesive orthodontic resin containing mesoporous bioactive glass and zwitterionic material. *Journal of Dental Sciences*, 2022. **17**(2): pp. 848–855.
56. Pupo, Y.M., et al., An innovative quaternary ammonium methacrylate polymer can provide improved anti-microbial properties for a dental adhesive system. *Journal of Biomaterials Science, Polymer Edition*, 2013. **24**(12): pp. 1443–1458.
57. Han, Q., et al., Anti-caries effects of dental adhesives containing quaternary ammonium methacrylates with different chain lengths. *Materials*, 2017. **10**(6): p. 643.
58. Imazato, S., et al., Incorporation of bacterial inhibitor into resin composite. *Journal of Dental Research*, 1994. **73**(8): pp. 1437–1443.
59. Czuba, L., Application of Plastics in Medical Devices and Equipment. In Kayvon Modjarrad and Sina Ebnesajjad. (eds.), Publisher: Elsevier. *Handbook of Polymer Applications in Medicine and Medical Devices*. Elsevier, 2014: p. 9–19.

60. Rebelo, R., et al. Poly Lactic Acid Fibre Based Biodegradable Stents and Their Functionalization Techniques. *In Raul Fangueiro and Sohel Rana. (eds.), Natural Fibres: Advances in Science and Technology Towards Industrial Applications.* 2016. pp. 331–342, Dordrecht: Springer Netherlands.

61. Chen, M.-C., et al., Mechanical properties, drug eluting characteristics and in vivo performance of a genipin-crosslinked chitosan polymeric stent. *Biomaterials*, 2009. **30**(29): pp. 5560–5571.

62. Skop, N.B., et al., Subacute transplantation of native and genetically engineered neural progenitors seeded on microsphere scaffolds promote repair and functional recovery after traumatic brain injury. *ASN Neuro*, 2019. **11**: p. 1759091419830186.

63. Jin, J., et al., Rectorite-intercalated nanoparticles for improving controlled release of doxorubicin hydrochloride. *International Journal of Biological Macromolecules*, 2017. **101**: pp. 815–822.

64. Borges, R., et al., New sol-gel-derived magnetic bioactive glass-ceramics containing superparamagnetic hematite nanocrystals for hyperthermia application. *Materials Science & Engineering C-Materials for Biological Applications*, 2021. **120**: p. 111692.

65. Murugesan, S. and T. Scheibel, Chitosan-based nanocomposites for medical applications. *Journal of Polymer Science*, 2021. **59**(15): pp. 1610–1642.

66. Nguyen, T.P., et al., Silk fibroin-based biomaterials for biomedical applications: A review. *Polymers*, 2019. **11**(12): p. 1933.

67. Mandal, B.B. and S.C. Kundu, Cell proliferation and migration in silk fibroin 3D scaffolds. *Biomaterials*, 2009. **30**(15): pp. 2956–2965.

68. Franck, D., et al., Evaluation of silk biomaterials in combination with extracellular matrix coatings for bladder tissue engineering with primary and pluripotent cells. *PLoS One*, 2013. **8**(2): p. e56237.

69. Zhao, Y.-H., et al., Novel conductive polypyrrole/silk fibroin scaffold for neural tissue repair. *Neural Regeneration Research*, 2018. **13**(8): p. 1455.

70. Davis, N.E., et al., Enhanced function of pancreatic islets co-encapsulated with ECM proteins and mesenchymal stromal cells in a silk hydrogel. *Biomaterials*, 2012. **33**(28): pp. 6691–6697.

71. Janani, G., S.K. Nandi, and B.B. Mandal, Functional hepatocyte clusters on bioactive blend silk matrices towards generating bioartificial liver constructs. *Acta Biomaterialia*, 2018. **67**: pp. 167–182.

72. Bandyopadhyay, A., et al., Silk: A promising biomaterial opening new vistas towards affordable healthcare solutions. *Journal of the Indian Institute of Science*, 2019. **99**(3): pp. 445–487.

73. DeStefano, V., S. Khan, and A. Tabada, Applications of PLA in modern medicine. *Engineered Regeneration*, 2020. **1**: pp. 76–87.

74. Tamai, H., et al., Initial and 6-month results of biodegradable poly-l-lactic acid coronary stents in humans. *Circulation*, 2000. **102**(4): pp. 399–404.

75. Li, G., et al., Synthesis and biological application of polylactic acid. *Molecules* (Basel, Switzerland), 2020. **25**(21): p. 5023.

76. Rebelo, R., M. Fernandes, and R. Fangueiro, Biopolymers in medical implants: A brief review. *Procedia Engineering*, 2017. **200**: pp. 236–243.

77. Jiang, J., et al., Novel amphiphilic poly (dimethylsiloxane) based polyurethane networks tethered with carboxybetaine and their combined antibacterial and anti-adhesive property. *Applied Surface Science*, 2017. **412**: pp. 1–9.

78. Zanini, S., et al., Development of antibacterial quaternary ammonium silane coatings on polyurethane catheters. *Journal of Colloid and Interface Science*, 2015. **451**: pp. 78–84.

79. Hsieh, F.-Y., H.-H. Lin, and S.-H. Hsu, 3D bioprinting of neural stem cell-laden thermoresponsive biodegradable polyurethane hydrogel and potential in central nervous system repair. *Biomaterials*, 2015. **71**: pp. 48–57.

80. Duxbury, P.J. and J.R. Harvey, Systematic review of the effectiveness of polyurethane-coated compared with textured silicone implants in breast surgery. *Journal of Plastic, Reconstructive & Aesthetic Surgery*, 2016. **69**(4): pp. 452–460.
81. Roina, Y., et al., ePTFE-based biomedical devices: An overview of surgical efficiency. *Journal of Biomedical Materials Research Part B: Applied Biomaterials*, 2022. **110**(2): pp. 302–320.
82. Cassady,   A.I.,   N.M.   Hidzir,   and   L.   Grøndahl,   Enhancing   expanded poly(tetrafluoroethylene) (ePTFE) for biomaterials applications. *Journal of Applied Polymer Science*, 2014. **131**(15): 1–14.
83. Insomphun, C., et al., Influence of hydroxyl groups on the cell viability of polyhy-droxyalkanoate (PHA) scaffolds for tissue engineering. *ACS Biomaterials Science & Engineering*, 2017. **3**(12): pp. 3064–3075.
84. Baptist, J.N. and J.B. Ziegler, *Method of Making Absorbable Surgical Sutures from Poly Beta Hydroxy Acids*. 1965, Google Patents.
85. Bugnicourt, E., Cinelli, P., Lazzeri, A., and Alvarez, V. A. Polyhydroxyalkanoate (PHA): Review of synthesis, characteristics, processing and potential applications in packaging, (2014).
86. Hoerstrup, S.P., et al., Functional living trileaflet heart valves grown in vitro. *Circulation*, 2000. **102**(suppl 3): pp. Iii-44–Iii-49.
87. Valappil, S.P., et al., Biomedical applications of polyhydroxyalkanoates, an overview of animal testing and in vivo responses. *Expert Review of Medical Devices*, 2006. **3**(6): pp. 853–868.
88. Abdullah, M.R., et al., Biomechanical and bioactivity concepts of polyetheretherketone composites for use in orthopedic implants—A review. *Journal of Biomedical Materials Research Part A*, 2015. **103**(11): pp. 3689–3702.
89. Scotchford, C.A., et al., Use of a novel carbon fibre composite material for the femoral stem component of a THR system: In vitro biological assessment. *Biomaterials*, 2003. **24**(26): pp. 4871–4879.
90. Qiu, H., et al., The mechanisms and the applications of antibacterial polymers in sur-face modification on medical devices. *Frontiers in Bioengineering and Biotechnology*, 2020. **8**: p. 910.

8 Tribological performance of polymeric materials for biomedical applications

Tannu Garg, Gaurav Sharma,
S. Shankar and S. P. Singh

CONTENTS

8.1   Introduction 121
8.2   Biomaterials.. 123
8.3   Tribology... 124
8.4   Biomedical engineering and types of biomaterials 125
     8.4.1   Metals 126
     8.4.2   Polymers 127
     8.4.3   Ceramics 127
     8.4.4   Composites... 127
     8.4.5   Natural biomaterials 127
8.5   Biomaterials: uses.. 128
8.6   Desired characteristics in biomaterials for use in medicine....................... 130
8.7   Polymer materials for biomedical application 131
8.8   Ultra-High Molecular Weight Polyethylene (UHMWPE) 132
8.9   Materials for hip arthroplasty 135
     8.9.1   Metal on plastic... 135
     8.9.2   Ceramic on plastic (or UHMWPE) 136
8.10 Crucial areas for biomaterial research in the future.................................... 136
References... 137

8.1   INTRODUCTION

A biomaterial is a synthetic material that is periodically or consistently in contact with body fluids and is used to replace or restore function to biological tissues. Biomaterials are employed in medical devices for a variety of purposes, including orthopaedic, cardiovascular, and wound healing. A body must fulfil the following conditions to implant biomaterials: biocompatible chemical composition to prevent negative tissue reactions, excellent resistance to degradation, adequate strength to endure the cyclic loading experienced by the joint, and high wear resistance.

A long, healthy life: thanks to developments in modern medicine, humanity has made great strides recently towards realising this age-old desire. But this

DOI: 10.1201/9781003319139-8

accomplishment also brings a whole new set of difficulties for medicine. A surge in age-related diseases is a result of our ageing population. Because of differences in our nutrition from that of our grandparents, obesity and metabolic illnesses are on the rise. Additionally, the popularity of high-risk leisure activities continues, with risks including internal bleeding and fractures. Future and current medical practises will need to adapt to these societal developments (Sahoo et al., 2019). Humans have worked to recover the functionality of bodily components damaged by sickness or trauma since the dawn of time. The biological systems linked with the human body

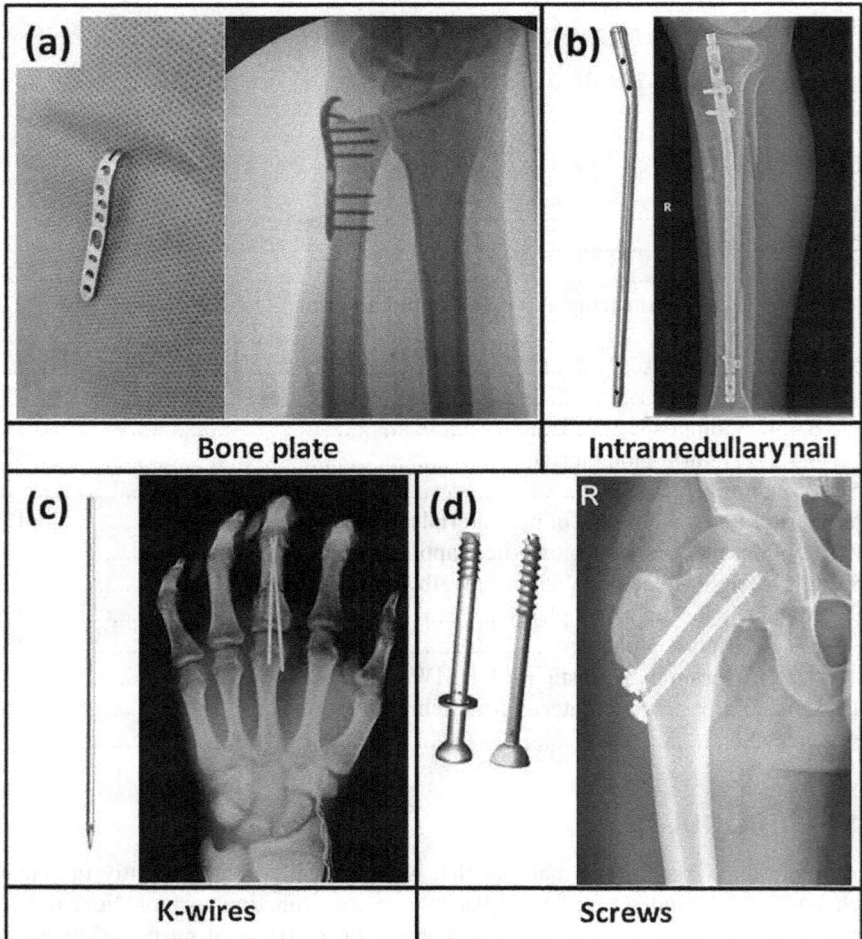

FIGURE 8.1   For internal fixation of fractures, common medical devices are employed. (a) A bone plate is used to stabilise an ulnar fracture; (b) An intramedullary nail is used to stabilise a tibial fracture; (c) A K-wire is used to stabilise a phalangeal fracture; and (d) Screws are used to stabilise a fractured femoral neck (*Common Medical Devices Used for Fracture Internal Fixation. (a) Bone... / Download Scientific Diagram*, n.d.).

are distinct. When commonly used substances directly interact with these biological systems, they may have a variety of negative consequences including harm to the body. As a result, unique substances known as biomaterials have been found to be compatible with live tissues and to perform the required engineering tasks. Implants and other medical devices frequently contain materials made up of metals and alloys, ceramics, and polymer-based materials (Figure 8.1).

The discipline of medicine also uses tribology, which is a science with applications beyond mechanical equipment. Most of the sliding and frictional contacts in the human body are found in the joints. Additionally, tribology encompasses friction on the skin, between the eyelids and the eyeball, and more. To pact with the claim of tribological values, such as resistance, wear, and lubrication among cooperating sides in a comparative signal, to biological and medical systems, a separate field known as biotribology was created. Biomaterials that have been created for use as medical devices (their apparatuses) and they remain typically intended as continued contact with living resources are referred to as biomedical materials.

Some examples of tribology in biomedicine are as follows:

1. Tribology of natural synovial joints and artificial replacements.
2. Use of dental implants.
3. Heart valve wear and replacement and lubrication of the pump in complete mechanical hearts.
4. Contact lens tribology and ocular tribology.
5. The use of screws and plates to heal bone fractures.
6. Friction with skin and garment contact with clothing.

The standard of human existence should also rise as more is learned about the tribological components of biomedicine (Sahoo et al., 2019).

8.2 BIOMATERIALS

Biomaterials can be made in the lab using metallic, polymer, ceramic, or composite materials or they can be obtained from nature. Biomaterials are frequently employed in medicinal instruments to supplement or change a normal function. Examples include hip replacements, heart valves, and supplies frequently used in surgery and dentistry. Today, biomaterials are crucial to medicine because they help patients recuperate from disease or injury by restoring function. To sustain and improve or replace damaged tissue or biological function, biomaterials are used in medical applications. They can be natural or manufactured. Biomaterials were first employed historically by the ancient Egyptians, who used sutures constructed from animal sinew. Medical science, biology, physics, chemistry, and more recently tissue engineering and materials science all influence the study of biomaterials today. The discipline has expanded over the last ten years as a result of advancements in regenerative medicine, tissue engineering, and other areas.

A biomaterial can be made from a variety of materials, including ceramics, glass, plastic, metals, and even living cells and tissues. These could be contact lenses, dental implants, hip replacements, or heart valves. They are often bio-degradable, and some are bio-absorbable; this means that after serving their purpose, they are gradually removed from the body (Marques et al., n.d.).

8.3 TRIBOLOGY

It is the learning of processes at the contact of two surfaces or on the surface of a solid. The tribological qualities include friction, wear, roughness, etc. Wear is the deformation of substantial or loss of a body when two surfaces in touch have comparative movement between them, whereas friction is the force preventing two surfaces from sliding against one another. Friction, one of the two deteriorating phenomena, determines how effectively mechanical assemblies work when sliding surfaces are in touch. It also causes wear, which is frequently the process that reduces the lifespan of a gadget. In friction and wear, sliding speed, temperature and applied load will be the influencing factors. Since corrosion causes surface degradation that encourages wear, the two fields of tribology and corrosion have recently become closely linked (Saravanan et al., n.d.).

Tribocorrosion, which considers the combined effect of corrosion and wear, has been coined because of the synergistic relationship between corrosion and wear. In a lot of technical domains, tribocorrosion is discovered to happen. The tribocorrosion effect that occurs when parts like pipelines, regulators, drives, excess incinerators, mining apparatus, medicinal implants, etc. are used might shorten their lifetime. In addition, tribocorrosion puts at risk the security of crucial arrangements such as nuclear-powered reactors and human transport schemes. The study of systems' tribological aspects is extremely important from an economic and technological standpoint. In industrialised nations, losses from energy waste and material wear amount to billions of dollars each year. Accurate comprehension of tribological processes can serve as a foundation for raising design standards and boosting engineering effectiveness. The future of humanity's energy conservation concerns has already been significantly impacted by this (Zhou & Jin, 2015).

The study of biological systems has benefited from understanding tribological principles, despite the field's traditional association with the surface contact of mechanical systems. One of the most recent subfields to develop within the subject of tribology is bio-tribology. All facets of tribology that relate to biological systems are covered by bio-tribology. It is acknowledged as one of the most crucial factors in many biological systems, which helps us understand how our natural systems function. It also aids in understanding the progression of diseases and the appropriate use of medicinal therapies.

One of the most fascinating fields of tribology research is bio-tribology, which has an impact on many elements of daily life, including contact lenses, artificial joints, and skin blisters. Tribology, in particular our reaction to perceived friction, often governs how we interact with our surroundings. An important example is the use of touch to assess surface roughness, moisture, and grip. Bio-tribology includes not only those fields related to tribology but also biomechanics, biochemistry, biology, physiology, clinical medicine, and pathology. Investigation in bio-tribology is increasingly having a positive impact on science, society, and healthcare, and there are many prospects (Shaun Berrien & Scott Eugene M Gregory, 1999) (Figure 8.2).

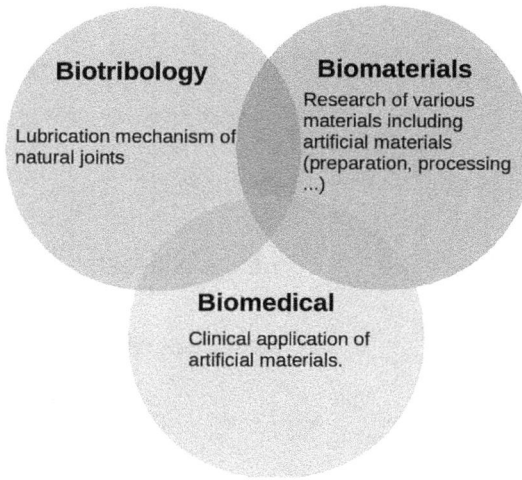

Biotribology

Lubrication mechanism of
natural joints

Biomaterials

Research of various
materials including
artificial materials
(preparation, processing
...)

Biomedical

Clinical application of
artificial materials.

FIGURE 8.2 Tribology's impact in biomedical engineering (*Biotribology.Jpeg (1056 ×*
816), n.d.).

It has long been the goal of biomechanical research of joints to better understand
the path mechanical processes connected to joint illnesses such as osteoarthritis
(Mow et al., 1993) as well as the structure–function relationship that provides joint
motion. The goal of bio-tribologists is to assess biological systems and comprehend
how they operate with such tribological efficiency, hence enhancing knowledge of
both their normal and pathologic states. A synovial joint's bearing system is made
up of articular cartilage, synovial fluid, and the supporting bone. The mechanical
properties of the materials that comprise the joint determine how well it performs.

It is obviously oversimplified to think of joint illness as the breakdown of bearing
lubricating mechanisms. However, it is reasonable to draw a comparison between a
synovial joint and an engineering bearing. Studies of synovial fluid lubrication, friction measurements in synovial junctions, causes of combined lubrication, measurements and analyses of cartilage wear and degradation, dual mechanics research, and
the progress of prosthetic junctions are a few examples of tribology in biomedicine.
Additionally, this topic encompasses the tribology of dental implantations and visual
tribology. The development of new materials appropriate for biomedical applications
is the result of research in this area. This has helped thousands of sick people around
the world, helping society as a whole (Sahoo et al., n.d.).

8.4 BIOMEDICAL ENGINEERING AND TYPES OF BIOMATERIALS

Biomedical engineering is the application of engineering concepts and principles
to biological and medical problems (e.g. diagnostic or therapeutic). Engineering
knowledge in medicine and the biological sciences is combined by biomedical engineers. These engineers use the principles of applied science (mechanical, electrical, chemical, and computer engineering) and physical science (physics, chemistry,

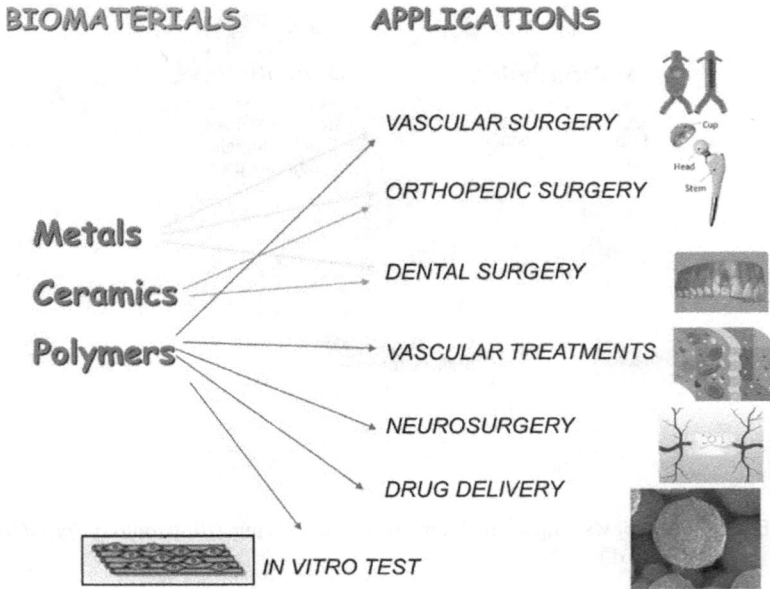

FIGURE 8.3   Type of biomaterials and their biomedical applications (*Type of Biomaterials and Their Biomedical Applications. /Download Scientific Diagram*, n.d.).

and mathematics) in life and medicine. Biological structures and diagnostic and therapeutic instruments can be constructed using many of the same principles that are used in creating and programming machines, despite the fact that the humanoid physique is a much more complicated structure compared to other devices, even the most innovative machines.

The creation of bio-compatible prosthetic devices, several investigative and therapeutic instruments, ranging from clinical tools to micro-implants, well-known imaging tools like MRIs and EEGs, tissue and stem cell engineering, clinical engineering, pharmaceuticals, and therapeutic biologicals are a few prominent biomedical engineering applications (Figure 8.3).

The majority of synthetic biomaterials used for implants are everyday substances that the ordinary materials engineer or scientist is familiar with. These substances can generally be broken down into the following groups: metals, polymers, ceramics, and composites (Kiran & Ramakrishna, 2021).

8.4.1   METALS

Metals are the most often used material class for load-bearing implants. For instance, metallic implants are implanted during some of the most popular orthopaedic procedures. Simple wires and screws, fracture fixation plates, and total joint prostheses (artificial joints) for the hips, knees, shoulders, ankles, and other joints are just a few examples. Metallic implants are employed in cardiovascular surgery, maxillofacial surgery, and dentistry in addition to orthopaedics. Stainless steels, commercially pure titanium and titanium alloys, and cobalt-base alloys are the most frequently utilised metals and alloys for medical device applications (Hussein et al., 2015).

8.4.2 POLYMERS

In medicine, a wide range of polymers are utilised as biomaterials. Their uses encompass everything from tracheal tubes to facial prostheses, heart and kidney parts to dentures, and hip and knee joints to dentures (Hussain et al., n.d.).

8.4.3 CERAMICS

Ceramics have historically been widely used in dentistry as restorative materials. These consist of cement, denture materials, and crown materials. Compared to metals and polymers, their usage in other biomedical sectors hasn't been widespread. For instance, ceramics' inadequate fracture toughness severely restricts their employment in load-bearing applications. For bone healing and augmentation as well as joint replacement, several ceramic materials are used.

8.4.4 COMPOSITES

The most effective composite biomaterials are utilised in dentistry as restorative materials or dental cements. Despite being highly sought after for bone healing and joint replacement due to their low elastic modulus levels, carbon–carbon and carbon-reinforced polymer composites have not yet demonstrated a combination of mechanical and biological qualities suitable for these applications. However, composite materials are often employed to create prosthetic limbs because of their low density/weight and excellent strength, which makes them the perfect choice for this function (Kiran & Ramakrishna, 2021).

8.4.5 NATURAL BIOMATERIALS

Several substances from the animal or plant kingdoms that are being explored for use as biomaterials deserve a brief mention, even though the biomaterials covered in this manual are synthetic. The fact that natural materials are comparable to those the body is accustomed to is one benefit of using them for implants. The study of biomimetics, or mimicking nature, is expanding in this respect. Natural materials typically do not have the toxicity issues that manufactured materials frequently do. Additionally, they might contain particular protein-binding sites and other biochemical signals that could help with tissue integration or healing. However, immunogenicity issues can arise with natural materials. These materials, particularly natural polymers, also have the potential to temperatures below denature or disintegrate their molten states. This significantly reduces their fabrication to create implants in various sizes and shapes. Collagen is an illustration of a natural substance. It is primarily found as fibrils, has a distinctive triple-helix shape, and is the most abundant, a common protein in animal life. Collagen, for instance, makes up over 50% of the protein in cowhide. It is a crucial part of connective tissue, which includes skin, tendons, ligaments, and bone. The human body has at least ten different kinds of collagen. Type I is mostly present in the skin, bones, and tendons, type II is in the articular cartilage of the joints, and type III is a significant component of blood vessels. A lot of research has been done on collagen's potential as a biomaterial. It is often implanted in the shape of a sponge, which lacks considerable stiffness or mechanical strength. It is marketed as a treatment for wound healing and has shown good promise as a scaffold for neo-tissue formation. For cosmetic purposes, dermal tissue can be expanded or built up using injectable collagen. Additionally, coral, chitin (from insects and crustaceans), keratin (from hair), and cellulose are all natural materials that are being considered (from plants).

Material	Application	Major properties
Alloy: titanium alloys, titanium aluminum vanadium alloy, cobalt chromium alloy, cobalt chromium molybdenum alloy	Total joint replacement	Wear and corrosion resistance
Inorganic: diamond-like carbon	Biocompatible coatings	Reduced friction and increased wear resistance
Ceramics: Al_2O_3, ZrO_2, Si_3N_4, SiC, B_4C, quartz, bioglass (Na_2O-CaO-SiO_2-P_2O_5), sintered hydroxyapatite ($Ca_{10}(PO_4)6(OH)_2$)	Bone joint coating	Wear and corrosion resistance
Polymers: ultrahigh molecular weight polyethylene, polytetrafluoroethylene (PTFE), poly(glycolic acid)	Joint socket interpositional implant temporomandibular joint (jaw) joint bone	Wear and corrosion resistance, low friction coefficient, elastics with less wear
Composites: specialized silicon polymers	Bone joint	Wear, corrosion, and fatigue resistance

INLINE FIGURE 1   Different types of material with major applications and properties (Zhou & Jin, 2015).

8.5   BIOMATERIALS: USES

To physically replace hard or soft tissues that have been harmed or destroyed by a pathological condition is one of the main uses for biomaterials. Although the body's tissues and structures work for a long time in most people, they are nonetheless subject to a number of harmful events, such as fracture, infection, and cancer, which can lead to discomfort, disfigurement, or loss of function. The damaged tissue may be able to be removed in some cases and replaced with a suitable synthetic material.

Orthopaedic implant devices are one of the most well-known uses for biomaterials. Rheumatoid arthritis and osteoarthritis both impact the structure of freely moving joints. Joints that move (have synovia), include the hip, knee, shoulder, ankle, and elbow. Such joints, especially weight-bearing joints like the hip and knee, might experience significant pain, which can have very negative impacts on ambulatory function. Since the invention of anaesthetic, antisepsis, and antibiotics, it has been able to replace these joints with prostheses, and hundreds of thousands of patients are aware of the pain alleviation and mobility restoration they provide.

Ophthalmics: Multiple disorders that affect the eye's tissues can cause impaired vision and, in the long run, blindness. For example, cataracts can make the lens cloudy. An artificial intraocular lens (polymer) can take its place. Materials for contact lenses are likewise regarded as biomaterials because they come into direct touch with the tissues of the eye. Similarly to intraocular lenses, they are used to maintain and improve eyesight (Kiran & Ramakrishna, 2021).

Applications in Cardiology: Heart valve and artery issues can occur in the cardiovascular, or circulatory, system (the heart and blood vessels that transport blood throughout the body), and both can be successfully addressed with implants. The structural changes in the heart valves prohibit them from fully opening or closing, and the sick valve can be replaced with a range of alternatives. Ceramics (carbons, metals, and polymers) are employed in building, just like orthopaedic implants. When fatty deposits (atherosclerosis) obstruct arteries, particularly the coronary arteries and the vessels in the lower limbs, it may be possible to replace individual segments with artificial arteries.

Applications in dentistry: In the mouth, bacterially controlled diseases can easily damage the tooth and the supporting gum tissues. Extensive tooth loss can result from dental caries (cavities), the demineralisation and breakdown of teeth brought on by the metabolic activity in plaque (a mucus-based film that traps bacteria on the surface of the teeth). A multitude of materials can be used to repair or reconstruct teeth in their whole as well as individual teeth or tooth parts.

Delivery systems for drugs: Devices for the controlled and targeted distribution of medications are one of the implant applications with the fastest expanding market. There have been numerous attempts to include drug reservoirs in implantable devices for a prolonged, ideally regulated release. Some of these technologies employ brand-new polymeric materials as drug delivery systems (Kiran & Ramakrishna, 2021).

Wound Recovery: Since sutures were first used to close wounds, they have been used in one of the earliest applications for implantable biomaterials. As early as 2000 B.C., the ancient Egyptians utilised linen as a suture. Polymers, the most common synthetic suture material, and various metals are examples of synthetic suture materials (e.g. stainless steels and tantalum). Fracture fixation devices are a key subset of wound healing technologies. These include bone plates, nails, screws, rods, and other tools used to treat fractures. Almost all fracture fixation devices used for orthopaedic applications are made up of metals, most notably stainless steels, even if some non-metallic materials (such as carbon–carbon composite bone plates) have been studied (Kiran & Ramakrishna, 2021) (Figure 8.4).

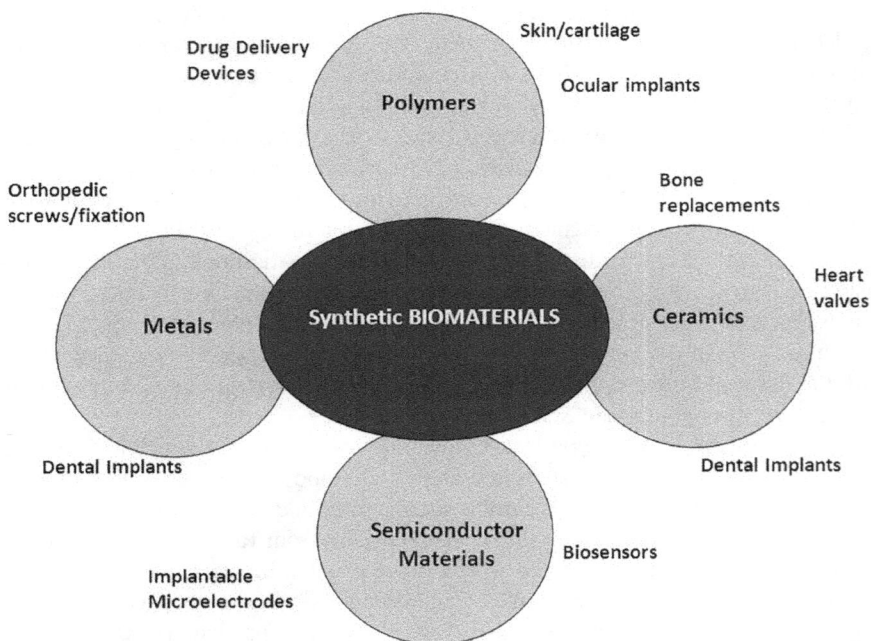

FIGURE 8.4 Type of biomaterials and their biomedical applications made up of different materials (Sahoo et al., n.d.).

8.6 DESIRED CHARACTERISTICS IN BIOMATERIALS FOR USE IN MEDICINE

Materials used inside the living human body should have specific combinations of qualities, some of which are listed in the following list, in order to survive with living tissues and other organic materials without degrading.

- Biocompatibility: The biomaterial must be biocompatible with living systems in order to prevent bodily injury, including any adverse impacts that a material may have on the biological system's constituent parts (bone, extra- and intracellular tissues, and ionic composition of plasma) (de Groot et al., 1987).
- Mechanical properties: The material should have a low modulus in addition to the high strength to increase the implant's service life and avoid loosening, which would necessitate revision surgery. Additionally, by matching the elasticity of biomaterials to that of bone, which ranges from 4 to 30 GPa, stress shielding – a reduction in bone density caused by an implant's removal of normal stress – can be avoided.
- High wear resistance: When rubbing against body tissues, the material should slide against them with little resistance. The implant may become loose due to an increase in friction coefficient or a decrease in wear resistance. Additionally, the wear debris produced can result in irritation that is harmful to the support of bone implants.

- Nontoxic: The substance shouldn't be harmful to living things like cells and organisms. There are two types of toxicity: cytotoxic (which damages individual cells) and genotoxic (which may alter the DNA of the genome). Implant rejection and other major health issues may result from failing to meet the biocompatibility and nontoxic requirements.
- Osseointegration: Osseointegration is described as "a direct structural and functional connection between organised, living bone and the surface of a load-carrying implant" in the original definition. Successful osseointegration is greatly influenced by the surface's roughness, chemistry, and topography. Implant loosening is caused by the implant surface's failure to osseointegrate with the surrounding bone. Some studies claim that the risk of being unable to eliminate the implant after usage makes osseointegration undesirable. A handful of things is shown that the implant can be safely detached.
- High corrosion resistance: The human body, which contains a highly oxygenated saline electrolyte with a pH value roughly of 7.4 and a temperature of 37°C, is hardly an atmosphere that one would consider friendly for an implanted metal alloy. Additionally, the high concentration of chlorine ions in body fluids causes metals to experience worsened corrosion conditions. When metal ions are released into the body by an implant consisting of a biomaterial with low corrosion resistance, hazardous reactions result. Thus, a desirable property of biomaterials is excellent corrosion resistance.
- Long fatigue life: Throughout a person's lifetime, the joints in their body are subjected to cyclic motion as well as cyclic fluctuation in loading. In order to avoid fatigue fracture, the material should have a strong resistance to fatigue failure. Hip prosthetic implants have been known to fail due to fatigue.

8.7 POLYMER MATERIALS FOR BIOMEDICAL APPLICATION

Due to their superior mechanical qualities, such as high moduli and rigidity, metallic and ceramic materials have been widely used in biomedical engineering as implants and devices. However, the metallic ions produced when metallic materials dissolve in body fluids can cause allergies, poisoning, cellular responses, and other problems that are frequently harmful to human health and lead to implant failure. Additionally, a lot of metallic materials have moduli that are higher than those of human bones; as a result, they might provide stress-shielding effects and cause implants to loosen. Additionally, ceramic materials have some drawbacks, like low fracture toughness.

As a result, biomaterials based on polymers are a possible replacement for metallic and ceramic materials in biomedicine. In comparison to metals and ceramics, polymer-based materials have a number of benefits, including low cost, ease of preparation, self-lubrication, and so on. They are frequently employed in the form of composites with additives to increase their tribological and mechanical characteristics. Because of their significant contribution to fundamental research and possible commercial uses, nanomaterials have recently captured the interest of scientists across many disciplines. Due to the fine qualities of nanomaterials, such as tiny size, wide surface areas, and increased activity, the incorporation of nanomaterial into polymers can also considerably improve their mechanical and tribological performances.

Researchers will keep finding novel biomimetic techniques for use in fundamental research and commercial applications such as ultra-hydrophobic surfaces, dry adhesives, and other spheres. It will take some time for the bionic research on the tribology of polymer-based composites used in biomedicine to advance significantly, but it has already started. The tribological properties of a number of polymer-based composites, including hydrogels used in biomedicine, epoxy resin, ultra-high molecular weight polyethylene (UHMWPE), and polyether ether ketone (PEEK), are discussed in the paragraphs that follow.

8.8   ULTRA-HIGH MOLECULAR WEIGHT POLYETHYLENE (UHMWPE)

Polyethylene, a polymer, is used to make the tibial and patellar components of knee replacements. Although normal polyethylene surfaces in hip implants have historically experienced wear, wear is less of an issue with knee implants because the bearing surfaces are flatter and do not produce the same kind of wear. Ultra-high cross-linked polyethylene (UHXLPE) or UHMWPE is used because it decreases even the smallest amount of wear, extending the lifespan of knee implants.

A total joint prosthesis has utilised UHMWPE as a bearing surface for more than 45 years. UHMWPE is used in the vast majority of joint replacement surgeries worldwide. Although there are rare literary examples of metal-to-metal contact joints, the most common contact in artificial joints is between metal (hard) and plastic (soft). Plastic replaces the soft cartilage in the joints, while metal replaces the surface of the bone. Due to its exceptional mix of physical and mechanical qualities, UHMWPE is currently the most used material in artificial joints. It is mainly notable for having qualities that make it chemically inert, lubricous, impact-resistant, and abrasion-resistant. UHMWPE's tribological characterisation is important, and this material has undergone extensive tribological testing. When compared to polytetrafluoroethylene (PTFE), UHMWPE exhibits significantly greater wear resistance (PTFE). Additionally, UHMWPE is discovered to have a low active resistance coefficient (mean value of 0.1) when used by alumina as the counter face in dry conditions (Shaun Berrien & Scott Eugene M Gregory, 1999).

UHMWPE is the most widely used polymer in orthopaedics. Most hip replacements still adhere to the Charnley and cubic paradigm of low frictional torque arthroplasty. Due to its superior wear resistance, ductility, and biocompatibility, UHMWPE is utilised in biomedical applications. Its mechanical and tribological qualities have been the subject of extensive research in recent years to provide patients with long-lasting implants. The tribological and mechanical performance of UHMWPE has been enhanced using a variety of techniques, such as irradiation, surface changes, and reinforcements (Hussain et al., 2020).

UHMWPE significantly reduces friction, which is thought to be caused by the material's ability to produce a lubricating coating in the contact zone. When compared to saline solution, bio-lubricants, such as sesame oil and nigella sativa oil, provide better friction and wear behaviour from UHMWPE than from stainless steel. Fatty acids, the primary constituent of all vegetable oils, may be responsible for the authors' prediction that using oils will reduce friction and wear loss (Guezmil et al., 2016).

High levels of biocompatibility, hardness, and wear resistance characterise UHMWPE. As a result, it is frequently utilised in joint arthroplasty as a bearing material with ceramic or metallic counter surfaces. Unquestionably, UHMWPE is important for getting exceptional results in complete joint arthroplasties. The tribological performance and longevity of the material are important factors for long-term clinical applications. However, UHMWPE implants have a short lifespan because of wear issues. Utilising UHMWPE in the periprosthetic environment causes osteolysis, which is followed by implant loosening. The aseptic loosening brought on by this implant loosening combined with fatigue finally results in the failure of the implant (Hussain et al., 2020). There are a variety of techniques, including increasing cross-linking, increasing the crystallinity percentage through irradiation, altering the surface through plasma treatment, or adding useful textures and reinforcements using particles or fibres (Ruggiero et al., 2015) (Figure 8.5).

UHMWPE can be cross-linked chemically using peroxides and irradiation or by utilising silane, which considerably enhances wear performance. These processes generate free radicals, which result in the creation of inter-chain covalent bonds and cross-linking. Due to ageing, deeper oxygen diffusion increases the reactivity of trapped free radicals with oxygen, which leads to increased oxidation. In UHMWPE, the active free radicals proceed through intramolecular and intermolecular breakdowns that cause time-dependent chain scission. Through this procedure, the cross-linking in the old UHMWPE is gradually reduced. As a result, the tie chain scission process promotes growth and further crystal perfection, increasing the crystallinity of aged UHMWPE.

The most typical technique for sterilising and/or cross-linking UHMWPE is irradiation. These processes generate free radicals, which result in the creation of inter-chain covalent bonds and cross-linking. A subsurface oxidised band might form as a result of the diffusion of free radicals into the polymer matrix or the diffusion of oxygen into the polymer as a result of irradiation. This subsurface oxidation zone can

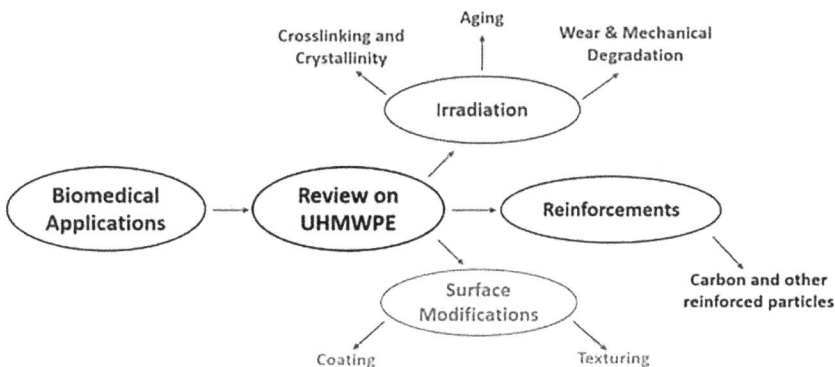

FIGURE 8.5   Ultra-high molecular weight polyethylene uses.

cause delamination, and failure frequently results from the beginning and spread of subsurface cracks (Hussain et al., 2020).

The findings demonstrated that all radiation-induced cross-linked UHMWPE has strong wear performance, although UHMWPE's mechanical performance is decreased by oxidation. The crystallinity and oxidation of UHMWPE are significantly influenced by the radiation dose and dose rate. At a higher radiation dose, the cross-link density and transvinylene concentration both increased. Wear and mechanical performance are altered by differences in crystallinity, oxidation, and cross-linking levels. The distribution and quantity of the oxidation products are also influenced by other factors, including temperature, packaging environment and packaging, and processing conditions. As UHMWPE components get older, oxygen diffuses deeply into them, interacts with free radicals that have been trapped there, and eventually leads to additional oxidation (Kurtz, 2009).

These radicals are removed by subjecting the irradiated polymer to an appropriate post-irradiation-induced cross-linking procedure. In order to maintain oxidative stability and stop long-term UHMWPE deterioration, a later remelting procedure removes free radicals. Oxidative deterioration can be lessened by sterilising UHMWPE in oxygen-depleted environments like vacuum packaging or inert gas. In order to slow down the oxidation and wear-related deterioration of the UHMWPE component, vitamin E has been regarded as a crucial antioxidant. Vitamin E interacts with free radicals that have been trapped inside of UHMWPE, causing them to react with oxygen. As a result, it stops UHMWPE from oxidising and raises its resilience to wear and fatigue (Kurtz, 2009).

The reinforcement of UHMWPE with other particles is a crucial way to improve its characteristics. A promising addition for improving the mechanical characteristics and wear resistance of UHMWPE is carbon nanoparticles. The ultra-high molecular weight polyethylene is reinforced primarily by the distribution state and concentration of carbon nanoparticles (UHMWPE). The integration of carbon nanoparticles into UHMWPE is extremely difficult and uniform dispersion is difficult because of the material's high melt viscosity. For improving the properties of UHMWPE, numerous other particles have been reported in the literature, including Nano ZnO, Fe-Al2O3/EVA, alendronate sodium (ALN), SiO_2 nanospheres, talc, zeolite, nanoclay, aramid, high-density polyethylene (HDPE), polyimide, PTFE, and polyethylene glycol (PEG). The dispersion method, size, fraction, and others have a significant impact on the wear and its mechanical properties (Hussain et al., 2020).

The most popular and effective joint replacements are total hip arthroplasties. Total hip replacement (THR) joints occasionally function well for 15 to 20 years. Because these younger people are now getting joints implanted more frequently, they need to be durable for 20 years or more (Wilches et al., 2008). The acetabular portion of a hip prosthesis is often constructed in UHMWPE. However, with time, as the wear decreases, the prolonged use of the prosthesis increases instability. Consequently, there has been an increase in recently realising that the body is the primary factor limiting the lifetime of complete joint replacement wear debris response (Marques & Davim, 2002) (Figure 8.6).

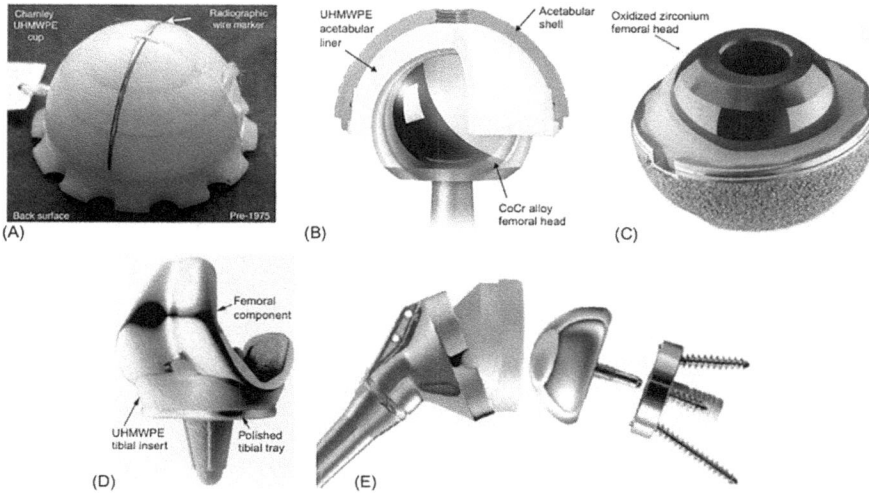

FIGURE 8.6   UHMWPE is used as biomedical implants in the following ways. (a) Cups, (b) liners, (c) head, (d) whole knee components, (e) shoulder prosthesis system components (Zhou & Jin, 2015).

8.9   MATERIALS FOR HIP ARTHROPLASTY

A ball-and-socket joint is the foundation of hip replacement. The femoral stem and ball fit into the cup or acetabular component and move in relation to it. Each of the components can be made from a wide range of materials.

8.9.1   METAL ON PLASTIC

At the beginning of hip substitutions in 1960 (when it was known as the low-friction arthroplasty, or LFA), this combination has been used in various versions. A few years later, the polyethylene's composition was improved. Ultra-strongly cross-linked polyethylene is the material now used in hip replacement implants. UHMWPE, sometimes known as (UHXLPE), is a very durable plastic substance with a very low risk of wear. Since the beginning of hip replacement procedures, metal on polyethylene has been the surgeons' material of choice for artificial hip components due to its performance and durability (McKellop et al., n.d.). Additionally, it is the most affordable bearing. As implants wear, they all shed debris. The body may eventually mistake polyethylene wear particles for pathogens or invaders. Osteolysis, or "dissolving of the bone," results in the body attacking them, which may necessitate replacing the implant (known as revision).

Technology advancements have, as previously mentioned, decreased the likelihood of wear in metal-on-polyethylene implants. They degrade quickly. They deteriorate at a rate of roughly 0.1 mm annually. Due to their more recent advances, metal and ceramic, the other materials already have great wear resistance built in (Figure 8.7).

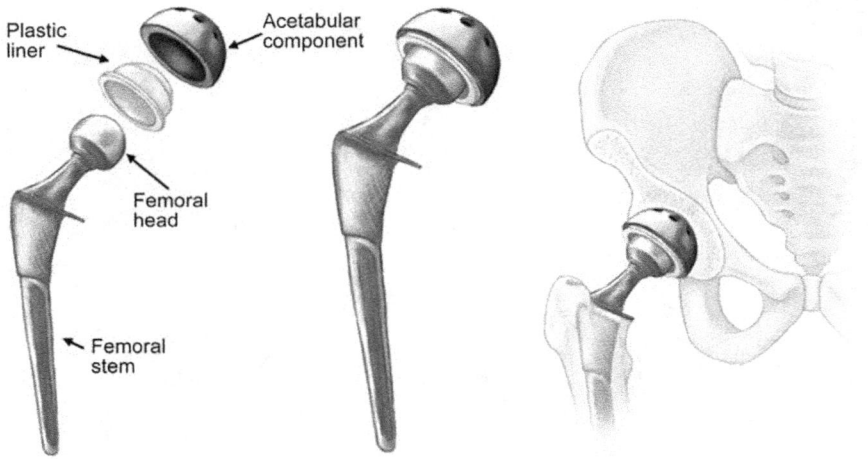

FIGURE 8.7   Individual parts of a total hip replacement are shown on the left; combined parts are shown in the centre; and the implant itself is shown on the right.

8.9.2   CERAMIC ON PLASTIC (OR UHMWPE)

A nice mix of two dependable materials is ceramic on UHMWPE. The most scratch-resistant implant material is ceramic, which is tougher than metal. The polyethylene bearing's wear rate can be significantly decreased by the firm, ultra-smooth surface (Ibrahim et al., 2017). Compared to metal on polyethylene, this form of implant has a lower potential wear rate. Although less expensive than ceramic on ceramic, ceramic on polyethylene is more expensive than metal on polyethylene. Ceramic components have occasionally fractured in the past, but newer, stronger ceramics have significantly reduced fracture rates (to 0.01%) compared to the older, more brittle ceramics. A very cross-linked, vitamin E-stabilised polyethylene-bearing material is used in some ceramic-on-polyethylene implants. Natural antioxidant vitamin E is anticipated to increase the implant bearings' lifetime when utilised in total joint replacements. In comparison to previous highly cross-linked polyethylene liners, these liners showed 95 to 99% reduced wear during laboratory testing.

Implants made up of ceramic on polyethylene have a possible wear rate of roughly 0.05 mm annually, which is 50% less than implants made up of metal on polyethylene. The more recent polyethylene liners with strong cross-linking have theoretical wear rates as low as 0.01 mm annually.

8.10   CRUCIAL AREAS FOR BIOMATERIAL RESEARCH IN THE FUTURE

The area of biomaterials is becoming more and more significant because of the high demands of ageing people and the rise in the average weight of persons. The utilisation of various implants and prostheses in the living human body is the subject of biomedical engineering (Viteri et al., n.d.). The usage of prosthetics, particularly joint replacements, has increased globally as human existence has become more complex. Therefore, thorough research into the tribological properties of the materials utilised, including friction and wear, is essential.

Additionally, tribology research has grown in importance as more and more young people are undergoing joint replacement surgeries, pushing the boundaries of these materials' effectiveness and service life. To reduce wear, researchers are constantly searching for the best arthroplasty materials. Additionally, other surface modification methods appropriate for biological applications have been created and are still being worked on. Even though this profession has recently witnessed significant advancements, there is still a lot of room for growth and progress.

Adjusting the immune response to a desirable level is known as immunomodulation. Widespread chronic disorders like type 1 diabetes, an autoimmune condition in which the body's defence kills insulin-producing cells in the pancreas, may be combated with the aid of immunomodulating biomaterials. An injectable synthetic biomaterial recently created by researchers corrected type 1 diabetes in non-obese diabetic mice. This is a significant step in creating a biodegradable platform to help control the disease's consequences. Medications, genetic materials, and proteins are all delivered therapeutically through the use of injectable biomaterials. They provide the opportunity to treat a range of illnesses by delivering medications precisely and preventing immune system absorption. Injectable biomaterials with both synthetic and naturally produced components are being studied for potential use in the treatment of heart attacks, cancer, and bone abnormalities.

Supramolecular biomaterials, which are collections of molecules that go beyond the capabilities of individual molecules, have the capacity to feel and react, making them perfect materials for treating disease or injury. Supramolecular biomaterials that may activate or deactivate in response to physiological inputs or that mimic biological signalling are being investigated by researchers.

REFERENCES

Biotribology.jpeg (1056 × 816). (n.d.). Retrieved July 20, 2022, from https://upload.wikimedia.org/wikipedia/commons/1/13/Biotribology.jpeg

Common medical devices used for fracture internal fixation. (a) Bone... | Download Scientific Diagram. (n.d.). Retrieved July 20, 2022, from https://www.researchgate.net/figure/Common-medical-devices-used-for-fracture-internal-fixation-a-Bone-plate-used-for-the_fig3_334661179

de Groot, K., Geesink, R., Klein, C. P. A. T., & Serekian, P. (1987). Plasma sprayed coatings of hydroxylapatite. *Journal of Biomedical Materials Research*, *21*(12), 1375–1381. https://doi.org/10.1002/JBM.820211203

Guezmil, M., Bensalah, W., & Mezlini, S. (2016). Effect of bio-lubrication on the tribological behavior of UHMWPE against M30NW stainless steel. *Tribology International*, *94*, 550–559. https://doi.org/10.1016/J.TRIBOINT.2015.10.022

Hussain, M., Naqvi, R. A., Abbas, N., Khan, S. M., Nawaz, S., Hussain, A., Zahra, N., & Khalid, M. W. (2020). Ultra-High-Molecular-Weight-Polyethylene (UHMWPE) as a promising polymer material for biomedical applications: A concise review. *Polymers*, *12*(2), 323. https://doi.org/10.3390/POLYM12020323

Hussein, M. A., Mohammed, A. S., & Al-Aqeeli, N. (2015). Wear characteristics of metallic biomaterials: A review. *Materials*, *8*(5), 2749–2768. https://doi.org/10.3390/MA8052749

Ibrahim, M. Z., Sarhan, A. A. D., Yusuf, F., & Hamdi, M. (2017). Biomedical materials and techniques to improve the tribological, mechanical and biomedical properties of orthopedic implants – A review article. *Journal of Alloys and Compounds*, *714*, 636–667. https://doi.org/10.1016/J.JALLCOM.2017.04.231

Kiran, A. S. K., & Ramakrishna, S. (2021). Biomaterials: Basic principles. In *An Introduction to Biomaterials Science and Engineering*, A Sandeep Kranthi Kiran and Seeram Ramakrishna, Eds., World Scientific, 82–93. https://doi.org/10.1142/9789811228186_0004

Kurtz, S. (2009). *UHMWPE Biomaterials Handbook: Ultra High Molecular Weight Polyethylene in Total Joint Replacement and Medical Devices*. Elsevier. https://books.google.com/books?hl=en&lr=&id=-50t0rdc0BgC&oi=fnd&pg=PP1&ots=_MrpoVmVxV&sig=a9zRDztdHdm2qUkYfi-hb5ThhEY

Marques, N., & Davim, J. P. (2002). Tribological comparative study of conventional and composite materials in biomedical applications. *Key Engineering Materials*, *230–232*, 487–490. https://doi.org/10.4028/www.scientific.net/KEM.230-232.487

Marques, N., & Davim, J. Paulo (n.d.). Tribological comparative study of conventional and composite materials in biomedical applications. *Trans Tech Publications*. Retrieved July 20, 2022, from https://www.scientific.net/KEM.230-232.487.pdf

McKellop, H., Campbell, P., Park, S. H., Schmalzried, T. P., Grigoris, P., Amstutz, H. C., Sarmiento A. (n.d.). The origin of submicron polyethylene wear debris in total hip arthroplasty. *Europepmc.Org*. Retrieved July 20, 2022, from https://europepmc.org/article/med/7634588

Mow, V. C., Ateshian, G. A., & Spilker, R. L. (1993). Biomechanics of diarthrodial joints: A review of twenty years of progress. *Journal of Biomechanical Engineering*, *115*(4B), 460–467. https://doi.org/10.1115/1.2895525

Ruggiero, A., D'Amato, R., & Gómez, E. (2015). Experimental analysis of tribological behavior of UHMWPE against AISI420C and against TiAl6V4 alloy under dry and lubricated conditions. *Tribology International*, *92*, 154–161. https://doi.org/10.1016/J.TRIBOINT.2015.06.005

Sahoo, P., Das, S., & Davim, J. Paulo (n.d.). Tribology of materials for biomedical applications. *Elsevier*. Retrieved July 20, 2022, from https://www.sciencedirect.com/science/article/pii/B9780081021743000012

Sahoo, P., Das, S. K., & Paulo Davim, J. (2019). Tribology of materials for biomedical applications. *Mechanical Behaviour of Biomaterials*, 1–45. https://doi.org/10.1016/B978-0-08-102174-3.00001-2

Saravanan, D., Sollapur, S., Anjappa, S., Malla, Chandrabhanu, Prasad, M. Satya, & Vignesh, S. (n.d.). Tribological properties of filler and green filler reinforced polymer composites. *Elsevier*. Retrieved July 20, 2022, from https://www.sciencedirect.com/science/article/pii/S2214785321063306?casa_token=TVxFYPgtg_8AAAAA:yOvxdrk3NOqIwWfKZcfNt07dILrDN7-m2k2FJy-q02HP9aj70p9ModUIqFeLIISY_X9IxrEWSA

Shaun Berrien, L. J., & Scott Eugene M Gregory, E. P. (1999). *Biotribology: Studies of the Effects of Biochemical Environments on the Wear and Damage of Articular Cartilage*. Virginia Tech. https://vtechworks.lib.vt.edu/handle/10919/28289

Type of biomaterials and their biomedical applications. / Download Scientific Diagram. (n.d.). Retrieved July 20, 2022, from https://www.researchgate.net/figure/Type-of-biomaterials-and-their-biomedical-applications_fig1_344942084

Viteri, Virginia Sáenz de, and, Elena Fuentes &, 2013, Jurgen Gegner. (n.d.). Titanium and titanium alloys as biomaterials. *Books.Google.Com*. Retrieved July 20, 2022, from https://books.google.com/books?hl=en&lr=&id=VGOfDwAAQBAJ&oi=fnd&pg=PA155&ots=-VfvGcOT7g&sig=GML-iczG8NLzYQ7AA1Q509f98CI

Wilches, L. V., Uribe, J. A., & Toro, A. (2008). Wear of materials used for artificial joints in total hip replacements. *Wear*, *265*(1–2), 143–149. https://doi.org/10.1016/J.WEAR.2007.09.010

Zhou, Z. R., & Jin, Z. M. (2015). Biotribology: Recent progresses and future perspectives. *Biosurface and Biotribology*, *1*(1), 3–24. https://doi.org/10.1016/J.BSBT.2015.03.001

9 Aspects of dynamic mechanical analysis in polymeric materials

Milanta Tom, Sabu Thomas, Bastien Seantier,
Yves Grohens, P. K. Mohamed,
S. Ramakrishnan and Job Kuriakose

CONTENTS

9.1 Introduction 140
9.2 Working principle 140
9.3 Instrumentation... 141
9.4 Measurements/experiments 142
    9.4.1 Amplitude sweep 142
    9.4.2 Temperature sweep 142
    9.4.3 Frequency sweep.. 143
    9.4.4 Time sweep 143
    9.4.5 Stress sweep 143
    9.4.6 Humidity sweep 144
        9.4.6.1 DMA operation modes.. 144
9.5 DMA analysis of polymeric materials... 144
    9.5.1 Rheology.. 147
    9.5.2 Creep and stress relaxation 148
    9.5.3 Tribological properties... 148
9.6 Practical applications of DMA data 148
    9.6.1 Filler–matrix interaction.. 148
    9.6.2 Curing behaviour 148
    9.6.3 Selection of ideal material 149
    9.6.4 Minimizing experimentation time.. 149
    9.6.5 Mechanical properties 149
    9.6.6 Structural property 149
9.7 Advantages and limitations 149
9.8 Conclusion 150
References... 150

DOI: 10.1201/9781003319139-9

9.1   INTRODUCTION

The technique of dynamic mechanical analysis can provide a great insight into researchers as well as industrialists to predict the performance of a material as the technique has the ability to mimic actual operating conditions. This analysis tool presents good perception of structure, morphology and viscoelastic behaviour of polymeric materials in an efficient way. The material's properties are characterized as a function of temperature, time, frequency, stress, strain, atmosphere or a combination of these parameters. The DMA analysis helps to confirm phase transitions occur in a material under certain set of parameters. The bulk properties as well as the interfacial characteristics, like the extent of interfacial interaction which determines the performance of a material, can be studied with the help of DMA (Schalnat et al., 2020).

The complex behaviour of polymers can be easily elucidated using DMA. The analysis of dynamic-mechanical performance of polymeric materials is required to confirm their suitability for specific high-performance applications. The transitions and relaxations occur in polymers with reinforcing agents have to be observed clearly as they have direct relation with the material performance. The DMA analysis is considered to be more sensitive when compared to other instruments like thermomechanical analyzer (Esmaeeli et al., 2019). Apart from analyzing the basic material properties of polymers and composite materials like glass transition and secondary transitions, molecular orientation, cold crystallization, optimization of curing process, effect of fillers, etc., DMA is able to quantify the characteristics of the finished part. DMA helps to correlate polymer structure, properties and processing conditions (Panwar & Pal, 2017).

9.2   WORKING PRINCIPLE

DMA applies an oscillatory force at a set frequency to the sample, then measures and reports the response of the material as changes in stiffness and damping. DMA data are used to obtain modulus information, which is a measure of stiffness of the material, calculated from the slope of stress/strain plot. The change in modulus as a function of specified parameter is the key for DMA analysis and the determination of viscoelastic properties of polymers (Menard, 1999).

DMA works by applying a sinusoidal oscillating stress causing sinusoidal deformation to a sample of known geometry. The relation between the stress and strain is important in determining viscoelastic properties of a material, and it can be expressed by Equation 9.1.

$$\sigma = \sigma 0 \sin(\omega t + \delta) \tag{9.1}$$

The stress applied can be described by a sine function where σ is the maximum stress applied, ω is the frequency of applied stress, and t is time. The phase difference between strain and stress is entirely dependent on the balance between viscous and elastic properties of the material. For ideal elastic systems, the strain and stress are completely in phase, and the phase angle (δ) is equal to 0. For viscous systems, the applied stress leads the strain by 90°. The phase angle of viscoelastic materials is somewhere in-between (Jayanarayanan et al., 2017). The phase angle between stress and strain gives a great insight about the viscoelasticity of the material. A small phase angle indicates that the material is highly elastic; a large phase angle indicates the material is highly viscous.

During a test in DMA, the input strain, the resulting stress and the lag between the two (phase angle δ) are measured. The complex moduli which represent the viscoelastic property can be automatically calculated:

- Storage Modulus, E' (MPa): $E' = $ stress/strain $\times \cos\delta$,
  Storage modulus represents the ability of the material to store energy and represents the elastic properties of a material.
- Loss Modulus, E'' (MPa): $E'' = $ stress/strain $\times \sin\delta$,
  Loss modulus is the heat dissipated by the material as a result of molecular motions (damping) and represents the viscous properties of a material.
- Complex modulus: $E^* = E' + iE''$,
  The storage modulus and loss modulus can be combined as a dynamic complex modulus E^*, representing the response of a viscoelastic material.
- Tan$\delta = E''/E'$ is the ratio of the dissipated energy to the energy stored per cycle of sample deformation and characterizes the material's damping properties. For purely elastic materials, Tan$\delta = 0$; for pure liquid, Tan$\delta = \infty$ (i.e., $\delta = 90°$); viscoelastic materials have intermediate values (Lee-Sullivan & Dykeman, 2000).

9.3   INSTRUMENTATION

The DMA instrument consists of several critical components including a drive motor to provide the sinusoidal deformation force, the drive shaft system to transfer the force from the drive motor to the clamps that hold the sample, the displacement sensor to measure the sample deformation, the temperature control system, an optical encoder displacement sensor to provide high resolution of oscillation amplitude, which results in excellent modulus precision ($\pm1\%$) and loss factor sensitivity (0.0001), and a bifilar-wound furnace complemented by a gas cooling accessory to allow a broad temperature range to be covered (Foreman, 1997).

The different types of fixtures that are available for a DMA instrument include the 3-point bending, single cantilever, dual cantilever, tension, compression, shear fixtures, sample holder for powders and soft samples. The selection of geometry for a particular test depends on sample's state, loading conditions and the experiment. The geometry or the fixture can affect the stress-strain data of DMA and must consider a geometry factor for calculations. Usually, a single cantilever is often used for thermoplastic polymer bar samples, and shear tests are used for thermosets. Thus, to get a reasonable and accurate data, the instrument has to be properly calibrated, sample should of proper dimensions, should use right geometry/fixtures, apply a reasonable stress/strain and maintain other testing parameters (Menard, 1999).

Although DMA can be either stress-controlled or strain-controlled, the choice always depends on the sample, testing parameters and end use. In strain-controlled analyzers, the probe is displaced to a set value, and a force transducer or a load cell is used to measure the stress. Stress-controlled analyzers work by applying a set force to the sample. These are cheaper to make because there is only one shaft, and it is found that many strain-controlled analyzers are really stress-controlled instruments with feedback loops. These analyzers are said to have good low force control to avoid the sample structure destruction, and they are more sensitive to material changes, thus duplicates practical conditions more accurately, as in most applications polymers are designed to resist load (Menard & Bilyeu, 2008).

Another selection criterion in DMA is the manner in stress or strain being applied. It can be either axial or torsional. In axial analyzers, the force is applied linearly and is mainly used for solids and semisolids. Torsional analyzers allow continuous shear to the material by applying force in a twisting manner. It can be used for analyzing polymer melts, liquids and even solids. The most commonly used geometry for axial analyzer is the tensile geometry, and for torsion, it is the parallel plate geometry. With a proper selection of geometry, both types of analyzers can handle similar samples with a limitation that axial instruments cannot handle very low viscous samples, and torsional analyzers are not suited for high-modulus samples (Menard & Menard, 2017).

9.4   MEASUREMENTS/EXPERIMENTS

A DMA measures stiffness as well as damping of a material. The stiffness is expressed as modulus and damping as tan δ value. The storage modulus, represented as either E′ or G′, is the in-phase component of modulus on applying the sinusoidal force. The out-of-phase component is the loss modulus, which is a measure of viscous behaviour of material, represented by E″ or G″. The ratio of the loss to the storage is the tan δ and is often called damping. It is a measure of the energy dissipation of a material. Damping varies with the state of the material, temperature and with the frequency.

There are different types of experiments in DMA, including amplitude sweep, temperature sweep, frequency sweep, time sweep and humidity sweep.

9.4.1   Amplitude sweep

This experiment is carried out to determine the linear viscoelastic range (LVE range) of a material (where elastic deformation occurs) under the set conditions of deformation. In this test, the strain amplitude is varied under constant temperature and frequency. It is usually observed that the storage and loss modulus show constant values at low strain amplitudes, i.e., within the linear viscoelastic range (Menard & Bilyeu, 2008).

9.4.2   Temperature sweep

This experiment is mainly used to analyze the dynamic behaviour of polymeric materials as a function of increasing temperature, where the amplitude and frequency of the stress are held constant. This helps in analyzing the structural changes that occur in polymers on varying temperatures, for example, curing process of epoxy composites. In addition, temperature sweeps gives useful information on molecular weight and distribution, transition temperatures, melting point, rubbery plateau modulus, crystallization, effect of crosslinker, etc. (Menard & Menard, 2017).

The changes in the modulus values that take place with temperature and transitions occur in a material account not only for the glass transition (T_g) and the melt but also for other transitions that occur in glassy and rubbery plateau which may be due to subtler changes in the material. The glass transition of the material is indicated as a large drop in the storage modulus on a log scale against a linear temperature scale. A concurrent peak in the tan δ is also observed. The curing of polymeric materials can be analyzed by DMA either by temperature ramps or isothermally. It is commonly used to get both the point of gelation and the point of vitrification for thermosetting materials (Mazurchevici et al., 2021).

9.4.3 FREQUENCY SWEEP

This experiment measures structural response of materials over range of frequencies under constant temperature and applied stress or strain. Frequency sweep generally provides time-dependent material behaviour and often combined with temperature sweep to study time-temperature superposition (TTS). The dominant modulus represents the structural behaviour, i.e., either elastic or viscous, and if there is any crossover, it indicates the transition from one behaviour to another. It is important to analyze materials over a range of frequencies as frequency can shift the glass transition values, which could even cause a material failure if the frequency factor is not considered in its design. The frequency sweep can also give information about molecular structure of polymers as the zero-shear plateau at low frequencies can be directly related to molecular weight according to the theory of Doi-Edwards (Ahmad Hazmi et al., 2017).

9.4.4 TIME SWEEP

In this experiment, the material behaviour is studied over a time scale while maintaining temperature and frequency parameters constant. This test is very useful to understand the property changes of material when transfers from one state to another. Polymeric materials show a number of time-dependent behaviour including setting of dispersions, curing and thixotropy (Bailly et al., 2010). Filled polymers show interesting time-dependent effects due to microstructural rearrangements during shearing process (Lee et al., 2004). Romeo et al. found that the time dependency of polymeric composites was prominent after a critical loading of fillers (Romeo et al., 2008).

9.4.5 STRESS SWEEP

In this experiment, the sample is subjected to small amplitude shear stress. The information about the stiffness of the material can be obtained from the linear viscoelastic region, i.e., during the early stages of the test. The disruption of polymer structures occurs at higher stresses and is indicated by a decrease in storage modulus. Yield stress – the stress that induces flow in viscoelastic material – is the other important measurement that we can obtain from stress sweep (Chowdhury et al., 2010).

9.4.6 HUMIDITY SWEEP

Properties of biopolymers are highly dependent on environmental conditions such as humidity. The water content in such polymers can act as plasticizers which can induce a reduction in the tensile properties. It should also be noted that the humidity values can influence the transition temperature of polymers (Bier et al., 2014). Bonnaillie and Tomasula observed decrease in storage modulus and an increase in loss modulus and tan δ values on increasing the relative humidity parameter (Bonnaillie & Tomasula, 2015).

9.4.6.1 DMA operation modes

As DMA can be utilized to analyze various types of materials, a number of loading systems have to be employed for accurate measurements. Different types of loads include, tension, bending, torsion/shear and compression. Usually, a linear drive can be used for most DMA tests with an exemption to torsion/shear loading where a rotational drive is necessary for the measurements.

The fundamental dynamic properties of viscoelastic materials include storage modulus, loss modulus and tan δ, whereas complex and dynamic viscosity, storage and loss compliance, transition temperatures, creep and stress relaxation are some of the secondary properties that can also be examined using DMA. The variation of dynamic properties under different testing conditions provides information about practical applicability (Correa et al., 2007; Oommen et al., 2000).

Parameters such as sample dimension and dimensional accuracy, type of fixture and its clamping and setting of measuring conditions are found to influence the accuracy of DMA measurements (Schalnat et al., 2020). Considering the sensitivity of the DMA instrument to different responses in polymers on deformation, DMA is a powerful tool for studying the structure–property relationships of polymeric materials.

9.5 DMA ANALYSIS OF POLYMERIC MATERIALS

Dynamic properties of viscoelastic materials are represented by complex modulus, which is the ratio of sinusoidal stress to strain. As discussed, DMA involves applying sinusoidal stress waves resulting in a strain wave. There will not be any phase difference between the stress and strain waves of purely elastic material, i.e., phase difference is 0°. For a purely viscous material, the phase difference is 90°. Polymers have characteristic viscoelastic behaviour and therefore have a phase angle between the two extremes (Kulkarni & Shaw, 2016). According to Mazurchevici et al., it is possible to predict the viscoelastic behaviour of polymeric materials from the shape of the storage modulus and loss modulus curves as it denotes the facts about the phase transitions. They also indicated that the ascending slope in damping curve denotes the beginning of material softening, and a sharp and narrow damping peak is an indication of homogeneity of the material (Mazurchevici et al., 2021).

Elastomers, being an important class of polymers, which has marked damping capacity, have been commercially used for applications requiring cyclic loading and continuous deformations. The viscoelastic properties of filled elastomers have been studied effectively by DMA. Dynamic mechanical properties of polymer materials depend on molecular structure, crystallinity and extent of crosslinking (Khonakdar, 2015). Several researchers have utilized this analyzing tool to understand the mechanism of exfoliation and intercalation, types of relaxations and approximation of morphology. The reinforcing effect of fillers in polymeric matrix can be claimed on the basis of increase in storage modulus and decrease in tan δ values. The thermomechanical stability of polymeric composites can be easily interpreted from the DMA graphs. Ning et al. utilized DMA to study the strain dependence of storage modulus known as "Payne effect" of filled natural rubber nanocomposites. They observed that filler-filler network formation and interfacial interaction have a great influence on the storage modulus. The higher value of storage modulus at the initial strain and higher the difference between initial strain modulus and ultimate dynamic storage are the results of the stronger filler–filler interaction. Higher filler–filler interaction can lead to easier agglomeration and weaker interfaces (Ning et al., 2018).

Akay studied the dynamic behaviour of carbon fibre-reinforced epoxy composites and observed a sharp transition that in longitudinal mode of testing which was attributed to the dominance of fibre property (Akay, 1993). Lin et al. observed the relation between the constrained region and mechanical properties in hybrid filler-reinforced rubber composites using DMA. They observed large increase in storage modulus for hybrid composites, which they attributed to enhanced constrained region which markedly contributed towards efficient load transfer from the matrix (Lin et al., 2016). Papageorgiou et al. discussed the reasons for high storage modulus in DMA experiments on graphene-reinforced elastomer composites. They consider the high interfacial area provided by nanocomposite which disrupts the matrix chain mobility and causes nano-confinement effect as the primary reason. In addition, the homogenous distribution of filler and its interaction with the matrix can also affect the viscoelastic properties (Papageorgiou et al., 2015). It is found that the driving amplitude used in the DMA has an influence on storage modulus and is marked by an increase in E' nonlinearly with amplitude irrespective of the sample span-to-thickness ratio used (Lee-Sullivan & Dykeman, 2000). Figure 9.1 represents typical DMA curve showing storage modulus of filled polymer (Yoon et al., 2020).

One of the important aspects that we can determine using dynamic mechanical analysis is the interfacial interaction in filled polymers. Interfaces play an important role in determining the bulk properties of polymeric materials (Sattar & Patnaik, 2020). Proper understanding of interfacial interaction is required in the case polymer nanocomposites, as the volume fraction of interfacial layer is higher. The peak value of tan δ can indicate the interfacial interaction by qualitatively representing internal friction of polymer chains. If the dispersion of filler particles is fair enough, the mobility of the polymer chains is less affected resulting in higher values of loss modulus and tan δ due to higher internal friction (Liang, 2011). If the interfacial interactions are strong enough, the peak value of tan δ will be minimum and there will be a shift in T_g value to higher temperature. The concentration of the added filler can also affect the interfacial interaction and hence the tan δ values of the polymer composite systems (Kubát et al., 1990). Figure 9.2 represents tan δ curve of polymer and polymer composite (Yoon et al., 2020).

Analysis and determination of glass transition temperature are critical for polymeric materials. Glass transition is considered as an alpha transition is considered as a major transition that occurs in polymers as a function of temperature. DMA is sensitive to other minor transitions (T_β and T_γ) over temperature which cannot be usually determined by differential scanning calorimetry (DSC) or thermomechanical analyzer (TMA) (Riga & Neag, 1991).

The glass transition of polymers (T_g) occurs within a certain temperature range, with abrupt change of physical properties which can be observed as dramatic drop in the storage (elastic) modulus, or as a peak in tan δ curve and loss modulus curve, where either onset or peak values can be used in determining T_g. On further increase in temperature, the material loses its structure and becomes rubbery in nature before its final melting.

According to Panwar et al., DMA can be utilized to study the agglomeration behaviour of nanofillers in polymeric matrices, role of percolation threshold, melt rheology and relaxation behaviour. The increase in storage modulus is usually an indication of better of dispersion of filler in polymeric matrix and interfacial adhesion of these fillers to polymer chains. The larger surface of fillers, especially nanofillers, restricts the chain mobility which results in decrease in damping factor (Panwar & Pal, 2017). The fundamental mechanical properties of polymeric composites can be confirmed by the stiffness values in terms of storage modulus and relaxation process.

The nature of filler such as elasticity in the case of natural fibres has an influence on the dynamic properties of polymer composites. It was observed that increase in frequency shifted T_g to higher temperature for optimum filler loading owing to good filler/matrix interaction (Pothana et al., 2003). DMA is suited to observe polymer chain motions associated with α and β relaxation processes in polymers. β relaxations are usually associated with phases present in polymeric composites or blends, and these transitions or relaxations cause a shift in corresponding temperature graph of DMA (Wilhelm et al., 2003). It is known that biopolymers are highly hydrophilic in

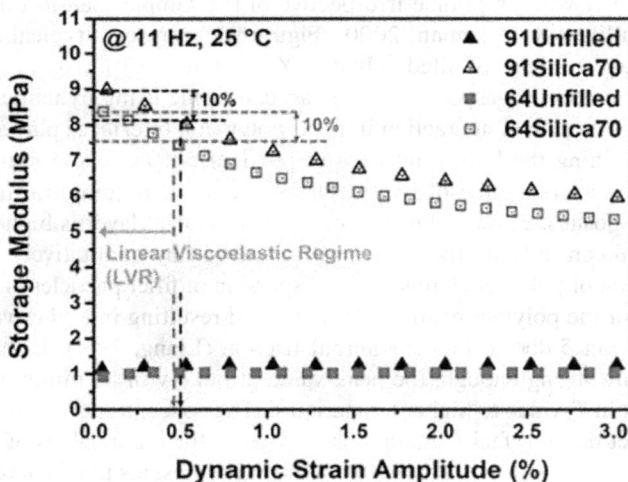

FIGURE 9.1 Typical DMA curve representing storage modulus of unfilled and filled polymer. Reprinted with permission (Yoon et al., 2020).

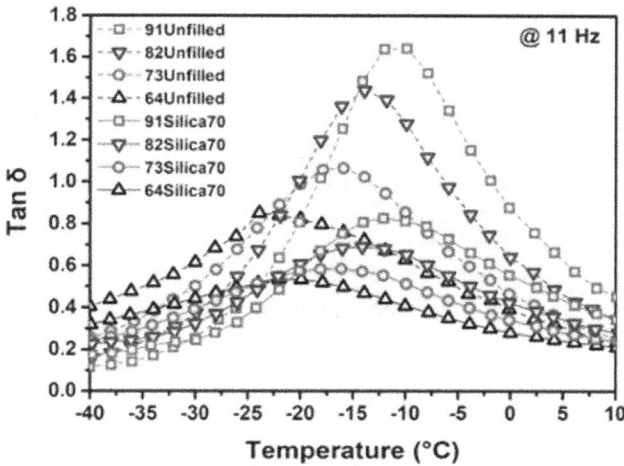

FIGURE 9.2 Typical tan δ curve from DMA analysis. Reprinted with permission (Yoon et al., 2020).

nature, and the physical and chemical properties are highly dependent on the moisture content. González observed that presence of water in chitosan films can cause plasticization and shifts the glass transition temperature to lower values (González et al., 2009).

It is possible to compute the filler distribution effectively using DMA. The filled elastomer dissipates energy during deformation. The elastomer-filler interaction can be estimated quantitatively by the difference in the storage modulus between high and low strain. According to Ajay et al., the filler–filler interaction was higher for lower particle size fillers (Ajay et al., 2021). Ghari and Jalali-Arani observed the relation between Young's modulus and complex modulus where the contribution from storage modulus as well as loss modulus has a significant contribution (Ghari & Jalali-Arani, 2016). The area under the tan δ peak can be related to the relaxation of polymeric chains (Kader & Bhowmick, 2003). The miscibility of polymer blends can be identified from the peak of tan δ. Higher peak height and full-width half-maxima signify reasonable miscibility of components in the polymer system (Panwar & Pal, 2017).

9.5.1 RHEOLOGY

The rheological analysis using DMA technique quantifies the dispersion of filler in polymeric matrices. This helps to analyze the filler–polymer interaction at different levels of dispersion. Another important aspect is using the principles of DMA to study the flow properties of polymeric liquids or melts. The response to stress/strain can be determined in short time compared to rheometers. In DMA measurements, there is no clear distinction between viscosity and modulus; also dynamic viscosity data can be used to approximate steady shear viscosity (Chartoff et al., 2008).

9.5.2 Creep and Stress Relaxation

The creep and stress relaxation cannot be considered as true dynamic analysis as the applied stress or strain held constant. Analysis of these viscoelastic properties is necessary as they can affect the performance of a polymeric material. In the creep analysis, the material is placed under constant stress and constant temperature until the sample equilibrates. Creep tests are used to analyze the ability of a material to recover internally induced stress within a specified period of time. Stress relaxation tests are carried by placing the sample under a constant strain, and the resulting stress is recorded as a function of time. Both creep and stress relaxation are important viscoelastic properties which can be studied by DMA (Chartoff et al., 2008).

9.5.3 Tribological Properties

Several researchers have used DMA as a tool to study the tribological behaviour of polymeric composites. Ge et al. studied the tribological behaviour in clay-rubber system containing different types of silane coupling agents. They observed that in the glassy region, the rubber composite containing mercapto-based silane coupling agent showed lower storage modulus than composites containing amino-based and tetra sulphide silanes. They have attributed this to the restriction of polymer chain mobility by the short sulphur bonds in mercapto-based composites. Also, it was observed that the peak of loss modulus was lower and broader owing to the good dispersion of clay and short sulphur bonds of mercapto-based silane coupling agent (Xin Ge et al., 2017). Joseph et al. observed the effect of hybrid filler system in the polymer matrix utilizing DMA. According to them, the filler content has a great influence on the storage modulus as agglomeration of fillers at higher loading resulted in lower values of storage modulus. They have attributed to the very high resistance offered by the filler system to the slipping of polymer chains (Joseph et al., 2020).

9.6 PRACTICAL APPLICATIONS OF DMA DATA

9.6.1 Filler–Matrix Interaction

Dynamic modulus and damping values can be used to interpret filler–matrix interaction. Improved adhesion between filler and matrix results in reduced mobility of polymeric chains, which decreases the adhesion factor. The decrease in adhesion factor decreases damping in polymeric composites (Bashir, 2021).

9.6.2 Curing Behaviour

Cure behaviour of thermosetting polymers and settling behaviour of adhesives and paints/coatings are important to determine their applicability. The curing behaviour is marked by a sudden increase in storage modulus, whereas vitrification is observed by a drop in tan δ peak and gel point is the intersection point of storage and loss modulus in modulus versus time graph (Forrest, 2008).

9.6.3 Selection of ideal material

To meet the multitude of technical requirements for various products and components, it is required to select the ideal material. The polymeric materials stem top most in the category of materials. It can be predicted from the DMA data the ideal material and/or possible alternatives. It is possible to identify which all polymer composites are suited for specific applications, for example, high deformation resistance, moderate damping capacity, etc., and therefore, the DMA analysis with suitable measuring systems and test specifications helps to make the right choice (Menard & Menard, 2017).

9.6.4 Minimizing experimentation time

It is important to analyze the long-term behaviour of materials used for structural applications under continuous cyclic loading. Time temperature superpositioning (TTS) in DMA reduces the experimentation time through coordination between temperature and time. The base of TTS lies on the fact that molecular transitions in polymeric material at elevated temperature can be directly related to time scale (frequency of measurement). The resultant data are shifted to master curve where the material behaviour is expressed at end-use temperature over a broad time scale. Usually, this material behaviour follows William-Landel-Ferry (WLF) equation (Foreman, 1997).

9.6.5 Mechanical properties

DMA provides an effective way to measure the stress–strain properties of thin films as well as fibres than conventional testing instruments. The available geometry and force range of DMA allow accurate measurements. In tyre industries, DMA can be utilized to study rolling resistance, wet and dry traction, and heat build-up. Therefore, higher stiffness in samples indicates smaller contact patch which implies better fuel efficiency and lower traction (Zhang et al., 2018).

9.6.6 Structural property

Structural properties of polymers like molecular weight distribution of polymers can be interpreted from the complex viscosity versus frequency curves. The important measurements that we can easily interpret from the DMA data are glass transition, secondary transitions, crystallinity, cross-linking, phase separation (polymer blends, copolymers, polymer alloys, composites), aging (physical and chemical), curing of networks, orientation and effect of additives (plasticizers, moisture) (Chartoff et al., 2008).

9.7 ADVANTAGES AND LIMITATIONS

Dynamic mechanical analysis is an important tool for determining the viscoelastic properties of polymers. DMA can provide information on major and minor transitions of materials; it is also more sensitive to changes after the glass transition temperature of polymers. Due to its use of oscillating stress, this method is able to quickly scan and calculate the modulus for a range of temperatures (Ürk et al., 2016). As a result, it is the only technique that can determine the basic structure of a polymer system while providing data on the modulus as a function of temperature. Finally, the environment of DMA tests can be controlled to mimic real-world operating conditions, so this analytical method is able to accurately predict the performance of materials in use (Menard, 1999).

DMA does possess limitations that lead to calculation inaccuracies. The modulus value is very dependent on sample dimensions, which means large inaccuracies are introduced if dimensional measurements of samples are slightly inaccurate. Additionally, overcoming the inertia of the instrument used to apply oscillating stress converts mechanical energy to heat and changes the temperature of the sample. Since maintaining exact temperatures is important in temperature scans, this also introduces inaccuracies. Because data processing of DMA is largely automated, the final source of measurement uncertainty comes from computer error (Menard & Bilyeu, 2008).

Although there are a number of limitations, the advancement in machine design and software helps to give a useful insight into the molecular structure of polymeric materials and to predict in-service performance makes it a necessary instrument for researchers.

9.8 CONCLUSION

The DMA plays a great part in the selection of ideal polymeric material for a specific application through precise indications of various responses of the material. DMA technology is the perfect solution to accurately predict the material behaviour. Rather than allowing the tests to be done over a range of parameters, it also allows the characterization of materials in various states. DMA is quite useful to explore thermo-mechanical properties of polymeric materials through the introduction of different modes of testing and providing a wide range of variable parameters.

REFERENCES

Ahmad Hazmi, A. S., Nik Pauzi, N. N. P., Abd. Maurad, Z., Abdullah, L. C., Aung, M. M., Ahmad, A., Salleh, M. Z., Tajau, R., Mahmood, M. H., & Saniman, S. E. (2017). Understanding intrinsic plasticizer in vegetable oil-based polyurethane elastomer as enhanced biomaterial. *Journal of Thermal Analysis and Calorimetry, 130*(2), 919–933. https://doi.org/10.1007/s10973-017-6459-1

Ajay, C., Das, R., & Gupta, S.D. (2021). Quantitative estimation of filler-filler interaction of rubber vulcanizates using dynamic mechanical analyzer. *Polymer Science Peer Review Journal, 1*(5), 1–4.

Akay, M. (1993). Aspects of dynamic mechanical analysis in polymeric composites. *Composites Science and Technology, 47*(4), 419–423. https://doi.org/10.1016/0266-3538(93)90010-E

Bailly, M., Kontopoulou, M., & El Mabrouk, K. (2010). Effect of polymer/filler interactions on the structure and rheological properties of ethylene-octene copolymer/nanosilica composites. *Polymer, 51*(23), 5506–5515. https://doi.org/10.1016/j.polymer.2010.09.051

Bashir, M. A. (2021). Use of Dynamic Mechanical Analysis (DMA) for characterizing interfacial interactions in filled polymers. *Solids, 2*(1), 108–120. https://doi.org/10.3390/solids2010006

Bier, J. M., Verbeek, C. J., & Lay, M. C. (2014). Thermal transitions and structural relaxations in protein-based thermoplastics. *Macromolecular Materials and Engineering*, *299*, 524–539.

Bonnaillie, L. M., & Tomasula, P. M. (2015). Application of humidity-controlled dynamic mechanical analysis (DMA-RH) to moisture-sensitive edible casein films for use in food packaging. *Polymers*, *7*(1), 91–114. https://doi.org/10.3390/polym7010091

Chartoff, R. P., Menczel, J. D., & Dillman, S. H. (2008). Dynamic Mechanical Analysis (DMA). *Thermal Analysis of Polymers: Fundamentals and Applications*, *1967*, 387–495. https://doi.org/10.1002/9780470423837.ch5

Chowdhury, S., Fabiyi, J., & Frazier, C. (2010). Advancing the dynamic mechanical analysis of biomass: Comparison of tensile-torsion and compressive-torsion wood DMA. *Holzforschung*, *64*. https://doi.org/10.1515/hf.2010.123

Correa, C. A., Razzino, C. A., & Hage, E. (2007). Role of maleated coupling agents on the interface adhesion of polypropylene-wood composites. *Journal of Thermoplastic Composite Materials*, *20*(3), 323–339. https://doi.org/10.1177/0892705707078896

Esmaeeli, R., Aliniagerdroudbari, H., Hashemi, S. R., Jbr, C., & Farhad, S. (2019). Designing a new Dynamic Mechanical Analysis (DMA) system for testing viscoelastic materials at high frequencies. *Modelling and Simulation in Engineering*, *2019*. https://doi.org/10.1155/2019/7026267

Foreman, J. (1997). Dynamic mechanical analysis of polymers. *American Laboratory*, January.

Forrest, M. J. (2008). Application to thermoplastics and rubbers. In Paul Gabbott (ed.), *Principles and Applications of Thermal Analysis*, John Wiley & Sons, 190–225. Hoboken, New Jersey, U.S. https://doi.org/10.1002/9780470697702.ch6

Ge, X., Zhang, Y., Deng, F., & Cho, U. R. (2017). Effects of silane coupling agents on tribological properties of bentonite/nitrile butadiene rubber composites. *Polymer Composites*, *38*(11), 2347–2357. https://doi.org/10.1002/pc

Ghari, H. S., & Jalali-Arani, A. (2016). Nanocomposites based on natural rubber, organoclay and nano-calcium carbonate: Study on the structure, cure behavior, static and dynamic-mechanical properties. *Applied Clay Science*, *119*, 348–357. https://doi.org/10.1016/j.clay.2015.11.001

González-Campos, J. B., Prokhorov, E., Luna-Bárcenas, G., Fonseca-García, A., & Sanchez, I. C. (2009). Dielectric relaxations of chitosan: The effect of water on the a-relaxation and the glass transition temperature. *Journal of Polymer Science: Part B: Polymer Physics*, *47*, 2259–2271. https://doi.org/10.1002/polb

Jayanarayanan, K., Rasana, N., & Mishra, R. K. (2017). Dynamic mechanical thermal analysis of polymer nanocomposites. In Sabu Thomas, Raju Thomas, Ajesh K. Zachariah, Raghvendra Kumar Mishra (eds.),*Thermal and Rheological Measurement Techniques for Nanomaterials Characterization* (Vol. 3). Chennai, India: Elsevier Inc. https://doi.org/10.1016/B978-0-323-46139-9.00006-2

Joseph, J., Munda, P. R., Kumar, M., Sidpara, A. M., & Paul, J. (2020). Sustainable conducting polymer composites: Study of mechanical and tribological properties of natural fiber reinforced PVA composites with carbon nanofillers. *Polymer-Plastics Technology and Materials*, *59*(10), 1088–1099. https://doi.org/10.1080/25740881.2020.1719144

Kader, M. A., & Bhowmick, A. K. (2003). Rheological and viscoelastic properties of multiphase acrylic rubber/fluoroelastomer/polyacrylate blends. *Polymer Engineering and Science*, *43*(4), 975–986.

Khonakdar, H. A. (2015). Dynamic mechanical analysis and thermal properties of LLDPE/ EVA/modified silica nanocomposites. *Composites Part B: Engineering*, *76*, 343–353. https://doi.org/10.1016/j.compositesb.2015.02.031

Kubát, J., Rigdahl, M., & Welander, M. (1990). Characterization of interfacial interactions in high density polyethylene filled with glass spheres using dynamic-mechanical analysis. *Journal of Applied Polymer Science*, *39*(7), 1527–1539. https://doi.org/10.1002/app.1990.070390711

Kulkarni, V. S., & Shaw, C. (2016). Rheological studies. In Vitthal S. Kulkarni, Charles Shaw (eds.), *Essential Chemistry for Formulators of Semisolid and Liquid Dosages*, Academic Press. https://doi.org/10.1016/b978-0-12-801024-2.00009-1

Lee, J. A., Kontopoulou, M., & Parent, J. S. (2004). Time and shear dependent rheology of maleated polyethylene and its nanocomposites. *Polymer*, *45*(19), 6595–6600. https://doi.org/10.1016/j.polymer.2004.07.017

Lee-Sullivan, P., & Dykeman, D. (2000). Guidelines for performing storage modulus measurements using the TA Instruments DMA 2980 three-point bend mode. I. Amplitude effects. *Polymer Testing*, *19*(2), 155–164. https://doi.org/10.1016/S0142-9418(98)00083-X

Liang, J. Z. (2011). Dynamic mechanical properties and characterization of inorganic particulate-filled polymer composites. *Journal of Thermoplastic Composite Materials*, *24*(2), 207–220. https://doi.org/10.1177/0892705710387254

Lin, Y., Liu, S., Peng, J., & Liu, L. (2016). The filler-rubber interface and reinforcement in styrene butadiene rubber composites with graphene/silica hybrids: A quantitative correlation with the constrained region. *Composites Part A: Applied Science and Manufacturing*, *86*, 19–30. https://doi.org/10.1016/j.compositesa.2016.03.029

Mazurchevici, S. N., Vaideanu, D., Rapp, D., Varganici, C. D., Cărăuşu, C., Boca, M., & Nedelcu, D. (2021). Dynamic mechanical analysis and thermal expansion of lignin-based biopolymers. *Polymers*, *13*(17), 2953. https://doi.org/10.3390/polym13172953

Menard, K. P. (1999). *Dynamic Mechanical Analysis: A Practical Introduction*. Boca Raton, FL: CRC Press.

Menard, K. P., & Bilyeu, B. W. (2008). Dynamic mechanical analysis of polymers and rubbers. In Kevin P. Menard, Bryan W. Bilyeu (eds.), *Encyclopedia of Analytical Chemistry*, Elsevier, 1–21. Amsterdam, Netherlands. https://doi.org/10.1002/9780470027318.a2007.pub2

Menard, K. P., & Menard, N. (2017). Dynamic Mechanical Analysis. In Kevin P. Menard & Bryan W. Bilyeu (eds.), *Encyclopedia of Analytical Chemistry*. John Wiley & Sons, Ltd., 1–22. https://doi.org/10.1002/9780470027318.a2007.pub3

Ning, N., Mi, T., Chu, G., Zhang, L. Q., Liu, L., Tian, M., Yu, H. T., & Lu, Y. L. (2018). A quantitative approach to study the interface of carbon nanotubes/elastomer nanocomposites. *European Polymer Journal*, *102*(November 2017), 10–18. https://doi.org/10.1016/j.eurpolymj.2018.03.007

Oommen, Z., Groeninckx, G., & Thomas, S. (2000). Dynamic mechanical and thermal properties of physically compatibilized natural rubber/poly(methyl methacrylate) blends by the addition of natural rubber-graft-poly(methyl methacrylate). *Journal of Polymer Science, Part B: Polymer Physics*, *38*(4), 525–536. https://doi.org/10.1002/(SICI)1099-0488(20000215)38:4<525:AID-POLB4>3.0.CO;2-T

Panwar, V., & Pal, K. (2017). Dynamic mechanical analysis of clay-polymer nanocomposites. In Vinay Panwar, Kaushik Pal (eds.), *Clay-Polymer Nanocomposites*. Chennai, India: Elsevier Inc. https://doi.org/10.1016/B978-0-323-46153-5.00012-4

Papageorgiou, D. G., Kinloch, I. A., & Young, R. J. (2015). Graphene/elastomer nanocomposites. *Carbon*, *95*, 460–484. https://doi.org/10.1016/j.carbon.2015.08.055

Pothana, L. A., Oommen, Z., & Thomas, S. (2003). Dynamic mechanical analysis of banana fiber reinforced polyester composites. *Composite Science and Technology*, *63*, 283–293. https://doi.org/10.1002/pc.750010109

Riga, A. T., & Neag, C. M. (1991). *Materials Characterization by Thermomechanical Analysis*, ASTM International, West Conshohocken, Pennsylvania, U.S.

Romeo, G., Filippone, G., Fernández-Nieves, A., Russo, P., & Acierno, D. (2008). Elasticity and dynamics of particle gels in non-Newtonian melts. *Rheologica Acta*, *47*(9), 989–997. https://doi.org/10.1007/s00397-008-0291-2

Sattar, M. A., & Patnaik, A. (2020). Role of interface structure and chain dynamics on the diverging glass transition behavior of SSBR-SiO2-PIL elastomers. *ACS Omega*, *5*(33), 21191–21202. https://doi.org/10.1021/acsomega.0c02929

Schalnat, J., Gómez, D. G., Daelemans, L., De Baere, I., De Clerck, K., & Van Paepegem, W. (2020). Influencing parameters on measurement accuracy in dynamic mechanical analysis of thermoplastic polymers and their composites. *Polymer Testing*, *91*(August), 106799. https://doi.org/10.1016/j.polymertesting.2020.106799

Ürk, D., Demir, E., Bulut, O., Çakıroğlu, D., Cebeci, F., Lütfi Öveçoğlu, M., & Cebeci, H. (2016). Understanding the polymer type and CNT orientation effect on the dynamic mechanical properties of high volume fraction CNT polymer nanocomposites. *Composite Structures*, *155*, 255–262. https://doi.org/10.1016/j.compstruct.2016.05.087

Wilhelm, H. M., Sierakowski, M. R., Souza, G. P., & Wypych, F. (2003). Starch films reinforced with mineral clay. *Carbohydrate Polymers*, *52*(2), 101–110. https://doi.org/10.1016/S0144-8617(02)00239-4

Yoon, B., Kim, J. Y., Hong, U., Oh, M. K., Kim, M., Han, S. B., Nam, J. Do, & Suhr, J. (2020). Dynamic viscoelasticity of silica-filled styrene-butadiene rubber/polybutadiene rubber (SBR/BR) elastomer composites. *Composites Part B: Engineering*, *187*(February), 107865. https://doi.org/10.1016/j.compositesb.2020.107865

Zhang, X., Cui, H., Song, L., Ren, H., Wang, R., & He, A. (2018). Elastomer nanocomposites with superior dynamic mechanical properties via trans-1, 4-poly (butadiene-co-isoprene) incorporation. *Composites Science and Technology*, *158*, 156–163. https://doi.org/10.1016/j.compscitech.2018.02.025

10 Additive manufacturing of artificial organs using polymeric materials

Asit Behera, R. R. Behera, S. K. Mohapatra, P. Jha, K. K. Joshi, Rahul, P. Sahu and S. K. Ghadei

CONTENTS

10.1 Introduction 156
10.2 History 156
10.3 List of patents... 157
10.4 Polymer-based additive manufacturing techniques for bioimplants............ 158
    10.4.1 Fused deposition modelling (FDM) 159
    10.4.2 Selective laser sintering (SLS).. 159
    10.4.3 Stereolithography (SLA)... 160
    10.4.4 Binder jetting 3D printing (BJP) 160
    10.4.5 3D plotting or polyjet printing (3DP) 161
    10.4.6 Laminated object manufacturing (LOM).. 161
    10.4.7 Inkjet bioprinting... 161
    10.4.8 Extrusion-based bioprinting 161
    10.4.9 Laser-assisted bioprinting 162
    10.4.10 Aerosol jet 3D printing 162
    10.4.11 Other techniques 163
10.5 Materials used (polymeric) for artificial organs 163
    10.5.1 Natural polymers 164
        10.5.1.1 Properties of natural polymers...................................... 164
        10.5.1.2 Applications of natural polymers.................................. 164
        10.5.1.3 Common natural polymers in 3D bioprinting.................. 164
    10.5.2 Synthetic polymers 167
        10.5.2.1 Properties of synthetic polymers 167
        10.5.2.2 Applications of synthetic polymers................................ 168
        10.5.2.3 Common synthetic polymers in 3D printing 169
10.6 Typical organ 3D printing techniques 173
10.7 Conclusion 174
References.. 174

DOI: 10.1201/9781003319139-10

10.1 INTRODUCTION

Human body possesses about 80 organs, and each organ contains multiple tissues having different physiological functions [1]. But when organ failure or defect takes place, there is a need for allograft transplantation which is the only therapy now available to deal with. But the long-term stability, expensive donor organ, side effects and nonavailability of donor limit the use of allograft transplantation. Hence, there is a surge in demand for manufacturing bioartificial organs. Bioartificial organs can be replaced for failed or damaged organs in the body, provided bioartificial organs must be biocompatible to the receiver's body.

Now, the question comes how to manufacture bioartificial organs. There are various ways by which bioartificial organs can be manufactured. But recently in past decade, 3D printing technology has emerged rapidly to be used in the biomedical industry.3D printing has many benefits like precise and rapid manufacturing of bioartificial organs. In addition to bioartificial organs, large scale-up scaffolds and living tissues can also be manufactured by using bio 3D printing. So, now, 3D printing technique is considered as the most reliable and efficient technique for manufacturing bioartificial organs [2].

Evolution of 3D printing emerged rapidly in the bioindustry when a bladder of real cells was manufactured by 3D printing in 1993 [3]. In the bioindustry, the process of 3D printing comprises 4 steps. First, 3D print materials were put for in vitro use without checking biocompatibility [4]. Second, biocompatible implants were developed and used permanently in vivo [5]. Third, biocompatible 3D-printed degradable implants were replaced in body which can start tissue regeneration in vivo [6]. Fourth, customized implants were manufactured using extracellular matrix and cells [7].

Polymers have a great impact on 3D printing of artificial organs. Polymers are the main constituent of bioink that is used in printing process. Bioinks are polymeric hydrogels that can be formed by cross-linking polymers through chemical, physical or biochemical ways. The polymeric hydrogels can be natural or synthetic one. These polymers contain bioactive groups, which facilitates the cells to provide stable environment. Compared to natural polymers, synthetic polymers provide better immunogenic responses and mechanical properties. But polymers used in biolinks should have some desirable properties like biostorable, biostable, biocompatible, and Biodegradable.

3D printing of polymeric materials can be useful for various artificial-organ manufacturing. It can be useful for the production of prosthesis, bioimplants and tissues. 3D printing technique of polymeric materials provides flexibility, customizable property, etc., by which rehabilitation devices and prosthetics can be manufactured. Implants including surgical fillers, implantable medical devices and degradable bioactive implants are commonly used in the human body. From porous 3D-printed polymers, scaffolds can be prepared that stimulate cellular responses and accelerate osteogenesis [8]. The artificial bone having sufficient porosity can also be prepared in vivo by using the above technique with the help of polymeric materials.

10.2 HISTORY

In this direction, a virtual model has been developed for bone reduction clamp using online available software, which can be used in finger fractures [9]. Similarly, an exoskeletal of cortex cast was designed by Jake Evill, which was used as a support for localized trauma zone. The prepared cortex cast is ultralight, recyclable, fully ventilated and hygienic [10]. In recent years, the scientific development in the technologies related to the prosthetics fabrication has provided a sustainable solution to fulfil the growing medical demands. Currently, additive manufacturing has been exploited for all possible applications using a variety of materials such as thermoplastic filaments, powder or liquid, and hydrogels.

10.3 LIST OF PATENTS

Table 10.1 depicts some of the innovations in the area of artificial organ manufacturing through the passage of time.

TABLE 10.1
List of patents published on artificial organ manufacturing

Sl. no.	Patent name	Patent no.	Year	References
1	Method and apparatus for biodegradable, osteogenic, bone graft substitute device	US5133755A	1992	[11]
2	Three-dimensional polymer matrices	US6471993B1	2002	[12]
3	Device for regeneration of articular cartilage and other tissue	US20030045943A1	2003	[13]
4	Controlled local/global and micro-/macroporous 3D plastic, polymer and ceramic/cement composite scaffold fabrication and applications thereof	US20030006534A1	2003	[14]
5	Implantable devices comprising biologically absorbable star polymers and methods for fabricating the same	US20060095122A1	2004	[15]
6	Tissue engineering scaffolds	US20040258729A1	2004	[16]
7	Modular tissue scaffolds	US10500053B2	2012	[17]
8	Method of manufacturing a porous polymer component involving the use of a dissolvable, sacrificial material	EP2826814A1	2013	[18]
9	Bone implants and method of manufacture	US20130131812A1	2013	[19]
10	Implants for soft and hard tissue regeneration	US20140200667A1	2014	[20]
11	A kind of toughness organizational structure and 3D printing-forming equipment thereof and method	CN103919629B	2016	[21]
12	Implantable medical devices fabricated from polymers with radiopaque groups	US9682178B2	2017	[22]
13	Medical stent based on 3D printing and printing method thereof	KR101920694B1	2019	[23]
14	A method of making an individual 3d printed ceramic bioresorbable bone implant for use in traumatology and orthopaedics	WO2022035854A1	2021	[24]

10.4 POLYMER-BASED ADDITIVE MANUFACTURING TECHNIQUES FOR BIOIMPLANTS

Artificial organs currently are being manufactured by 3D printing which can be classified into three processes: (1) Inkjet-based 3D printing, (2) Extrusion-based 3D printing and laser-assisted 3D printing. From all these 3D printing processes, fused deposition modelling (FDM) and stereolithography (SLA) are the most used process for manufacturing of artificial organs. Again, polyglycolic acid (PGA), polylactic acid (PLA), etc., are the most commonly printed polymers in the artificial organ manufacturing industry. When polymers are used in 3D printing, the end materials possess porosity which can be controlled by varying parameters of printing. Thus, it's much helpful in the bioprinting process. Figure 10.1 depicts different processes of 3D printing of polymers.

As per ASTM standards, AM can be divided into the following seven categories based on creating individual layer. Due to the rapid progress of 3D bioprinting in the

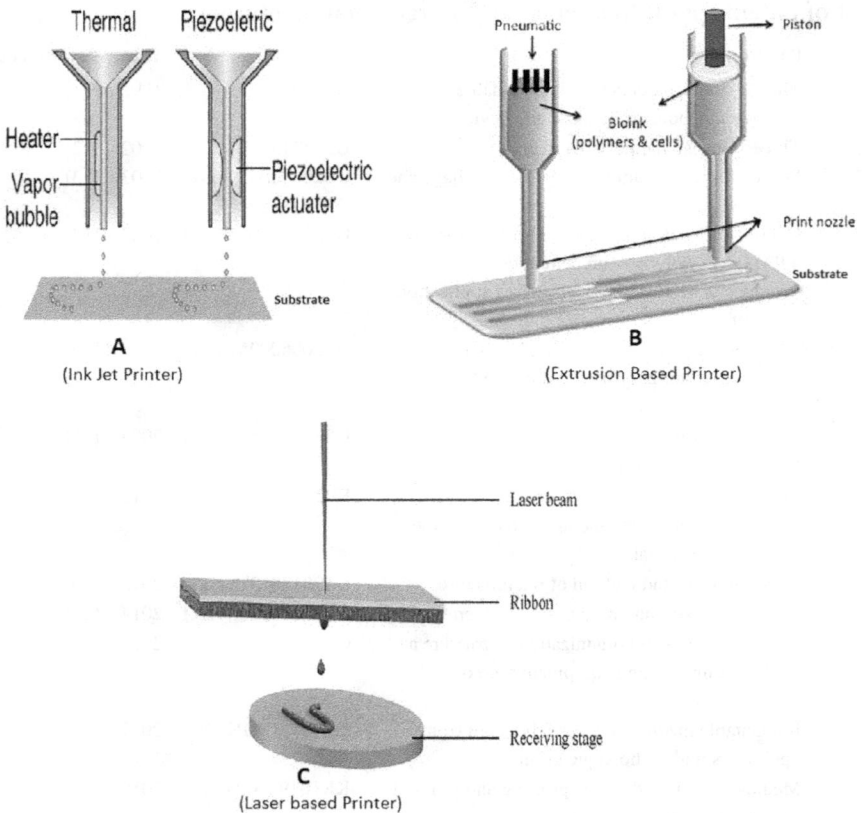

FIGURE 10.1 Types of 3D printing of artificial organs. (a) Inkjet bioprinting. (b) Extrusion-based bioprinting. (c) Laser-assisted bioprinting.

medical industry, the 3D-printed artificial organs production has increased. For the manufacturing of artificial organs, 3D manufacturing techniques are used individually or in mixed mode. Some of the 3D printing processes related to bioprinting have been discussed below.

10.4.1 Fused deposition modelling (FDM)

Fused deposition modelling is an oldest additive manufacturing process as a whole. Basically, in this process of printing, a thermoplastic polymer is fed into a liquefier and the filament is extruded simultaneously [25]. For bioinks, FDM produces melted thermoplastics. Various process parameters affect the property of the parts manufactured by FDM. Working process parameters (air pocket, frame angle, layer thickness), FDM machine process parameters (choice of temperature, nozzle diameter, scanning rate), polymer properties (viscosity, morphology, heat capacity, thermal conductivity), etc., act as influencing parameters in bioprinting in FDM.

The FDM printer has certain regions like hot end, cold end and print bed. The semimolten material that comes out of the printer solidifies on the bed, and simultaneously, another fresh layer gets deposited automatically. The bond between two layers provides strength to the product. Rheologically and mechanically balanced raw materials are utilized for 3D printing. Some binder materials are also mixed so as to balance homogeneity, rheological properties and mechanical friction. The resolution and performance of the produced products depend on various parameters such as processing temperature, raster angle, raster thickness, layer height, layer density, and printing velocity [26].

For artificial organ manufacturing by FDM process, some limited materials like PVC, PCL, and polyacrylamide are commonly employed. For instance, due to low melting temperature, PCL is used normally for tissue engineering scaffold preparation. By FDM process, complex scaffolds with good mechanical strength and geometric accuracy can be prepared but one drawback is that bioprinting activity can't be done directly under high melting temperature.

10.4.2 Selective laser sintering (SLS)

Selective laser sintering process is a very common 3D printing process used for artificial organ manufacturing. It may use fossil-based polymeric materials in the porous state that is neither nonbiodegradable nor recyclable. Sometimes, dry blending process is adopted in order to produce biomass plastic. Carl Deckard patented the SLS process in the year of 1988 [27]. Polymers such as polyaryletherketones (PAEK), polystyrene, and polyamides can be used for SLS process.

This process utilizes a laser beam to sinter powdered materials. First of all, the powdered materials are deposited on the bed. Then, according to the 3D design, the laser source is incident on the selected areas of the powder, thus sintering and binding the powder. After sintering, the binded materials form a solid structure of desired shape. Sintering takes place with the help of heat produced by laser source.

10.4.3 Stereolithography (SLA)

This process was developed by Chuck Hull in 1986 [28]. It can use polymeric materials like resins and elastomers that can be combined with various biocompatible materials to be 3D-printed. The SLA technique is based on photopolymerization. It requires an intense digital light projector to initiate the photolytical cross-linking of bioinks which enables cross-linking one layer in single printing plane [29]. In this process, ultraviolet light is incident on photopolymerizable polymer in liquid form followed by cross-linking it into a hardened layer. This is repeated layer by layer to form the 3D structure.

The SLA technique does not heat the donor polymer. It has higher resolution, greater cell viabilities and reduced printing time. Stereolithography is used in bio-medical applications, for example, to make computerized tomography (CT)-based molds for producing artificial heart valves [30]. In SLA process, as light source controls the printing, so light-sensitive bioinks are generally utilized to build the structure. Hyperbranched polymers, functionalized oligomers, star/branched polymers, etc., are used as the building blocks for getting the desired geometry [31]. In layer-by-layer manner, methacrylated gelatin (GelMA), polyethylene glycol diacrylate (PEGDA), etc., can also be printed by SLA. Cell viability can be up to 90%. Cytotoxicity of the lights and photoinitiators in SLA supress the use of SLA in artificial organ 3D printing [32] (Figure 10.2).

10.4.4 Binder Jetting 3D Printing (BJP)

Binder jet printing is the combination of powder and liquid. It is generally used for the design of muscle cells, fibroblast and scaffolds. It uses a programmable file to

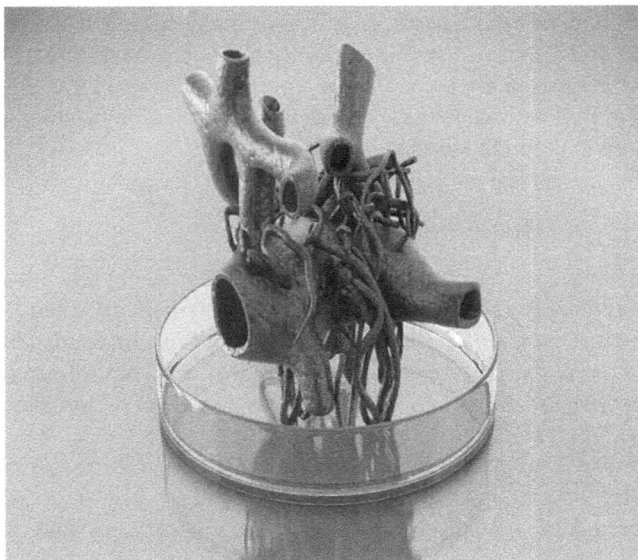

FIGURE 10.2 Artificial organ manufactured by SLA [33].

print a structure. Here, liquid binder is used to facilitate the printing process. First of all, a layer of powder is sprinkled on the bed. Then, as per the design requirement, the binder is dropped over the powder bed from the print head. This produces a 2D object. As the single layer formation completes, then the build platform moves down side and again fresh layer of powder is incident over the bed. The excess materials are moved to an overflow box [34].

10.4.5 3D PLOTTING OR POLYJET PRINTING (3DP)

3D plotting is more or less similar to binder jet printing. Only difference is that here in 3D plotting, resin is dropped instead of binder. The resin must be UV-sensitive photocurable resins. Like BJP, here in this process, print heads jet resins over the selective predefined locations, and the charge is hardened by the use of UV light. After the first layer, the built platform moves in the downward direction. 3DP is able to create a multimaterial complex-shaped object. It is utilized to create anatomical models that are useful for presurgical planning [35]. Due to the use of multipolymer resins, the strength of 3D-printed part increases. Various photopolymer resins like verodent, veroclear, fullcure, etc., can be used in polyjet printing [36].

10.4.6 LAMINATED OBJECT MANUFACTURING (LOM)

This is a unique process in which sheet lamination technique is used. In this process, thin sheets of materials are taken and binded together by the application of heat-activated glue that produces a layer-by-layer assembly [37]. The end product is formed by cutting extra materials by laser source, but compared to other techniques, the resolution of the end product is low and also internal tension produced is low. But due to the lack of diversity of biomaterials, this technique is least useful in the biomaterial application.

10.4.7 INKJET BIOPRINTING

Inkjet-based 3D printing technique is very much adopted in biomedical fields. In this process, droplets of the building materials are selectively deposited. The building material generally includes photopolymers. As the inkjet-printed materials are compatible with living beings, its use has a surge in the bioindustry. The inkjet-bioprinted materials are generally used in printing tissue scaffolds for cell seeding.

It is a noncontact process in which 2D inkjet printers are used. This technique can be classified into electrostatic inkjet bioprinting, thermal inkjet bioprinting and piezoelectric inkjet bioprinting [38]. In this process, acoustic waves get generated through the bioink chamber [39]. Again, droplets are generated by means of voltage production as pressure is applied between two surfaces.

10.4.8 EXTRUSION-BASED BIOPRINTING

Extrusion-based bioprinting has been widely used for tissue engineering and biofabrication [40]. The extruded bioinks are distributed over the building substrate by pneumatic force or by mechanical force (Pneumatic or screw driven). Extrusion-based bioprinting has control over porosity and distribution of cells in fabricated parts. It has the capacity for high cell-density deposition. So, nowadays, living cells are being deposited with biocompatible polymers. Through a series of events like sol-gel transformation, polymerization, chemical cross-linking, and enzymatic reaction, solidification of polymer solutions is achieved [41].

A large number of biomaterials, including cells, growth factors, and other bioactive agents, can be simultaneously deposited with polymeric solutions or hydrogels. The products can be useful for pathological mechanism analyses, cell transplantation, regenerative medicine preparation, etc. A critical limitation of the 3D-printed living cells/natural polymers for the bioartificial organ manufacturing is the notorious weak mechanical properties of the products.

10.4.9 LASER-ASSISTED BIOPRINTING

Laser-assisted bioprinting was developed in the year of 2004 to print biomaterials with high resolution [42]. Bioink is the cell in gel or liquid solution. It is deposited over the metal plate. When the metal plate gets heated by a laser source, then the solution gets vapourized as bioink droplets [43]. But the main drawback of this process is that cell death occurs due to the thermal damage occurred by the laser source. Femtosecond lasers can be utilized to eliminate this damage [44].

10.4.10 AEROSOL JET 3D PRINTING

Aerosol jet 3D printing has vast application in the electronics industry. In this process, the aerosol is transported by the carrier gas to the substrate [45]. Recently, interest in flexible, stretchable and wearable electronics has motivated the development of this kind of technique to customizable healthcare devices, such as implantable bionic ears, as shown in Figure 10.3. The printed bionic ears can intricately merge biological and nanoelectronic functionalities with enhanced auditory sensing for radio-frequency reception and stereo-audio music reproduction [46].

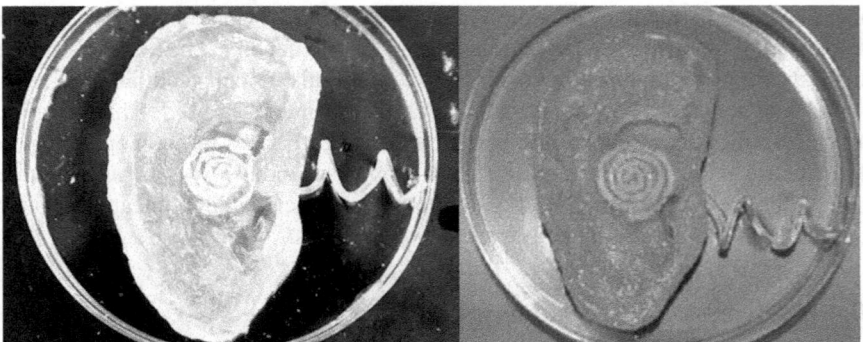

FIGURE 10.3 3-Dimensional printed bionic ear [47].

10.4.11   OTHER TECHNIQUES

For the manufacturing of artificial organs, various other techniques are also developed, for example, magnetic flotation-based magnetic bioprinting. Magnetic bioprinting works on two strategies: (1) incubation of cells with nanoparticles using Fe_3O_4 magnetic field to perform a gel by electrostatic interactions and (2) combination of a label-free cell with paramagnetic buffer in an external magnetic field [48].

For tissue engineering/tissue regeneration, bioplotting is employed. It employs a syringe for extruding tubes of material. UV radiation may be employed for healing when layer-by-layer material deposition takes place.

Acoustic bioprinting is another technique that works on the principle of acoustic wave technology. It works on depositing cells on the substrate that are condensing picolitre droplet of bioinks in an acoustic field [49].

10.5   MATERIALS USED (POLYMERIC) FOR ARTIFICIAL ORGANS

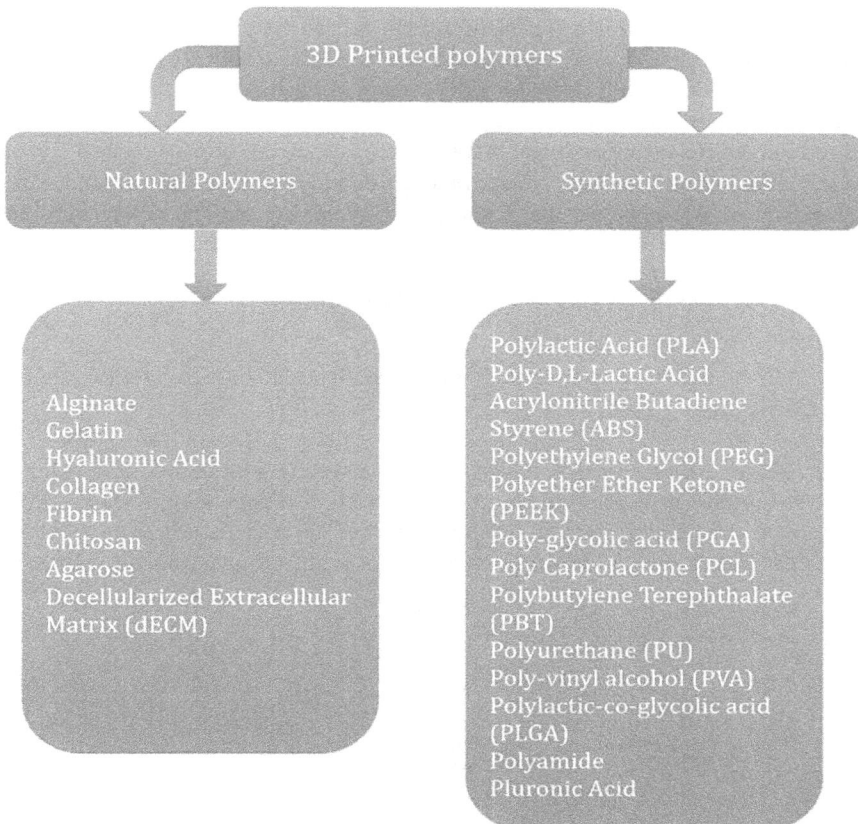

FIGURE 10.4   Classification of polymers useful in 3D printing of artificial organs.

10.5.1 NATURAL POLYMERS

10.5.1.1 Properties of natural polymers

Natural polymers are bio-derived polymers that are present in nature. Silk, DNA, proteins, and cellulose are the examples of natural polymers. These polymers can be used in different industries. Among natural polymers, some polymers are there that can be dissolved in cell-friendly inorganic solvents, namely fibrinogen, hyaluronic acid, gelatin, and alginate. These polymers when dissolved in solvent form hydrogels or solutions. The hydrogel has sufficient fluidity that allows it to be printed layer-by-layer with the help of additive manufacturing [50]. After the 3D printing, the hydrogel or polymeric solution provides proper biomimic environment and facilitates cellular activities. Then, natural polymers perform certain functions like bioartifical organ generations and homogeneous/heterogeneous histogenesis modulations. These activities promote biomolecular/cellular activities, biophyscial/chemical cues for tissue/organ morphologies and provide vascular/neural network settings.

10.5.1.2 Applications of natural polymers

Natural polymers have extensive use in various biomedical applications, particularly in artificial-organ manufacturing. Natural polymers such as collagen, gelatin, decellularized extracellular matrix (dECM), and fibrinogen are printed individually or within themselves or with other polymers so as to form a principal component of bioink. These natural polymers have great cell–material interaction which helps it to be used in manufacturing artificial organs.

Good biocompatibility and greater biodegradability help the natural polymers to be used in the human body as the 3D-printed artificial organs. The following section depicts the use of various natural polymers to be used in bioprinting process.

10.5.1.3 Common natural polymers in 3D bioprinting

10.5.1.3.1   Alginate

10.5.1.3.1.1   Origin   It is derived from brown algae. It is anionic polysaccharide, also called as algin.

10.5.1.3.1.2   Properties   Alginate is actually a synonym for alginic acid. Alginate is able to dissolve in water and can cross-link with divalent cations such as barium (Ba^{2+}) ions, calcium (Ca^{2+}) and strontium (Sr^{2+}). These cross-linked products are very much useful in drug delivery, regenerative medicine and wound healing [51].

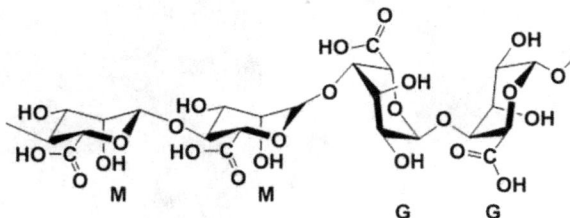

FIGURE 10.5   Structure units of alginate molecule [52].

The viscosity of the alginate hydrogel depends on the polymer concentration. If polymer concentration increases in hydrogel, then bioactivity reduces and vice versa. Figure 10.5 depicts the structure of alginate.

10.5.1.3.1.3 Applications Because of the rapid biodegradability, good biocompatible alginate is frequently used as bioinks in 3D printing process [53]. In history, first, alginate was applied in 3D bioprinting in the year 2003. Here, as an additive, gelatin hydrogel was printed with sodium alginate [54]. Later for soft tissue biprinting, Park et al. emphasized on the suitable concentration of alginate hydrogel. They found that alginate hydrogel containing 3wt% alginate shows good cell viability, proliferation capability and good printability. It is evident that oxidized alginate has a more potential usage in organ 3D printing. Jia et al. investigated on oxidizing alginate molecules to control printability. It is proved that 5%–15% conc. alginate is very much recommended for 3D bioprinting.

10.5.1.3.2 Gelatin

10.5.1.3.2.1 Origin Gelatin is a partially hydrolyzed protein by breaking the triple helix of collagen into single-strain molecules.

10.5.1.3.2.2 Properties Gelatin is a water-soluble, biodegradable, noncytotoxic polymer. This polymer is widely applied in 3D bioprinting due to the property of excellent biocompatibility and high water-absorbing capacity. Gelatin has amphoteric behaviour for amino acid. Figure 10.6 shows the molecular structure of gelatin.

10.5.1.3.2.3 Applications Hybrid hydrogel (gelatin/methacrylate, GelMA) can be formed when gelatin molecules are mixed with the methacrylamide group. In the presence of UV ray and photoinitiator, the GelMA hydrogel can be photopolymerized [56]. Increase in gelatin concentration in solution can increase viscosity. Hence, this can be efficiently used in bioprinting of artificial organs.

10.5.1.3.3 Hyaluronic acid

10.5.1.3.3.1 Origin Hyaluronic acid (HA) is the mixture of N-acetyl-d-glucosamine and d-glucuronic acid. It is a polysaccharide existing in living organisms [57].

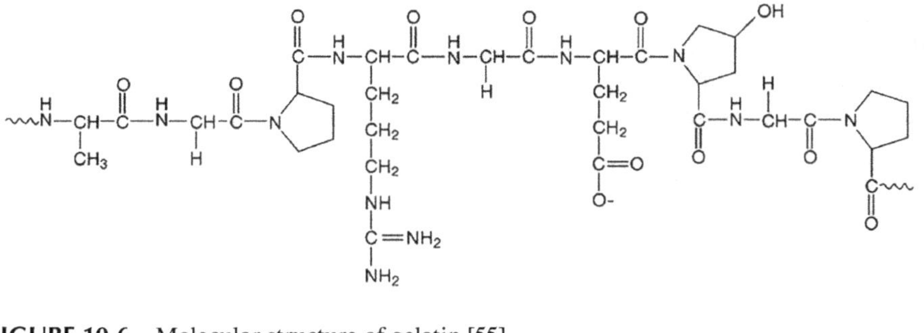

FIGURE 10.6 Molecular structure of gelatin [55].

10.5.1.3.3.2 Properties HA participates in angiogenesis, cell proliferation, etc., for being biodegradable and biocompatible. It has poor mechanical property which shows fidelity in 3D printing. HA can be degraded into low-weight molecules when reacts with hyaluronidase and β-glucuronidase [58]. It is a lubricating hydrophilic polymer that can form highly viscous hydrogels at low concentrations.

10.5.1.3.3.3 Applications By cross-linking HA with methacrylate in UA-light source, hyaluronic acid methacrylate (HAMA) is formed [59]. Hybrid HAMA-GelMA 'bioinks' are generally applied in tissue engineering applications like cartilage, neural and cardiovascular tissues. Due to greater biocompatibility and bio-degradability, HA is very much useful in tissue engineering. It can be used in 3D bioprinting in hydrogel forms [60].

10.5.1.3.4 Collagen
10.5.1.3.4.1 Origin It exists naturally and is a triple-helical biocompatible protein.

10.5.1.3.4.2 Properties Collagen is helpful in cell growth, and collagen scaffolds have less immunological reactions. It is used as a scaffold material for tissue engineering. For porous scaffolds, it can increase proliferation, adhesion, etc.

10.5.1.3.4.3 Applications It is generally useful for bone and cartilage scaffold repair in 3D printing. By combining collagen with other polymers like hyaluronic acid, fibrin, and alginate, viscosity, printability and degradation rate can be altered which can be very useful in artificial-organ 3D printing. It is evident that 3D bio-printed collagen scaffold can increase the neurological function recovery of axons and can provide good mechanical strength to injured spinal cord [61].

10.5.1.3.5 Fibrin
10.5.1.3.5.1 Origin It is blood-derived fibrous protein. It is formed by polymerizing fibrinogen in the presence of the protease thrombin.

10.5.1.3.5.2 Properties As proteolytic enzymes are present in fibrin, fibrin generally degrades rapidly.

10.5.1.3.5.3 Applications For cell encapsulation, fibrin hydrogel has good cytocompatibility. It has good cell viability and biocompatibility. It is used largely in biomedical fields such as wound healing, pharmacy and tissue repair. For artificial-organ 3D printing, fibrin is chosen to be an optimal constituent [62]. Quick degradation velocity, low viscosity and rapid gelation process make fibrin more suitable for organ 3D printing. Bioactive agents and cells can be incorporated with fibrin without any reduction in cell viability.

10.5.1.3.6 Chitosan
10.5.1.3.6.1 Origin It is a natural polysaccharide formed by deacetylation of chitin.

10.5.1.3.6.2 Properties It has poor mechanical strengths and slow gelation properties.

10.5.1.3.6.3 Applications Due to biodegradable and antibiotic properties, chitosan is applied in most of the biomedical areas like the skin, bone and cartilage. It has high viscosity which promotes it to be used in extrusion-based 3D printing of artificial organs. Chitosan is very popular to be used in tissue engineering and scaffold manufacturing. Cheng et al. [63] synthesized composite chitosan for 3D printing; Wu et al. [64] used chitosan for cell growth and Lee et al. [65] fabricated scaffolds by using chitosan.

10.5.1.3.7 Agarose

10.5.1.3.7.1 Origin It is derived from the cell wall of red algae. It is a linear polysaccharide and is composed of 3,6-anhydro-α-l-galactopyranose and β-d-galactopyranose.

10.5.1.3.7.2 Properties Cell encapsulation capacity of agarose is very poor. The gelling temperature of agarose depends on the polymer concentration.

10.5.1.3.7.3 Applications It is suitable for the extrusion-based 3D bioprinting processes [66]. It is used as a modified polymer in 3D bioprinting. It is possible by cross-linking and bending with other components in the polymeric hydrogel [67].

10.5.1.3.8 Decellularized Extracellular Matrix (dECM)

10.5.1.3.8.1 Origin It is a mixture of natural polymers that is obtained from decellularization of animal tissues [68].

10.5.1.3.8.2 Properties The decellulization process involves the original tissues to be remained inside. It provides tissue-specific microenvironments. The decellularization processes may be biochemical, physical or chemical.

10.5.1.3.8.3 Applications In the tissue 3D bioprinting, procine-liver-derived dECM acts as a functional substrate [69]. As dECM is of lower viscosity, it needs another supportive material for 3D bioprinting. For organ 3D bioprinting, dECM can provide cells with customized milieus. dECM is very much useful for tissue-/organ-specific function preservation in artificial organ 3D printing. Some of the applications of natural polymers are discussed in Table 10.2.

10.5.2 Synthetic polymers

10.5.2.1 Properties of synthetic polymers

Synthetic polymers are synthesized by chemical reactions between two or more elements. Almost all synthetic polymers have superior mechanical properties than natural polymers. But these polymers are relatively bioinert. Because during the processing due to the application of heat and external stimuli, its bioactivity

TABLE 10.2

Natural polymers and their applications

Bioink type	Outcomes	Application
Alginate	Bioprinting and cartilage matrix development, and 3D neural tissue construction	Tissue engineering, neural tissue
Gelatin	Influence of parameters on printability	A resource for bioink designing
Hyaluronic acid	Dual-cross-linking hyaluronic acid hydrogel	Tissue engineering
Hyaluronic acid	Development of 3D bioprinted tissues	Cartilage bioprinting
Collagen	Novel bioinks of various tissues	Tissue engineering
PU-gelatin	Complex tissue for muscle-tendon	Muscle unit
Alginate-chitosan	3D neural tissue construction	Neural tissue
Collagen-gelatin	Print of cell-laden hydrogel	Tissue engineering
Hyaluronic acid-gelatin	Development of stable bioinks	High viable liver construct
Collagen-chitosan	Influence of printing parameters on quality	Tissue engineering
Gelatin-methacrylamide	Improvement of mechanical and rheological properties	Tissue engineering
Alginate-hyaluronic acid	Bioprinting and cartilage matrix development	Tissue engineering
Alginate-PCL	Investigation of layer effect on cell proliferation in vitro and in vivo	Tissue engineering
PEG-gelatin	Characterization of gel-phase bioinks	Tissue engineering
PLA-gelatin	Development of gelatin-based bioinks	Living tissue constructs
Gelatin-PE	Development of bioinks using FFF process	Tissue engineering
Alginate-PCL fibers	Mechanical in-vitro and in-vivo analysis	Bone organ engineering

reduces. Again, these polymers may be biodegraded by microorganisms, but their strong mechanical properties lead to be used in artificial organ 3D printing process. Mechanical properties such as tensile strength, elastic modulus, fatigue, and fracture toughness help the polymer to withstand internal stresses developed in bioimplants. These polymers are stress-tolerant, low cost and light weight. Sol-gel temperatures of these polymers are also low.

10.5.2.2 Applications of synthetic polymers

Synthetic polymers are utilized in muscle tissue printing. As these materials have better elastic property and good strength, these materials are used in the muscle tissue printing [70]. Again, synthetic polymers are very much useful in printing scaffold for the bone tissue. The printing process includes melt molding, phase separation, gas foaming and solvent casting. In fact, scaffold manufacturing is a prerequisite for bone tissue engineering [71].

3D bioprinting of artificial organs by synthetic polymer is very much useful. Regeneration or repair of organs can be done by means of these polymers. Inception of organ printing is synchronized by using some polymers (e.g. PCL) as a scarified layer, supplying sufficient strength while printing, which is then removed by immersing the printed structure in a solution without destroying the structure [72].

10.5.2.3   Common synthetic polymers in 3D printing

10.5.2.3.1   Polylactic acid (PLA)

10.5.2.3.1.1   Origin   PLA is hydrolytically degradable aliphatic polyester.

10.5.2.3.1.2   Properties   It is degradable, biocompatible and printable for which it is usually used as polymeric bioink [73].

10.5.2.3.1.3   Applications   PLA is well equipped with FDM 3D printing technique. FDM-generated filaments can be integrated with PLA to be used in musculoskeletal tissue engineering for fabrication of ligaments. But, sometimes, PLA degrades releasing by-products that cause inflammation and cell demise [74]. Again, brittleness of PLA also restricts the use of PLA in bioprinting. In order to overcome this limitation, PLA is mixed with ceramics to form artificial organs of higher strength [75].

10.5.2.3.2   Poly-D,L-Lactic Acid

10.5.2.3.2.1   Origin   It is of amorphous structure. It is a polymer with a lactic acid origin.

10.5.2.3.2.2   Properties   It is biocompatible and hydrophobic in nature. Its elevated strength lets it to be used for the manufacturing of scaffolds in SLA techniques.

10.5.2.3.2.3   Applications   It is widely used in forming porous and biocompatible scaffolds. Hence, most of its applications include tissue engineering and orthopaedic rehabilitation [76]. Due to the hydrophobicity of PDLLA, water does not enter into matrix, thus the decaying process is extended.

10.5.2.3.3   Acrylonitrile Butadiene Styrene (ABS)

10.5.2.3.3.1   Origin   It is a petrochemical product and is a triblock copolymer. It is amorphous in nature. It is prepared in the presence of polybutadiene by the polymerization between acrylonitrile and styrene [77].

10.5.2.3.3.2   Properties   Due to the presence of 3 different monomers, ABS is heat-endurant and has good impact strength and toughness. For good printability, ABS is a commonly used polymer in 3D printing. It is chemically resistant to alkalis, phosphoric acid, vegetable oils and alcohols [78].

10.5.2.3.3.3   Applications   ABS is used as a printing material in FDM and SLS techniques. Chen et al. [79]. found that by adding some quantities of poly(methyl methacrylate) (PMMA) to ABS, mechanical performance and scratch resistance increase rapidly. Addition of methacrylate-butadiene-styrene (MBS) also increases toughness to the highest level.

10.5.2.3.4   Polyethylene Glycol (PEG)

10.5.2.3.4.1   Origin   It is prepared by radical polymerization reaction. It is hydrophilic in nature.

10.5.2.3.4.2   Properties   It has a linear or branched structure that contains asymmetric or dissymmetric hydroxyl ion as its tail groups. PEG is resistant to protein adsorption and mainly forms hydrogel. These have lower mechanical strength and are nonbiodegradable.

10.5.2.3.4.3   Applications   It's biocompatibily allows it to be used in scaffold manufacturing and drug-delivery system [80]. It is mostly used in soft tissue repair. PEH has less cell adhesion and tissue formation. Hence, PEG is generally modified with acrylate groups to create the photopolymerizable PEGDA. For manufacturing artificial organs and scaffolds, PEGDA is photopolymerized by UV-light in 3D-printed area. Some researchers have combined PEG with GelMA to generate optimal hybrid 'bioinks' to improve the mechanical properties of the engineered hard tissues.

10.5.2.3.5   Polyether Ether Ketone (PEEK)

10.5.2.3.5.1   Origin   PEEK can been synthesized by using nucleophilic substitution of 4,4′-difluorobenzophenone with hydroquinone in the presence of anhydrous potassium carbonate under microwave irradiation to produce good yield.

10.5.2.3.5.2   Properties   Polyether ether ketone (PEEK) is a synthetic polymer having low heat conductivity, good chemical stability and superior biocompatibility. Its elasticity and strength are similar to the bone material.

10.5.2.3.5.3   Applications   PEEK is used in SLS and FDM 3D printing techniques for producing the prototype of bone replacement. By allowing radiographic evaluation, PEEK has the advantage in orthopaedic applications.

10.5.2.3.6   Poly-glycolic acid (PGA)

10.5.2.3.6.1   Origin   PGA is synthesized from glycolic acid monomers through polycondensation or ring-opening polymerization.

10.5.2.3.6.2   Properties   Because of its chemical versatility, poly-glycolic acid (PGA) is mainly used in 3D scaffold manufacturing. Mechanical properties and physical properties of PGA can be withheld by copolymers. PGA can be biodegraded to glycolic acid monomer that can be removed by some catalytic action.

10.5.2.3.6.3   Applications   PGA is used in bone internal fixation devices and in preparation of resorbable sutures. Compared to PDLLA, the degradation products of PGA are not toxic.

10.5.2.3.7   Polycaprolactone (PCL)

10.5.2.3.7.1   Origin   PCL is prepared by ring-opening polymerization of ε-caprolactone using the catalyst such as stannous octoate.

10.5.2.3.7.2   Properties   It is less expensive, nontoxic, bio degradable and semi-crystalline polyester that degrades by hydrolysis. But the biodegradation rate of PCL is much slower compared to other synthetic polymers.

10.5.2.3.7.3   Applications   PCL is well suited for FDM 3D printing techniques. PPL lacks binding sites for cells. Hence, PCL is combined with various functional biomaterials to create hybrid structures for cell viability. Cho et al. [81] prepared PCL-alginate scaffold encapsulating chondrocytes for cartilage regeneration. PCL is more often used as an additive for various biomedical uses. PCL is used as a polymeric plasticizer to thermoplastic PVC, used as an additive for resins to improve their processing characteristics and used with starch to increase biodegradability. PCL is used in the manufacturing of biodegradable polyurethanes (PUs) for manufacturing implantable biomaterials.

10.5.2.3.8   Polybutylene terephthalate (PBT)

10.5.2.3.8.1   Origin   Polybutylene terephthalate (PBT), a strong and highly crystalline synthetic resin, is produced by the polymerization of butanediol and terephthalic acid.

10.5.2.3.8.2   Properties   PBT has permissible toughness, strength and elasticity. It is mainly employed in FDM techniques.

10.5.2.3.8.3   Applications   It is used in the preparation of bone scaffolds of canine trabecular bones and in tissue regeneration. It is also used as a filler in orthopaedic surgery.

10.5.2.3.9   Polyurethane (PU)

10.5.2.3.9.1   Origin   PU is composed of oligodiol and organic units through carbamate links. It is a linearly segmented polymer.

10.5.2.3.9.2   Properties   PU is a biodegradable elastomer having excellent biocompatibility, good mechanical strength and thermosetting characteristics.

10.5.2.3.9.3   Applications   It is mainly used in the manufacturing of cartilage tissue engineering, fabrication of nerve and muscle scaffolds and bones. It can be contracted and expanded repetitively to be used as a choice for muscle generation [82]. Due to the excellent chemical and mechanical properties, biodegradable PUs have been employed for use in bioartificial-organ 3D printing.

10.5.2.3.10   Poly-vinyl alcohol (PVA)

10.5.2.3.10.1   Origin   Poly-vinyl alcohol (PVA) is synthesized in the environment of acetate and vinyl alcohol.

10.5.2.3.10.2   Properties   PVA is a water-soluble polymer and is used in SLS printing technique. These are semicrystalline, biocompatible and bioinert polymer. For bone cell ingrowth, PVA can produce a proper matrix. Its semicrystalline structure allows efficient oxygen and nutrients passage to the cell.

10.5.2.3.10.3   Applications   PVA is widely useful in numerous load-bearing treatments including craniofacial defect treatment and bone tissue engineering applications.

10.5.2.3.11   Polylactic-co-glycolic acid (PLGA)

10.5.2.3.11.1   Origin   Two monomers, lactic acid and glycolic acid, when copolymerized together form PLGA. Aluminium isopropoxide, tin (II) 2-ethylhexanoate and tin (II) alkoxides are the catalysts used for the synthesis of PLGA.

10.5.2.3.11.2   Properties   It is a good cytocompatible polymer having biodegradable nature [83]. It has same mechanical features like the human bone.

10.5.2.3.11.3   Applications   PLGA is more often used in tissue-restoring system and in bone regeneration. But its poor mechanical strength and rapid degradation rate limit its usage as a scaffold material. In biomedical applications, PLGA is used as hydrogels, films and scaffolds. PLGA has better mechanical properties in load-bearing applications. But it has less bioactivity for which mainly PLGA is used as a supportive material.

10.5.2.3.12   Polyamide (PA)

10.5.2.3.12.1   Origin   It is synthesized using step-growth polymerization. By amide bonds, repeating units are connected to form polyamide.

10.5.2.3.12.2   Properties   It has good strength and durability. Polyamides are more often used in 3D printing.

10.5.2.3.12.3   Applications   It is used where strength requirement is more in bio-implants. It is used for the manufacturing of artificial organs in small quantity.

10.5.2.3.13   Pluronic acid (or Poloxamer)

10.5.2.3.13.1   Origin   Pluronic acid is a triblock copolymer having two hydrophilic poly ethylene oxide and one hydrophobic polypropylene oxide segment.

10.5.2.3.13.2   Properties   It is best suited for extrusion-based 3D printing. It is used as a scaffold material due to good thermal response characteristics [84]. It can be mixed with other materials homogeneously due to low viscosity and can be used as bioink.

10.5.2.3.13.3   Applications   Pluronic acid has low cell-survival capability. Diacrylation of pluronic acid and incorporation of bioactive molecules into the pluronic acid can improve cell viability. Michael et al. [85] mixed pluronic acid with acrylate in the bioink and did UV cross-linking. The new hydrogel increased its cell viability to 86%.

10.6 TYPICAL ORGAN 3D PRINTING TECHNIQUES

An artificial organ 3D printing includes 3 major steps: 1, material preparation; 2, 3D printing using natural hydrogels and supportive materials; 3, maturation of tissues in the 3D-printed part.

In the first step, biocompatible cells and implantable polymers are prepared. Prior to which information for defective organs is collected and transferred to CAD models. In the second step, 3D printing is done as per the instruction of CAD model through a 3D printer. In the third step, multicellular organization and homogeneous/heterogeneous tissue modulation/coordination/maturation for the expected physiological or pathological functionality realization. The bioartificial organs are temporarily cultured in vitro or in vivo after 3D printing. Then they are connected directly to the host blood vessels to restore the missing physiological functions. Table 10.3 depicts 3D printing of polymers in biomedical use.

TABLE 10.3
3D printing in biomedical field using polymers

Sl. no.	Advancements	Description	References
1	Human organ	Human organs can be prepared by polymer 3D printing. The printed organ can work similar to original organ. Tissues of nerves, heart, liver, blood vessels, etc., can be manufactured by using polymers.	[86]
2	Cells printing	3D printing is very much useful for cell tissue printing. Personalized 3D heart with human tissue and human cells can be printed through 3D printing by using polymer.	[87]
3	Heart tissue	Artificial heart transplantation can occur in cardiac patient; cardiac tissues can be restored for blood perfusion.	[88]
4	Printing of heart	Cardiac tissues can be fabricated like original by which blood vessels, cells and chambers, and heart using human tissue can be built.	[89]
5	Bone tissue engineering	AM can repair bone defects and trauma. It can provide good environment for tissue growth.	[90]
6	Skin printing	It can create natural structure of skin by which protection from external environment can be obtained.	[91]
7	Vascular channels	Vascular channels and biological matrices can be created by this technology.	[92]
8	Printing of smart material	It can be used to manufacture smart materials like implants, smart stent, and smart medical devices which can change shape according to requirement.	[93]

10.7 CONCLUSION

In this chapter, various 3D printing techniques for artificial organ 3D printing were discussed. FDM and SLA methods were found to be the most popular 3D printing process for bioprinting. Various compatible polymers, their origin, properties and applications in organ manufacturing were discussed briefly in this chapter. It was evident that both natural polymers and synthetic polymers are very much essential in bioprinting of artificial organs.

REFERENCES

1. Blanchard, Susan, (2005) 3- Anatomy and Physiology. In: Enderle, John D., Blanchard, Susan M., & Bronzino, Joseph D. (eds.) *Biomedical Engineering, Introduction to Biomedical Engineering* (Second Edition). Academic Press, Pages 73–125, ISBN 9780122386626, doi: 10.1016/B978-0-12-238662-6.50005-7
2. Gu, Zeming, Fu, Jianzhong, Lin, Hui, & He, Yong, Development of 3D bioprinting: From printing methods to biomedical applications, *Asian Journal of Pharmaceutical Sciences*, 2020;15(5):529–557, ISSN 1818–0876, doi: 10.1016/j.ajps.2019.11.003
3. Munaz, A., Vadivelu, R. K., John, J. S., Barton, M., Kamble, H., & Nguyen, N. T., Three-dimensional printing of biological matters, *Journal of Science: Advanced Materials and Devices*, 2016;1(1):1–17, ISSN 2468-2179, doi: 10.1016/j.jsamd.2016.04.001
4. Gross, B. C., Erkal, J. L., Lockwood, S. Y., Chen, C., & Spence, D. M., Evaluation of 3D printing and its potential impact on biotechnology and the chemical sciences, *Analytical Chemistry*, 2014;86(7):3240–3253, doi: 10.1021/ac403397r
5. Sidambe, A. T., Biocompatibility of advanced manufactured titanium implants-a review. *Materials (Basel)*, 2014;7(12):8168–8188, Published 2014 Dec 19, doi: 10.3390/ma7128168
6. Liu, Guo, He, Yunhu, Liu, Pengchao, Chen, Zhou, Chen, Xuliang, Wan, Lei, Li, Ying, & Lu, Jian, Development of bioimplants with 2D, 3D, and 4D additive manufacturing materials, *Engineering*, 2020;6(11):1232–1243, ISSN 2095–8099, doi: 10.1016/j.eng.2020.04.015
7. Tan, F., & Al-Rubeai, M., Customizable implant-specific and tissue-specific extracellular matrix protein coatings fabricated using atmospheric plasma, *Frontiers in Bioengineering and Biotechnology*, 2019;7:247, Published 2019 Sep 27, doi: 10.3389/fbioe.2019.00247
8. Wang, Chong, Huang, Wei, Zhou, Yu, He, Libing, He, Zhi, Chen, Ziling, He, Xiao, Tian, Shuo, Liao, Jiaming, Lu, Bingheng, Wei, Yen, & Wang, Min, 3D printing of bone tissue engineering scaffolds, *Bioactive Materials*, 2020;5(1):82–91, ISSN 2452-199X, doi: 10.1016/j.bioactmat.2020.01.004
9. Fuller, Sam, Butz, Daniel, Vevang, Curt, & Makhlouf, Mansour, Application of 3-dimensional printing in hand surgery for production of a novel bone reduction clamp, *The Journal of Hand Surgery*, 2014;39:1840–1845, doi: 10.1016/j.jhsa.2014.06.009
10. Pal, Akhilesh Kumar, Mohanty, Amar K., & Misra, Manjusri, Additive manufacturing technology of polymeric materials for customized products: Recent developments and future prospective, *RSC Advances*, 2022, 2021;11:36398.
11. Brekke, John H., Method and apparatus for diodegradable, osteogenic, bone graft substitute device, 1992, Patent no: S5133755A
12. Shastri, Venkatram R., Martin, Ivan, Langer, Robert S., & Seidel, Joachim, Three-dimensional polymer matrices, 2002, Patent no: US6471993B1
13. Brekke, John, Bradica, Gino, & Goldman, Scott, Device for regeneration of articular cartilage and other tissue, 2003, Patent no: US20030045943A1

14. Taboas, Juan, Maddox, Rachel, Krebsbach, Paul, Hollister, Scott, & Chu, Tien-Min, Controlled local/global and micro/macro-porous 3D plastic, polymer and ceramic/cement composite scaffold fabrication and applications thereof, 2002, Patent no: US20030006534A1

15. Pacetti, Stephen, Implantable devices comprising biologically absorbable star polymers and methods for fabricating the same, 2004, Patent no: US20060095122A1

16. Czernuszka, Jan, Sachlos, Eleftherios, Derby, Brian, Reis, Nuno, & Ainsley, Christopher, Tissue engineering scaffolds, 2004, Patent no: US20040258729A1

17. Hollister, Scott J., Feinberg, Stephen E., Murphy, William L., Jongpaiboonkit, Leenaporn, Adox, James R., & Migneco, Francesco, Modular tissue scaffolds, 2012, Patent no: US10500053B2

18. Mohanty, Soumyaranjan, Emnéus, Jenny, Wolff, Anders, Dufva, Martin, Larsen, Layla Bashir, Skolimowski, Maciej, & Amato, Letizia, Method of manufacturing a porous polymer component involving use of a dissolvable, sacrificial material, 2013, Patent no: EP2826814A1

19. Ganey, Timothy, Bone implants and method of manufacture, 2013, Patent no: US20130131812A1

20. Carter, Andrew J., Implants for soft and hard tissue regeneration, 2014, Patent no: US20140200667A1

21. 王小红 许雨帆, A kind of toughness organizational structure and 3D printing-forming equipment thereof and method, 2014, Patent no: CN103919629B

22. Wang, Yunbing, Gale, David C., & Gueriguian, Vincent J., Implantable medical devices fabricated from polymers with radiopaque groups, 2008, US9682178B2

23. 하동헌조동우김병수채수훈, Medical stent based on 3d printing and printing method thereof, KR101920694B1

24. Bohdan, Arkadii, Volkov, Vadim, & Rogankov, Oleg, A method of making an individual 3d printed ceramic bioresorbable bone implant for use in traumatology and orthopedics, WO2022035854A1

25. Shaqour, B., Abuabiah, M., Abdel-Fattah, S. et al., Gaining a better understanding of the extrusion process in fused filament fabrication 3D printing: a review. *Introduction of Advanced Manufacturing Technology* 2021;114:1279–1291, doi: 10.1007/s00170-021-06918-6

26. Mostafaei, Amir, Elliott, Amy M., Barnes, John E., Li, Fangzhou, Tan, Wenda, Cramer, Corson L., Nandwana, Peeyush, & Chmielus, Markus, Binder jet 3D printing—Process parameters, materials, properties, modeling, and challenges, *Progress in Materials Science*, 2021;119:100707, ISSN 0079–6425, doi: 10.1016/j.pmatsci.2020.100707

27. Wang, Yue, Xu, Zhiyao, Wu, Dingdi, & Bai, Jiaming, Current status and prospects of polymer powder 3D printing technologies, *Materials*, 2020:13:2406, doi: 10.3390/ma13102406

28. Ngo, Tuan D., Kashani, Alireza, Imbalzano, Gabriele, Nguyen, Kate T.Q., & Hui, David, Additive manufacturing (3D printing): A review of materials, methods, applications and challenges, *Composites Part B: Engineering*, 2018;143:172–196, ISSN 1359–8368, doi: 10.1016/j.compositesb.2018.02.012

29. Bagheri, Ali, & Jin, Jianyong, Photopolymerization in 3D printing, *ACS Applied Polymer Materials*, 2019;1(4):593–611, doi: 10.1021/acsapm.8b00165

30. Nikolova, M.P., & Chavali, M.S., Recent advances in biomaterials for 3D scaffolds: A review, *Bioactive Materials*, 2019;4:271–292, Published 2019 Oct 25, doi: 10.1016/j.bioactmat.2019.10.005

31. Gungor-Ozkerim, P.S., Inci, I., Zhang, Y.S., Khademhosseini, A., & Dokmeci, M.R., Bioinks for 3D bioprinting: An overview, *Biomaterials Science*, 2018;6(5):915–946, doi: 10.1039/c7bm00765e

32. Tetsuka, H., & Shin, S.R., Materials and technical innovations in 3D printing in biomedical applications, *Journal of Materials Chemistry B*, 2020;8(15):2930–2950, doi: 10.1039/d0tb00034e

33. https://www.statnews.com/2021/06/18/3d-bioprinting-organ-transplant-waitlists-fda-delay/

34. Zhou, Xuan, Feng, Yihua, Zhang, Jiahui, Shi, Yanbin, & Wang, Li., Recent advances in additive manufacturing technology for bone tissue engineering scaffolds, *The International Journal of Advanced Manufacturing Technology*, 2020;108:3591–3606. doi: 10.1007/s00170-020-05444-1

35. Cheng, Y.L., & Huang, K.C., Preparation and characterization of color photocurable resins for full-color material jetting additive manufacturing, *Polymers (Basel)*, 2020;12(3):650, Published 2020 Mar 12, doi: 10.3390/polym12030650

36. Tappa, K., & Jammalamadaka, U., Novel biomaterials used in medical 3D printing techniques, *Journal of Functional Biomaterials*, 2018;9(1):17, Published 2018 Feb 7, doi: 10.3390/jfb9010017

37. Park, Joon, Tari, Michael, & Hahn, H., Characterization of the laminated object manufacturing (LOM) process, *Rapid Prototyping Journal*, 2000;6:36–50, doi: 10.1108/13552540010309868

38. Kumar, Piyush, Ebbens, Stephen, & Zhao, Xiubo, Inkjet printing of mammalian cells – Theory and applications, *Bioprinting*, 2021;23:e00157, ISSN 2405–8866, doi: 10.1016/j.bprint.2021.e00157

39. Li, Xinda, Liu, Boxun, Pei, Ben, Chen, Jianwei, Zhou, Dezhi, Peng, Jiayi, Zhang, Xinzhi, Jia, Wang, & Xu, Tao, Inkjet bioprinting of biomaterials, *Chemical Reviews*, 2020;120:10793–10833, doi: 10.1021/acs.chemrev.0c00008

40. Hospodiuk, M., Moncal, K.K., Dey, M., & Ozbolat, I.T. (2018) Extrusion-Based Biofabrication in Tissue Engineering and Regenerative Medicine. In: Ovsianikov, A., Yoo, J., & Mironov, V. (eds.) *3D Printing and Biofabrication. Reference Series in Biomedical Engineering.* Springer, Cham, doi: 10.1007/978-3-319-45444-3_10

41. Xie, Z., Gao, M., Lobo, A.O., & Webster, T.J., 3D Bioprinting in tissue engineering for medical applications: The classic and the hybrid, *Polymers*, 2020;12:1717, doi: 10.3390/polym12081717

42. Guillotin, B., Souquet, A., Catros, S., Duocastella, M., Pippenger, B., Bellance, S., Bareille, R., Rémy, M., Bordenave, L., Amédée, J., & Guillemot, F. Laser assisted bioprinting of engineered tissue with high cell density and microscale organization, *Biomaterials*, 2010 Oct;31(28):7250–7256, doi: 10.1016/j.biomaterials.2010.05.055, Epub 2010 Jul 2, PMID: 20580082

43. Montero, Félix E., Rezende, Rodrigo A., da Silva Jorge, V. L., & Sabino, Marcos A., Development of a smart bioink for bioprinting applications, *Frontiers in Mechanical Engineering*, 2019:5, doi: 10.3389/fmech.2019.00056

44. Guillotin, Bertrand, Ali, Muhammad, Ducom, Alexandre, Sylvain, Catros, Keriquel, Virginie, Souquet, Agnès, Remy, Murielle, Fricain, Jean-Christophe, & Guillemot, Fabien, Laser-Assisted Bioprinting for Tissue Engineering, In: Gabor Forgacs and Wei Sun (eds.) *Biofabrication Micro- and Nano-fabrication, Printing, Patterning and Assemblies.* Elsevier, Amsterdam, Netherlands. 2013, doi: 10.1016/B978-1-4557-2852-7.00006-8

45. Hales, Samuel, Tokita, Eric, Neupane, Rajan, Ghosh, Udayan, Elder, Brian, Wirthlin, Douglas, & Kong, Yong, 3D printed nanomaterial-based electronic, biomedical, and bioelectronic devices, *Nanotechnology*, 2019;31, doi: 10.1088/1361–6528/ab5f29

46. Sebastian Mannoor, Manu, Jiang, Ziwen, James, Teena, Kong, Yong, Malatesta, Karen, Soboyejo, W., Verma, Naveen, Gracias, David, & McAlpine, Michael, 3D printed bionic ears. *Nano Letters*, 2013;13, doi: 10.1021/nl4007744

47. https://www.chemistryworld.com/news/3d-printer-churns-out-bionic-ear/6177.article

48. Buyukhatipoglu, Kivilcim, Chang, Robert, Sun, Wei, & Clyne, Alisa, Bioprinted nanoparticles for tissue engineering applications, *Tissue Engineering. Part C, Methods*, 2009;16:631–642, doi: 10.1089/ten.TEC.2009.0280

49. Vanaei, Saeedeh, Parizi, Sam, Vanaei, Shohreh, Salemizadehparizi, Fatemeh, & Vanaei, Hamidreza, An overview on materials and techniques in 3D bioprinting toward biomedical application, *Engineered Regeneration*, 2020;2, doi: 10.1016/j.engreg.2020.12.001

50. Pradhan, S., Brooks, A.K., & Yadavalli, V.K., Nature-derived materials for the fabrication of functional biodevices, *Materials Today Bio*, 2020;7:100065, ISSN 2590-0064, doi: 10.1016/j.mtbio.2020.100065

51. Abasalizadeh, F., Moghaddam, S.V., Alizadeh, E. et al., Alginate-based hydrogels as drug delivery vehicles in cancer treatment and their applications in wound dressing and 3D bioprinting, *Journal of Biological Engineering*, 2020;14:8, doi: 10.1186/s13036-020-0227-7

52. Liu, Fan, Chen, Qiuhong, Liu, Chen, Ao, Qiang, Tian, Xiaohong, Fan, Jun, Tong, Hao, & Wang, Xiaohong, Natural polymers for organ 3D bioprinting, *Polymers*, 2018;10:1278, doi: 10.3390/polym10111278

53. Axpe, E., & Oyen, M.L., Applications of alginate-based bioinks in 3D bioprinting, *International Journal of Molecular Sciences*, 2016;17(12):1976, Published 2016 Nov 25, doi: 10.3390/ijms17121976

54. Kakarla, Akesh B., Kong, Ing, Turek, Ilona, Kong, Cin, & Irving, Helen, Printable gelatin, alginate and boron nitride nanotubes hydrogel-based ink for 3D bioprinting and tissue engineering applications, *Materials & Design*, 2022;213:110362, ISSN 0264–1275, doi: 10.1016/j.matdes.2021.110362

55. Kommareddy, Sushma, Shenoy, Dinesh, & Amiji, Mansoor, *Gelatin Nanoparticles and Their Biofunctionalization*. Elsevier, Amsterdam, Netherlands. 2007, doi: 10.1002/9783527610419.ntls0011

56. Sun, M., Sun, X., Wang, Z., Guo, S., Yu, G., & Yang, H. Synthesis and properties of Gelatin Methacryloyl (GelMA) hydrogels and their recent applications in load-bearing tissue, *Polymers (Basel)*, 2018;10(11):1290, Published 2018 Nov 21, doi: 10.3390/polym10111290

57. Gupta, R.C., Lall, R., Srivastava, A., & Sinha, A. Hyaluronic acid: Molecular mechanisms and therapeutic trajectory, *Frontiers in Veterinary Science*, 2019;6:192, Published 2019 Jun 25, doi: 10.3389/fvets.2019.00192

58. Park, Yongdoo, Tirelli, Nicola, & Hubbell, Jeffrey, Photopolymerized hyaluronic acid-based hydrogels and interpenetrating networks, *Biomaterials*, 2003;24:893–900, doi: 10.1016/S0142–9612(02)00420-9

59. Liu, F., Chen, Q., Liu, C., et al., Natural polymers for organ 3D bioprinting, *Polymers (Basel)*, 2018;10(11):1278, Published 2018 Nov 16, doi: 10.3390/polym10111278

60. Han, X., Chang, S., Zhang, M., Bian, X., Li, C., & Li, D. Advances of hydrogel-based bioprinting for cartilage tissue engineering, *Frontiers in Bioengineering and Biotechnology*, 2021;9:746564, Published 2021 Sep 29, doi: 10.3389/fbioe.2021.746564

61. Pugliese, Raffaele, Beltrami, Benedetta, Regondi, Stefano, & Lunetta, Christian, Polymeric biomaterials for 3D printing in medicine: An overview, *Annals of 3D Printed Medicine*, 2021;2:100011, ISSN 2666–9641, doi: 10.1016/j.stlm.2021.100011

62. Antezana, P.E., Municoy, S., Álvarez-Echazú, M.I., et al., The 3D bioprinted scaffolds for wound healing. *Pharmaceutics*, 2022;14(2):464, Published 2022 Feb 21, doi: 10.3390/pharmaceutics14020464

63. Cheng, Y.-L., et al., Enhanced adhesion and differentiation of human mesenchymal stem cell inside apatite-mineralized/poly(dopamine)-coated poly(?-caprolectone) scaffolds by stereolithography, *Journal of Materials Chemistry B*, 2016;4(38):6307–6315.

64. Lin, Y.C., Chen, G.T., & Wu, S.C., Carbohydrates-chitosan composite carrier for Vero cell culture. *Cytotechnology*, 2016;68(6):2649–2658, doi: 10.1007/s10616-016-9989-7

65. Pezeshki-Modaress, Mohamad, & Zandi, Mojgan, 2 3 Fabrication of a porous wall and higher interconnectivity scaffold comprising gelatin/chitosan via combination of salt-leaching and lyophilization methods, *Iranian Polymer Journal*, 2012;21, doi: 10.1007/s13726-012-0019-0

66. Genicot-Joncour, S., Poinas, A., Richard, O., et al., The cyclization of the 3,6-anhydro-galactose ring of iota-carrageenan is catalyzed by two D-galactose-2,6-sulfurylases in the red alga chondrus crispus, *Plant Physiology*, 2009;151(3):1609–1616, doi: 10.1104/pp.109.144329

67. Gong, C., Kong, Z., & Wang, X., The effect of agarose on 3D bioprinting, *Polymers*, 2021;13:4028, doi: 10.3390/polym13224028

68. Choudhury, D., Yee, M., Sheng, Z.L.J., Amirul, A., & Naing, M.W., Decellularization systems and devices: State-of-the-art, *Acta Biomaterialia*, 2020 Oct 1;115:51–59, doi: 10.1016/j.actbio.2020.07.060, Epub 2020 Aug 7, PMID: 32771593.

69. Wang, X., Advanced polymers for three-dimensional (3D) organ bioprinting, *Micromachines*, 2019;10:814, doi: 10.3390/mi10120814

70. Dhandayuthapani, Brahatheeswaran, Yoshida, Yasuhiko, Maekawa, Toru, & Sakthi Kumar, D., Polymeric scaffolds in tissue engineering application: A review, *International Journal of Polymer Science*, 2011; 2011. Article ID 290602, 19 pages, doi: 10.1155/2011/290602

71. Chocholata, P., Kulda, V., & Babuska, V., Fabrication of scaffolds for bone-tissue regeneration, *Materials (Basel)*, 2019;12(4):568, Published 2019 Feb 14, doi: 10.3390/ma12040568

72. Place, Elsie, George, Julian, Williams, Charlotte, & Stevens, Molly, Synthetic Polymer scaffolds for tissue engineering, *Chemical Society Reviews*, 2009;38:1139–1151, doi: 10.1039/b811392k

73. Rydz, J., Sikorska, W., Kyulavska, M., & Christova, D., Polyester-based (bio)degradable polymers as environmentally friendly materials for sustainable development, *International Journal of Molecular Sciences*, 2014;16(1):564–596, Published 2014 Dec 29, doi: 10.3390/ijms16010564

74. Singh, Daljeet, Babbar, Atul, Jain, Vivek, Gupta, Dheeraj, Saxena, Sanjai, & Dwibedi, Vagish, Synthesis, characterization, and bioactivity investigation of biomimetic bio-degradable PLA scaffold fabricated by fused filament fabrication process, *Journal of the Brazilian Society of Mechanical Sciences and Engineering*, 2019;41, doi: 10.1007/s40430-019-1625-y

75. Balla, E., Daniilidis, V., Karlioti, G., Kalamas, T., Stefanidou, M., Bikiaris, N.D., Vlachopoulos, A., Koumentakou, I., & Bikiaris, D.N., Poly(lactic Acid): A versatile biobased polymer for the future with multifunctional properties—From monomer synthesis, polymerization techniques and molecular weight increase to PLA applications, *Polymers*, 2021;13:1822, doi: 10.3390/polym13111822

76. Chen, V.J., & Ma, P.X., Nano-fibrous poly(L-lactic acid) scaffolds with interconnected spherical macropores, *Biomaterials*, 2004 May;25(11):2065–2073, doi: 10.1016/j.biomaterials.2003.08.058, PMID: 14741621.

77. Britannica, The Editors of Encyclopaedia. "acrylonitrile-butadiene-styrene copolymer". Encyclopedia Britannica, 20 Mar. 2019, https://www.britannica.com/science/acrylonitrile-butadiene-styrene-copolymer. Accessed 15 April 2022.

78. Zhang, Huiliang, Liu, Nanan, Ran, Xianghai, Han, Changyu, Han, Lijing, Zhuang, Yugang, & Dong, Lisong, Toughening of polylactide by melt blending with methyl methacrylate–butadiene–styrene copolymer, *Journal of Applied Polymer Science*, 2012;125, doi: 10.1002/app.36952

79. Chen, Siyuan, Lu, Jiabao, & Feng, Jiachun, 3D-printable ABS blends with improved scratch resistance and balanced mechanical performance, *Industrial & Engineering Chemistry Research*, 2018;57, doi: 10.1021/acs.iecr.7b05074

80. Kong, X.B., Tang, Q.Y., Chen, X.Y., Tu, Y., Sun, S.Z., & Sun, Z.L., Polyethylene glycol as a promising synthetic material for repair of spinal cord injury, *Neural Regeneration Research*, 2017;12(6):1003–1008, doi: 10.4103/1673–5374.208597

81. Kundu, J., Shim, J.H., Jang, J., Kim, S.W., & Cho, D.W., An additive manufacturing-based PCL-alginate-chondrocyte bioprinted scaffold for cartilage tissue engineering, *Journal of Tissue Engineering and Regenerative Medicine*, 2015 Nov;9(11):1286–1297, doi: 10.1002/term.1682. Epub 2013 Jan 24, PMID: 23349081.

82. Ikada, Y., Challenges in tissue engineering, *Journal of the Royal Society Interface*, 2006;3(10):589–601, doi: 10.1098/rsif.2006.0124

83. Félix Lanao, R.P., Jonker, A.M., Wolke, J.G., Jansen, J.A., van Hest, J.C., & Leeuwenburgh, S.C., Physicochemical properties and applications of poly(lactic-co-glycolic acid) for use in bone regeneration, *Tissue Engineering Part B: Reviews*, 2013;19(4):380–390, doi: 10.1089/ten.TEB.2012.0443

84. Lee, Y., Park, S.Y., Mok, H., & Park, T.G., Synthesis, characterization, antitumor activity of pluronic mimicking copolymer micelles conjugated with doxorubicin via acid-cleavable linkage, *Bioconjugate Chemistry*, 2008 Feb;19(2):525–531, doi: 10.1021/bc700382z, Epub 2007 Dec 29, PMID: 18163537.

85. Müller, Michael, Becher, Jana, Schnabelrauch, Matthias, & Zenobi, Marcy, Nanostructured pluronic hydrogels as bioinks for 3D bioprinting, *Biofabrication*, 2015;7:035006, doi: 10.1088/1758–5090/7/3/035006

86. Agarwal, S., Saha, S., Balla, V.K., Pal, A., Barui, A., & Bodhak, S., Current developments in 3D bioprinting for tissue and organ regeneration–A review, *Frontiers of Mechanical Engineering*, 2020;6:589171, doi: 10.3389/fmech.2020.589171

87. Kim, J., Kong, J.S., Han, W., Kim, B.S., & Cho, D.W., 3D cell printing of tissue/organ-mimicking constructs for therapeutic and drug testing applications, *International Journal of Molecular Sciences*, 2020;21(20):7757, Published 2020 Oct 20, doi: 10.3390/ijms21207757

88. Khan, S., & Jehangir, W., Evolution of artificial hearts: An overview and history, *Cardiology Research*, 2014;5(5):121–125, doi: 10.14740/cr354w

89. Alonzo, M., AnilKumar, S., Roman, B., Tasnim, N., & Joddar, B., 3D bioprinting of cardiac tissue and cardiac stem cell therapy, *Translational Research*, 2019;211:64–83, doi: 10.1016/j.trsl.2019.04.004

90. Amini, A.R., Laurencin, C.T., & Nukavarapu, S.P., Bone tissue engineering: Recent advances and challenges, *Critical Reviews in Biomedical Engineering*, 2012;40(5):363–408, doi: 10.1615/critrevbiomedeng.v40.i5.10

91. Augustine, R., Skin bioprinting: A novel approach for creating artificial skin from synthetic and natural building blocks, *Progress in Biomaterials*, 2018;7:77–92, doi: 10.1007/s40204-018-0087-0

92. Lee, V.K., Kim, D.Y., Ngo, H., Lee, Y., Seo, L., Yoo, S.S., Vincent, P.A., & Dai, G., Creating perfused functional vascular channels using 3D bio-printing technology, *Biomaterials*, 2014 Sep;35(28):8092–8102, Epub 2014 Jun 23, PMID: 24965886; PMCID: PMC4112057, doi: 10.1016/j.biomaterials.2014.05.083

93. Wang, Zhenzhen, & Yang, Yan, Application of 3D printing in implantable medical devices, *BioMed Research International*, 2021;2021. Article ID 6653967, 13 pages, doi: 10.1155/2021/6653967

11 An investigation of polymeric materials for hip joint

Ranjeet Kumar Singh, Swati Gangwar and D. K. Singh

CONTENTS

11.1 Background information... 181
    11.1.1 Reason for failure synthesis hip joint inside human body.............. 183
    11.1.2 Role of bearing surfaces in hip joint implant 184
        11.1.2.1 Metal-on-polyethylene (MoP)... 184
        11.1.2.2 Metal-on-metal (MoM)... 185
        11.1.2.3 Ceramic-on-ceramic (CoC) 185
        11.1.2.4 Ceramic-on-polyethylene (CoP).. 185
11.2 Material selection in articulating surface for bearing in hip joint............... 186
    11.2.1 Matrix material: ultra-high-molecular-weight polyethylene
        (UHMWPE) 187
        11.2.1.1 Effect of hydroxyapatite (HA) with ultra-high-
               molecular-weight polyethylene (UHMWPE).....................188
        11.2.1.2 Effect of carbon nanomaterials or other additive
               with ultra-high-molecular-weight polyethylene
               (UHMWPE)...192
11.3 Conclusion 196
References.. 196

11.1 BACKGROUND INFORMATION

Hip joint is one of the most important bearing joint after knee joint in humanoid body, which support body weight having the task of linking the femur with pelvis [1]. The hip joint is connecting link between acetabulum of pelvis and the head of femur. These two segments are seen like a ball-on-socket joint which is covered by the joint capsule [2, 3]. Stability is provided to the hip joint by different types of structures, including a system of ligaments and muscles. This type of arrangement allows motion as well as supports the body weight in both static and dynamic conditions. During normal walking, a compressive load acts on the hip joint, and this load is approximately equal to three times the body weight. This compressive load may increase up to ten times the body weight during running, jumping, or climbing stairs [4]. Nowadays, hip joint problems affect not only the elderly but also younger people.

DOI: 10.1201/9781003319139-11

Hip patients suffer from pain or stress during walking, standing, sleeping, sitting, and climbing stairs [5]. So hip joint replacement is required for this type of patients to decrease or eliminate pain and improve the range of leg motion.

Hip replacement is common surgery performed in the world today. The total number of patients who undergo this type of surgery is set to increase every year [6, 7]. One million hip replacement surgeries are carried out every year (till 2016), and it is expected this number will double until 2025 [3]. Hip replacement surgery does not give permanent solution, but it eliminates pain for certain period of time (10–15 years). The first attempt at hip surgery dates back to 1750 in England without any replacement. In 1840, first idea for the treatment of hip was to replace it with synthetic prosthesis. After prosthesis, wear debris particles release into the body, and these particles produce adverse effects (toxic effects) in the human body, causing this idea to end.

After that, biological elements can be used as prosthesis to reduce this problem. In 1880, Prof. Themistocles Gluck inserted the first socket with an ivory ball in a hip prosthesis, and this prosthesis fixed into the bone by screws. This type of prosthesis structure is used with some modification nowadays. Sir John charley attempted the first resurfacing procedure in 1950. Sir John Charnley also gives the concept of low friction arthroplasty (LFA) [1, 8]. This low-friction concept gives a better idea of the selection of material for artificial hip joint.

Hip joint replacement is a process where natural hip joint is replaced by synthesis hip joint [9, 10]. The aim of this surgery is to provide a better life for the patient and eliminate pain. A good design and good material selection of synthesis hip joint increase the durability of the implant by transferring the load with minimum friction and wear, which increases the period of time for implantation. A typical artificial hip joint consists of four parts, such as acetabular cup (socket), liner, femoral head (ball), and stem [11, 10].

Hip joint replacement process is also known as hip joint prosthesis [12]. There are mainly three types of joint prosthesis used in the human body. Hip joint prosthesis may be cemented, cementless, or hybrid. In cemented prosthesis, patients after surgical operation are able to walk without support. Generally, this type of surgery has been chosen for weak and elderly patients. But cementless prosthesis used for young patient who have more physical movement involved [13, 14].

In cemented prosthesis, poly (methyl methacrylate) (PMMA) is used to fix the prosthesis into bone, and this type of prosthesis fails because of delamination of the femoral stem. In cementless or uncemented prosthesis, hydroxyapatite or porous coating avoids the need for cement. Hybrid prosthesis occurs when one component is cemented and other is uncemented [14]. Nowadays, surgeons use

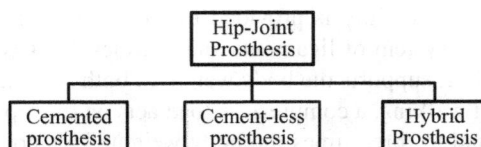

FIGURE 11.1 Type of hip joint prosthesis.

cemented prosthesis for elderly patients and cementless prosthesis for young patients. Sometimes, a synthesis hip implant fails inside the human body and requires surgery again. Failure of this synthesis hip is due to many reasons, including manufacturing or design defects of component of the hip joint, fracture, infection, or osteolysis.

11.1.1 REASON FOR FAILURE SYNTHESIS HIP JOINT INSIDE HUMAN BODY

Failure of synthesis means synthesis hip inside the human body does not work properly or affects other organs, so it requires surgery again. This synthesis hip joint fails in the human body after implantation in a short period of time or after some time due to some reason, but there are three main reasons for failure of implantation: (a) low biocompatibility (b) wear debris and (c) low yield stress

Biocompatibility means material used for synthesis hip joint does not produce adverse effects inside the human body and is compatible with the bone, tissue, and surrounding environment. The biocompatible material must be bio-active, bio-inert, and biodegradable. The biocompatibility of hip joint materials includes surface compatibility, mechanical compatibility, and osteocompatibility [15]. Low biocompatible wear debris materials produce infection inside the human body and affect other organs of the human body.

In all these processes, wear debris generates and produces adverse effects in the human body. Wear debris can result in inflammation, osteolysis, and losing the synthesis hip [16]. Wear debris from the implanted material is one main cause for required revision surgery [117, 18]. Due to wear debris, particles affect the human cell or start the osteolysis and bone resorption [19]. The osteolysis process is started by phagocytosis

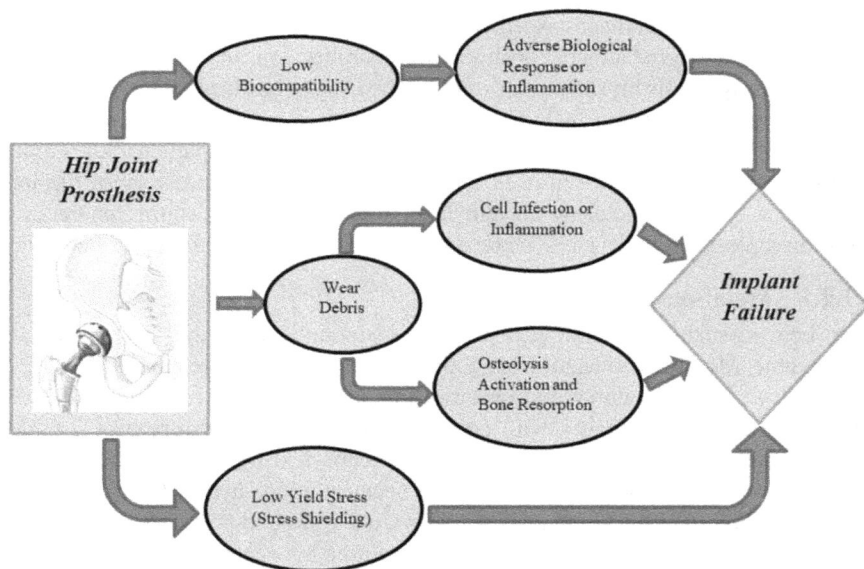

FIGURE 11.2 Mechanical, biological, and tribological drawback of hip implant.

of wear debris particulate, and this debris is produced due to the articulation motion between two bearing components, the initiation of macro-phase, and external body giant cells [20, 21]. External body giant cells are involved in bacterial infection. So osteoarthritis is one of the most important factors in joint degradation [7].

Low yielding of implant material increases the stress shielding effect. Bone resorption or aseptic loosening results in increased stress shielding, which can lead to more stress in bone cement [22, 23]. Stress shielding is the main cause of the sudden failure of hip joint prosthesis. Originally, load is supported by bone but after implantation this load is distributed between bone and implant. As a result, impact of stress on bone is reduced, and this phenomenon is known as stress shield. So, the selected material's Young modulus must be approximately equal to the bone's Young modulus. Changing the stem geometry, such as cross section, length, taperness, and curvature along the femoral stem, reduced the stress shield effect in hip joint replacement. An optimal parameter design helps reduce stress shield effect [24–26]. Most hip implant failures are due to wear debris generated from the bearing surface. The life of an implant also depends on the life of bearing surface [27, 28]. So the study of bearing surface for hip joint prosthesis is a crucial factor.

11.1.2 ROLE OF BEARING SURFACES IN HIP JOINT IMPLANT

Bearing surface for hip joint is the meeting area where the femoral ball and linear are connected. Material selection for this bearing surface may be different for different patients mainly depends on age, activity, weight, etc. So, the development of new alternate bearing material for hip implant is the main challenge for the researcher to increase the life of implant. So, the less friction and less wear are the critical parameter for selecting the materials for bearing surface for hip joint prosthesis. The ideal bearing couple for hip joint replacement means excellent structural strength, excellent biocompatibility, high resistance to degradation or corrosion, minimum friction, and minimum wear [29].

Mainly, in synthesis hip either hard-on-hard bearing or hard-on-soft is bearing couples. Hard-on-hard bearing includes metal-on-metal or ceramic-on-ceramic, which are regarded as the optimal choice for the younger and active patient [30]. Finally, four types of combination been used as bearing surfaces in the history of hip joint replacement, such as metal-on-polyethylene, metal-on-metal, ceramic-on-ceramic, and ceramic-on-polyethylene [1]. These different bearing couples are described below.

11.1.2.1 Metal-on-polyethylene (MoP)

In this bearing surface, femoral head prepared by metal and acetabular is prepared by polyethylene. Metal-on-conventional PE bearing surface has more possibility of revision surgery compared with metal-on-cross-linked PE [31]. So cross-linked PE have greater significance compared with conventional PE. Micro-texture on Co-Cr-Mo disc decrease PE wear about 50% compared with non-texture CoCrMo polished disc in different shear situation. This is possible because micro-hydro-dynamic bearing enhance the lubricant film thickness between Co-Cr-Mo and polyethylene [32]. This hydro-dynamic lubricant film decreases contact area between two surfaces, so wear decreases. Polyethylene wear is one of the main causes of artificial bearing failure because of late dislocation (after 5 year) [33].

11.1.2.2   Metal-on-metal (MoM)

In this bearing surface, femoral head and acetabular cup both are made by metal. Metal-on-metal bearing surface is not suitable for those patients who are metal sensitive [34]. There are some materials, such as stainless steel, cobalt and titanium-based alloys, that are popularly used as biocompatible materials [35]. Wear and friction are less in thermal-oxidized-texture titanium alloy compared with untreated titanium alloy because of formation of titanium oxide layer [36]. MoM bearing surfaces have a higher chance of failure compared with MoP [37]. Metallic ion release and debris can cause metal loses and the formation of pseudo tumours [16]. Metal ion wear particle reaction with protein and change the value of P_H [38]. These metals wear particle developing cancer in future [39].

11.1.2.3   Ceramic-on-ceramic (CoC)

In this bearing surface, femoral head and acetabular cup both are made by ceramic. Aluminium oxide and zirconia are the popular choice as CoC bearing material [40–42]. The advantages of these materials are high corrosion resistance, high wear resistance, low wettability, and high biocompatibility. Low wetting angle (45°) of alumina makes its extremely good wear resistance property [40]. These ceramic materials also show least friction and better lubrication compared with metal or polyethylene [43, 44]. Poor lubrication is one of the major causes of squeaking noise [45]. This type of bearing surface is generally used for young and active patient [30]. COC reduces osteolysis, dislocation, risk of revision, and aseptic loosening but also enhances the squeaking and intraoperative ceramic fracture compared with MOP [46]. This type of bearing decrease the risk of revision surgery for late dislocation [47, 48]. Disadvantages of ceramic are possibility of crack. Ceramic materials are hard and brittle in nature so it can crack. This crack propagates, and finally component fails [49, 50].

11.1.2.4   Ceramic-on-polyethylene (CoP)

In this type of bearing surface, femoral head of hip is made by ceramic and acetabular cup is made by polyethylene. This type of bearing surface minimizes the risk of fracture. Polyethylene cups joined with ceramic or metallic materials are commonly used in synthesis bearing because of their outstanding tribological property and elastic properties, which reduce stress shielding [50]. Here, the problem with PE is the wear of debris particles.

The other problems related to PE use as implantation include average mechanical property, lack of adhesion to living tissue and surface, etc. [51]. Reduce friction and wear resistance improve its material property (cross linkage) and surface property [19]. Consider friction and wear property of materials, cross-linked polyethylene (PE) may be the best choice for use as bearing material for articulating surface or linear of the acetabular component [52].

Nowadays, surgeon does not prefer the metal inside the human body. So, CoP bearing and CoC bearing use in synthesis hip joint. CoP bearing decreases the durability of hip joint, but at the same time, it decreases the chance of sudden failure compared with CoC bearing. CoP bearing decreases fracture rate and hip noise compared with CoC bearing but increases osteolysis and aseptic loosening [53, 54].

TABLE 11.1

Advantage and disadvantage of different types of bearing couples uses in artificial hip joint

Type of bearing	Advantage	Disadvantage
Metal-on-polyethylene (MoP)	• Good long-term results in elderly patients • Higher rate of liner wear	• More wear rates • PE liner wear particle produced the occurrence of osteolysis.
Metal-on-metal (MoM)	• Decreases wear rate • Increase range of motion	• Bone, soft tissue reacts with metal wear particles cause of pseudo-tumour creation. • Cobalt or chromium ions can affect the body. • High rate of osteolysis cause of early implant failure.
Ceramic-on-ceramic (CoC)	• Less wear rates • Less osteolysis • Very high survival rate during long-term outcomes. • Wear particles in human body is Harmless.	• Ceramic fracture, Squeaking noise and sudden fail synthesis hip.
Ceramic-on-polyethylene (CoP)	• Decrease fracture rate and hip noise compared to CoC bearing • Lower wear rate	• Durability of synthesis hip is less compared to CoC bearing

CoP bearing produces more wear compared with CoC bearing. Average wear rate of CoP was 0.92% per year and for CoC was 0.018% per year [29]. So, CoC and CoP both are better option for bearing couple for total hip joint replacement [55–57]. Here, there is no single material that can remove all types of problems related to hip implant. So, the hybrid biopolymer composite is one choice to develop new alternate biomaterial, which is used as articulating surface in bearing for hip joint.

Acetabular component mainly fails in bearing couple of hip joints. This articulation surface of bearing mainly made by either ceramic or polymer materials. Polymer materials choose over ceramic material because decrease the chance of sudden failure. High wear rate of polymer decreases the durability of implant and synthesis hip joint fails due to osteolysis and aseptic loosening.

11.2 MATERIAL SELECTION IN ARTICULATING SURFACE FOR BEARING IN HIP JOINT

Polymer is the first choice for low friction bearing surface for hip implant compared with metal or ceramic. Other important property of polymer is highly corrosion resistance [51]. Highly stable polymers, such as polytetrafloraethylene (PTFE), polyether etherketone (PEEK) and ultra-high-molecular-weight polyethylene (UHMWPE), are important for hip joint prosthesis [58]. In all these polymers, UHMWPE has been likely as appropriate bearing material for articulating surface for hip joint since 1960s [59, 60]. UHMWPE-created hybrid composites play a main role in articulating the surface of bearing couple in hip joint [61, 62]. Therefore, good materials for acetabular component have high mechanical properties, high biocompatibility, and minimum wear with low coefficient of friction [63, 64]. Nowadays, UHMWPE uses as linear in CoC bearing to decrease the chance of sudden failure or uses as acetabular component in CoP bearing.

So many researchers attempt to increase wear resistance of UHMWPE by using radiation of cross linkage and heat treatment [60]. Hybrid composite materials using UHMWPE as a matrix material are now a popular choice to enhance mechanical and wear resistance. Nowadays, hybrid biopolymer composites based on UHMWPE are a noble choice for use as linear or acetabular component in hip joint prosthesis.

11.2.1 MATRIX MATERIAL: ULTRA-HIGH-MOLECULAR-WEIGHT POLYETHYLENE (UHMWPE)

UHMWPE is a thermoplastic polymer contains only hydrogen and carbon. It have simple chemical structure but its order of directorial structure at molecular level makes it much more complex [65]. UHMWPE is one type of polymer which is used as articulating surface or linear of bearing in hip joint prosthesis because of many advantages. This thermoplastic is tough with predominant impact strength. Other important properties such as no water immersion, high corrosion resistance, non-toxic, non-sticking as well as self-lubricating make a better material for the articulating surface of bearing in hip joint replacement [66–68]. This material also provides tremendous mechanical properties in cryogenic environment. It decreases noise and vibration, harmful effect of chemical reaction [68, 10]. So, UHMWPE offers a combination of exceptional properties compare to other polymer.

Mechanical properties of UHMWPE have also been depending upon percentage of crystalline nature of the polymer and morphology of the crystalline region. This percentage of crystalline nature of UHMWPE related to the real polymer yield strength by a quadratic relationship meaningfully [69]. Linear semi-crystalline UHMWPE polymer can be divided into two phase: (a) crystalline phase and (b) amorphous phase. This semi-crystalline polymer has deformation, possibility of fragmentation as well as degradation of crystalline region. UHMWPE has superior wear resistance with low coefficient of friction and chemical resistance compare to other polymer [70–72]. Wear of UHMWPE produce long-term failure due to osteolysis. Means, wear debris particles of this material over certain period of time start inflammation and bone loss. Other disadvantage of this material is poor wettability result low interfacial bond strength [73–75]. Melting point of this material is approximate 144°C but mechanical properties degrade at 70°C. So UHMWPE bend with high heat resistance material to increase thermal resistance property [76].

Finally, one of the major problems of UHMWPE is related to wear debris particles when use as a linear for bearing surface in hip joint implant. So, the researcher developed different type of UHMWPE. Nowadays, attention of researcher communities has been developing new alternate UHMWPE by (a) increase the cross linkage in polyethylene, (b) hybrid biopolymer composite [77, 78]. Crosslinking and its subsequent use as reinforcing filler are the best known methods to improve polymer performance. Crosslinking is an extensively used technique to reduce wear, by means of electron beam and gamma irradiation. This effects the reorientation of the polymer

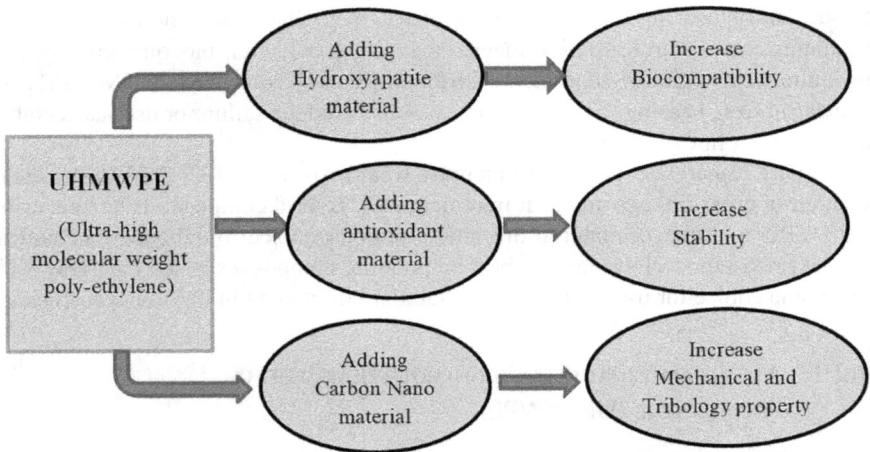

FIGURE 11.3   The objective of hydroxyapatite, antioxidant, and carbon nanomaterial using as filler material in ultra-high-molecular-weight polyethylene.

chains along shear stress, leading to weakened polymer upon perpendicular sliding along the direction of orientation [79].

Juan Carlos et al. [80] conclude that hardness and wear property of UHMWPE vary with respect to temperature. Here, temperature is taken for hardness analysis at (20°C, 25°C, 30°C, 35°C, 40°C, 45°C, 50°C, 55°C, 60°C) and wears analysis at (20°C, 30°C, 40°C, 50°C). In this experiment, hardness value decreases with increase temperature and wear resistance property also decreases. Here, the rate of reduction of wear property much more compared with rate of reduction of hardness value. So, the temperature variation is one of the important factors to provide the stability of material's properties.

Few organic oxides such as zirconia oxide, Vitamin E provide stability during wear process. UHMWPE with different type of reinforcement filler material developed different types of composite for industrial, aerospace and biomedical application. The aim of developed composite material increases the wear resistance and mechanical performance of materials compare to pure UHMWPE [81]. So, UHMWPE used as linear for bearing surface in hip joint implant improves its wear resistance property, decreases friction coefficient, increases mechanical strength, and provides stability in human environment. All these problems reduced by single reinforced in UHMWPE are not possible. So, the hybrid biopolymer composite is the better option compared to single material.

11.2.1.1   Effect of hydroxyapatite (HA) with ultra-high-molecular-weight polyethylene (UHMWPE)

Hydroxyapatite (HA) is good bio-active ceramic materials but brittle nature has been restricted in scope of medical application [82]. HA structure analogous to the mineral parts of human bone so its increase the biocompatibility of composite [83]. Mechanical property of HA is low like strength, fatigue resistance, toughness, and

TABLE 11.2

Effect of hydroxyapatite (HA) use as filler material in ultra-high-molecular-weight polyethylene (UHMWPE)

Sl. no	Matrix/filler	Fabrication process	Result	Ref.
1.	UHMWPE/HA (0, 13.3%, 23.5 v % and 31.5% by volume	Compression moulding/ Ultrasonication and stirred/Hot oven	Friction coefficient and wear minimum at 31.5% volume of HA at 150°C compared with 150°C. Flexural yield stress, flexural modulus, flexural yield strain, and maximum strain up to breaking are high at 180°C (moulding temperature) compared with 150°C. Maximum crystallinity obtains at 150°C and 31.5% volume of HA.	[82]
2.	UHMWPE/HA	Review	High modulus of elasticity cause of implant failure due to stress shielding effect. Polymer wear rate is inversely proportional to surface strength such as hardness and creep strength.	[83]
3.	UHMWPE/HA	swelling/ball milling/hot compression moulding	Ball milling and swelling treated composite sample have perform better mechanical properties compare to other sample. Here, Young's modulus of elasticity increase up to 90% and yield strength double compared with pure UHMWPE.	[85]
4.	UHMWPE/HA	Twin-screw extrusion and compression moulding (230°C, 10 MPa).	Young moduli increase up to nine percent (HA content 50 wt.%) compared to pure UHMWPE. Percentage of elongation and tensile strain continuous decrease up to 50 wt.% HA contents. Composite exhibited superior ductility compared to pure UHMWPE because of percentage of plastic strain more in composite	[86]
5.	HDPE/HA in ethanol	Compression- moulding (145°C, 5 MPa).	Whisker HA /HDPE increase 4–5 times fatigue life compared with HDPE/20 volume % HA but 20 volumes % HA reinforced HDPE have more fatigue life compared with 40 volumes % HA. HA whisker has low stiffness loss, less permanent deformation as well as low dissipation of energy at a given no. of cycle related to HA powder.	[87]
6.	HDPE/HA	Twin-screw extruder and Gamma radiation/Gamma Irradiation	Tensile storage, creep-recovery behaviour, and modulus improve with increasing the HA nanoparticles ratio. Crystallinity, creep recovery, viscoelastic, and relaxation behaviour of HDPE nanocomposite improved due to gamma irradiation.	[88]
7.	UHMWPE/Vitamin E	Review	Vitamin E in matrix material react with free radical, decrease the oxidation and wear degradation of UHMWPE. Finally, Vitamin E in UHMWPE increases resistance to wear and fatigue. Coating on surface of UHMWPE increases mechanical as well as wear resistance properties. Effective texturing improves the friction and wear on mating surfaces	[89]

(Continued)

TABLE 11.2
Continued

Sl. no	Matrix/filler	Fabrication process	Result	Ref.
8.	UHMWPE/ Vitamin E	Blending and diffusion of vitamin E into UHMWPE during irradiation	Vitamin E reduces oxidative degradation of UHMWPE. Diffusion of UHMWPE into UHMWPE after radiation crosslinking have more wear resistance and mechanical property compared to blend vitamin E with UHMWPE powder before consolidation.	[90]
9.	UHMWPE/ ULPWPE/ Xylene	compression moulding (10 MPa, 200°C, 2h) and injection moulding (200–230°C)	Yield strength, ultimate tensile strength, Young's modulus, impact strength, fatigue strength more in injection moulding ultra-high-molecular-weight polyethylene in controlled manner (MP-UHMWPE) compared with compression moulding ultra-high-molecular-weight polyethylene (CM-UHMWPE). Break to elongation in MP-UHMWPE were less but in permissible limit of knee joint application. Wear resistance property also improve in MP-UHMWPE compared with CM-UHMWPE.	[91]
10.	UHMWPE/HA (0 to 5 volume %)	-	Increase the volume % of HA in UHMWPE increase the mass density. Young's modulus, yield strength maximum at 3% volume fraction of HA whereas ultimate strength decreases continuously.	[84]
11.	UHMWPE/HA (20 wt.%) /BO (5 and 10 wt.%) UHMWPE (M. W = 3 × 10⁶g/mol) and HA (2–3 µm)	Planetary ball milling and compression moulding (300°C, 10 MPa). Sample is U, UH, UHB 5, UHB 10.	Degree of crystallinity continuous decrease and less in UHMWPE/HA/BO-(10 wt.%) composite. Tensile strength of composite material (UHMWPE/HA/BO) compared with pure UHMWPE was less but more than UHMWPE/HA. Young's modulus maximum in UHMWPE/HA/BO compared with UHMWPE and UHMWPE/HA Wear, Surface roughness and friction coefficient minimum in UHMWPE/HA/BO compared to UHMWPE and UHMWPE/HA. Wear and friction coefficient of UHMWPE/HA less compared to pure UHMWPE, but Surface roughness more compared with pure UHMWPE.	[3]
12.	UHMWPE/HA (0, 1 and 7 wt.%)	Vacuum-hot pressing, Ball mill, radiated and irradiated sample	The irradiated UHMWPE/7% nano-HAP also had a synergistic function of wear reduction. Crystallinity, density of non-irradiated sample is greater than irradiated sample. This crystallinity and density increase with increase filler content. Ultimate stress and strain decrease with increase filler content but modulus of elasticity increase. These ultimate stress, strain and modulus of elasticity have been lower value in irradiate sample compared with non-irradiated.	[92]
13.	UHMWPE/HA	Vacuum hot press moulding	Higher surface density of HA resulted lower contact angle of micro-composite.	[93]
14.	UHMWPE/HA	Vacuum hot press moulding	Wear resistance property increase with increase filler content into UHMWPE (approximate 40%). Tensile property of this new micro-composite did not give satisfactory result.	[94]

brittleness although high degree of crystalline nature and high structure stability make it more attractive. Degree of crystalline nature of material is directly proportional to hardness and stiffness. Structure of HA close to the bone tissue therefore HA is the important material for the human bone and mineral. So, HA use in bio-degradable (PLGA, PLL, PHB) as well as non-biodegradable (HDPE, PMMA, PA, UHMWPE) materials to increase the stiffness [84].

UHMWPE has limitation related to Young's modulus and wear resistance property. It produces permanent deformation and cause of revision surgery [2]. UHMWPE have very high melt viscosity and also dissolve in very few solvents such as paraffin oil, xylene, and decline. So, the uniform dispersion of HA powder in UHMWPE matrix is difficult [1 to 3]. J. Crowley [95] concludes that hydroxyapatite (HA) is one type of mineral that is close to component of bone. So, it has the ability to integrate into the bone structure and support to bone growth. In this experiment, authors conclude that increasing the volume % of HA in UHMWPE increases the mass density. Here, Young's modulus and yield strength are maximum at 3% volume fraction of HA whereas ultimate strength decreases continuously. Since mixing and uniform dispersion of HA in UHMWPE and different types of fabrication method effect on the quality of UHMWPE/HA composite. So, there are different fabrication processes for UHMWPE/HA composite have been proposed such as solid-state mixing, thermal forming, UHMWPE in paraffin oil using twin-screw extrusion, and compression mounding [1]. Moulded UHMWPE is more wear resistant compared with extruded UHHMWPE [89].

UHMWPE/HA composite material properties depend on moulding temperature. Wear-resistant and friction coefficient of UHMWPE/HA gradient composites moulded at 150°C are better than gradient composite moulded at 180°C, although flexural property is slightly poor. Advantage of gradient composite avoids the cracking under flexural stress. Here, flexural yield stress, flexural yield strain, maximum strain up to breaking and flexural modulus are high at 180°C compared with 150°C [82].

UHMWPE/HA mixing in paraffin oil by twin-screw extrusion and fabricated the composite material by compression moulding (230°C, 10 MPa). Here, % of elongation and tensile strain decrease continuous up to 50 wt% HA content. Yield strength give approximate the same value [86]. UHMWPE/HA composite prepared by using swelling/ball milling/hot compression moulding (180°C and 100 MPa) perform better mechanical and wear resistance property compared with non-swelling composite. Weight percentage of HA (50 nm) powder was 30 wt% in UHMWPE increase Young's modulus of elasticity up to 90% and yield strength double compare to pure UHMWPE [85].

A.V. Maksimkin et al. [96] fabricate the composite material by UHMWPE and varying percentage of HA (0 wt%, 10 wt%, 20 wt%, 30 wt%, 40 wt%, 50 wt%, 60 wt%). In this experiment, the degree of crystallinity and modulus of elasticity both increased continuously with increasing wt.% of HA. Friction coefficient of composite have minimum at 50 wt% of HA. Ultimate strength has increases up to 10 wt.% of HA after that its decrease. Maximum value of yield strength of composite obtained at 20 wt.% of nano-HA. Author concludes that optimal concentration of HA in the UHMWPE matrix is 50% and better mechanical properties obtained at 20 wt.% of HA.

Mechanical strength obtained in injection moulding (IM) of UHMWPE at (200–230°C) more compared with compression moulding (CM) of UHMWPE at (10 MPa, 200°C, 2 h). Break to elongation in IM-UHMWPE were less compared with CM-UHMWPE. Wear resistance property also improve in IM-UHMWPE compared with CM-UHMWPE [91]. In this experiment, authors conclude that mechanical property and tribological property improve in injection moulding process compared with compression moulding process. HA (20 volume %) reinforced HDPE have more fatigue life compared with HA (40 volume %) using compression moulding (145°C, 5 MPa) [87]. Ultimate stress and strain decrease with increase filler content HA (up to 7 wt.%) in UHMWPE but modulus of elasticity increase. Higher surface density of HA resulted lower contact angle of micro-composite. So the water wetted surface obtained [94]. Wear resistance property increase with increase filler content (HA) into UHMWPE (approximate 40%). Tensile property of this new micro-composite did not give satisfactory result [93].

11.2.1.2 Effect of carbon nanomaterials or other additive with ultra-high-molecular-weight polyethylene (UHMWPE)

Low interaction between UHMWPE and HA has been one of the complications that effects of low mechanical and low tribological performance in a this composite material due to the development of microstructural defects and agglomeration [97]. Due to this reason, HA nanoparticle use with other reinforcement such as carbon nano particle, graphene nanoplates, graphene oxide, zirconium oxide, organophilic bentonite, etc. in UHMWPE. There are different author fabricates the hybrid biopolymer composite and conclude that mechanical as well as tribological property improve compared to biopolymer composite (UHMWPE with HAp). Many researchers are found that when HAp use with small amount of carbon nano particle; drastically change in mechanical as well as tribological properties.

Carbon nanotubes (CNTs), graphene oxide (GO) and graphene nano-platelets (GNP) are allotrope of carbon belong to carbon family. These material can be consider as biomedical implant because of their mechanical, thermal and electrical properties [98, 7]. Carbon nano tubes have higher Young's modulus and aspect ratio [99].

There are many researchers who work with carbon-nanoparticle-reinforced UHMWPE composite and find that the wear resistance and mechanical properties largely improve in comparison with pure (pristine) UHMWPE.

Jawed K. Oleiwi et al. [104] compares the mechanical and tribological properties of HA and CNT with UHMWPE. Here wt.% of each reinforced is 1,2,3,5 wt.% in UHMWPE. Mechanical properties such as compression strength, Flexural strength, flexural modulus, flexural strain, max shear stress and impact strength give best result at 3 wt.% of CNT in UHMWPE but in case of HA flexural strength, flexural modulus, max shear stress increase up to 5 wt.% but Flexural modulus, and impact strength increase up to 3 wt.% after that its decrease. In this experimental analysis, volumetric wear rate decrease in both type of nanocomposite continuous up to 5 wt.%.

So, advance ceramic materials, such as CNT (carbon nanotube), graphene oxide or graphene use in fewer amounts reinforce with UHMWPE give better wear-resistant and mechanical properties compare to pure UHMWPE. The nanoadditives in

TABLE 11.3
Effect of different type of filler material in ultra-high-molecular-weight polyethylene (UHMWPE)

Sl. no	Matrix material	Reinforcement material	Method	Result	Ref.
1.	UHMWPE	Multi-walled CNTs (1 wt.%, 3 wt.% and 5 wt.%)	Compression moulding	Hardness increase (4, 18, 25 %) Creep displacement decrease (18, 21 & 29 %) Elastic modulus increase (7, 3 & 16.7 %)	[100]
2.	UHMWPE	CNT (0.5 wt.%)	Ball Milling, Sonication, and compression moulding	Sonication method is identified as superior, but ball milling and sonication attained similar COF and hardness value.	[80]
3.	UHMWPE	CNT (0.05 and 0.1 in wt.%)	Sonication and Ball milling, compression moulding	Composite have higher aspect ratio has shown greater hardness, greater elastic modulus, greater tribological behaviour and also thermal stability compared with composite having lower aspect ratio. Addition of 0.05 wt.% of HARC in PE reduces the wear rate by 76% as compared to PE but addition of 0.1 wt.% reinforcement reduces the wear rate by 53%.	[101]
4.	UHMWPE	CNT and HA Each contain (1, 2, 3 and 5 wt.%)	20 MPa and 61.6 shore D for UHMWPE	Highest value of compression strength and Hardness is 40.5 MPa (3% n-HAP) and 66 shore D (3% CNT).	[102]
5.	UHMWPE	CNT and HA Each contain (1, 2, 3 and 5 wt.%)	.0285 MPa flexural strength of UHMWPE	Flexural strength continuous increase up to 5 wt.% in case of HA [.0382 MPa] but in case of CNT increase up to 3 wt.% and further decrease. Flexural strength, flexural modulus, flexural strain, max shear stress and impact strength give best result at 3 wt.% of CNTs. Flexural strength, flexural modulus max shear stress increases up to 5 wt.%. Flexural modulus and impact strength increase up to 3 wt.% after that its decrease.	[103]

(Continued)

TABLE 11.3
Continued

Sl. no	Matrix material	Reinforcement material	Method	Result	Ref.
6.	UHMWPE	CNT and HA Each contain (1 wt.%, 2 wt.%, 3 wt.% and 5 wt.%.)		Volumetric wear rate decreases in both type of nano composite. Volumetric wear rate in UHMWPE+ HA is less.	[104]
7.	UHMWPE	GO (0.1, 0.3, 0.7, 1, 2, 3) in wt.%	Stirring and hot pressing	Wear rates decrease up to 1 wt.% of GO. Frictional coefficient slight increase continuous.	[105]
8.	UHMWPE	GO (.1, .3, .7, 1) in wt.%	Ultrasonic disperse--on, High speed ball mixing, Hot pressing moulding	Coefficient of friction, scratch depth, wear rate decreases continuous with increase of GO, but Micro- hardness increase continuous.	[106]
9.	UHMWPE	fluorinated graphene (0.1, 0.3, 0.5, 1) in wt.%	Ultrasonication, stirring and Hot pressing, MTT assay	Micro hardness increases continuous up to 64% and wear rate decrease up to 43%. The toxicity of graphene was detected by osteoblast. Graphene showed toxicity when the grapheme concentration reached to 1 wt.% in composite	
10.	UHMWPE	HA (10 wt.%) and GNP (0.1 wt.%, 0.5 wt.% and 1 wt.%) Sample is [U, UH, UHG (.1), UHG (0.5), UHG [1]	Ultrasonication with ethanol, Stirred and Hot pressing	Yield strength and Tensile strength increase with increase Filler content. Average coefficient of friction decreases with increase Filler content Except for UHG [1] (54% friction coefficient decrease) Wear rates decrease with increase Filler content. (80% wear reduction).	[107]
11.	UHMWPE	Zirconia-nanoparticle/ hydroxyapatite	Tensile, Vickers hardness and pin on desk test	Improve wear resistance, increase tensile strength and hardness.	[11]

composite materials decrease coefficient of friction as well as increase wear resistance. This is possible because of thin tenacious transfer film developed at counter surface of composites [108]. In particulate reinforce composite, size, shape, type, and content of filler material play an important role to improve the tribological property in sliding as well as wear resistance.

Meysam Salari et al. [11] fabricate the hybrid biopolymer composite with UHMWPE-reinforced zirconia nanoparticle and hydroxyapatite. In this experiment, authors conclude that wear resistance and mechanical properties such as tensile strength and hardness of composite improve compared to pure form of UHMWPE. Crystalline nature, viscoelastic and creep recovery for HDPE nanocomposite improved due gamma irradiation as compare to gamma radiation [88]. Irradiation sample have low wear and low coefficient of friction. These ultimate stress, strain and modulus of elasticity have been lower value in irradiate sample compare to non-irradiated [92]. Finally, Irradiation sample have greater significance compare to radiation sample for articulating surface of bearing couple in hip joint.

During Irradiation, oxidative degradation of UHMWPE increases in air means increase wear and decrease the mechanical strength. So, it decreases the life of implant. Vitamin E is one type of antioxidant in UHMWPE which stabilized the UHMWPE [109, 90]. Vitamin E in matrix material reacts with free radical and decreases the oxidation and wear degradation of UHMWPE. Finally, Vitamin E in UHMWPE increases resistance to wear and fatigue [89].

There are two methods to incorporating vitamin E in UHMWPE (1) Blend vitamin E with UHMWPE powder before consolidation (2) diffusion of UHMWPE into UHMWPE after radiation crosslinking. Vitamin E blends UHMWPE powder before consolidation during irradiation protects the polymer from oxidation but reduce the efficiency of crosslinking. So it increases wears resistance property but decreases the mechanical property [90]. Diffusion of UHMWPE into UHMWPE after radiation crosslinking increases wear resistance property. Here, mechanical property is less than pure UHMWPE but much more than Vitamin E blend UHMWPE [90].

Bentonite is one type of a clay material (2:1 type alumina-silicate) used in biomedical applications such as adsorption of pollutants. Wear resistance and mechanical property also improve adding organic bentonite (BO) in UHMWPE/HA composite [84]. Some organic molecules use with bentonite to decrease the hydrophilic nature of bentonite. This modified and new biomaterial is known as organophilic bentonite. Here, the degree of crystallinity continuous to decrease and is less in UHMWPE/HA/BO-(10 wt.%) composite. Young's modulus of elasticity is higher in BO and HA contain composite. Wear, surface roughness, and friction coefficient is minimum in UHMWPE/HA/BO compared with UHMWPE and UHMWPE/HA [84]. Tensile strength of composite material (UHMWPE/HA/BO) is less compared with pure UHMWPE but more than UHMWPE/HA. Mechanical and tribological properties improve when 10 wt.% BO use in UHMWPE/HA [84]. Means, using BO in UHMWPE/HA decrease wear and coefficient of friction as well as improve Young's modulus, tensile property.

Addition of nano zinc oxide particle in UHMWPE/HA composite had not significantly affect its mechanical properties but obtained good antibacterial properties in the sample [110]. Al_2O_3 containing composite show better densification compared with HA and CNTs reinforcement composite because sub-micron size of Al_2O_3 [111]. The follow-up period which use ceramic-on-PE mean 8.22 year on total CoP based hip implant and ceramic-on-ceramic mean 9.23 year for CoC hip implant [112]. This difference is very small and in future CoP may be performed better compared with CoC.

11.3 CONCLUSION

Nowadays, hip joint replacement becomes a talk of medical application due to increasing issues in human hip joints. Majorly most effective part of synthesis hip who get affected with time is bearing couple. Ceramic-on-ceramic and ceramic-on-polyethylene are largely available in the market. But focus of the researcher is to increase the life of synthesis hip (greater than 15 year) and reduce the sudden fracture of the prosthesis (brittle fracture in ceramic). Ultra-high-molecular-weight polyethylene (UHMWPE) uses either linear in CoC bearing or acetabular component in CoP bearing uses by surgeon.

Compared with other type of polymer, UHMWPE uses as articulating surface of bearing in synthesis hip joint. But disadvantage of this material low yield strength, high wear as well as low compatibility with bone and tissue. Improve the mechanical compatibility and wear resistance properties ceramic nanomaterial use as filler material is better option.

Hydroxyapatite (HA) uses as filler material in UHMWPE improve compatibility as well as wear resistance properties but low interaction between UHMWPE and HA has been one of the complications that effects mechanical and tribological performance of composite. This is due to the development of microstructural defects and agglomeration of nano particle.

Increasing interaction between HA and UHMWPE, there are some materials used, such as organophilic bentonite (BO), Aluminium oxide (Al_2O_3) nanoparticle, zinc oxide (ZnO_2), and carbon nanoparticles. All these nanomaterials adding into UHMWPE/HA improve mechanical compatibility as well as wear resistance properties. But ceramic nanomaterials drastically change mechanical and tribological properties of UHMWPE/HA composite compared with other types of additive use in composite material.

REFERENCES

1. Merola, M., & Affatato, S. (2019). Materials for hip prostheses: a review of wear and loading considerations. *Materials, 12*(3), 495.
2. Benzon, H. M., Rathmell, J. P., Wu, C. L., Turk, D. C., Argoff, C. E., & Hurley, R. W. (2022). *Practical Management of Pain E-Book*. Elsevier Health Sciences, New York, USA.
3. Ghalme, S. G., Mankar, A., & Bhalerao, Y. (2016). Biomaterials in hip joint replacement. *International Journal of Materials Science and Engineering, 4*(2), 113–125.
4. Das, S. S., & Chakraborti, P. (2018, June). Development of biomaterial for total hip joint replacement. In *IOP Conference Series: Materials Science and Engineering* (Vol. 377, No. 1, p. 012177). IOP Publishing.
5. Xu, H., Zhang, D., Chen, K., & Zhang, T. (2019). Taper fretting behavior of PEEK artificial hip joint. *Tribology International, 137*, 30–38.
6. Wyles, C. C., Jimenez-Almonte, J. H., Murad, M. H., Norambuena-Morales, G. A., Cabanela, M. E., Sierra, R. J., & Trousdale, R. T. (2015). There are no differences in short-to mid-term survivorship among total hip-bearing surface options: a network meta-analysis. *Clinical Orthopaedics and Related Research®, 473*(6), 2031–2041.
7. Affatato, S., Ruggiero, A., & Merola, M. (2015). Advanced biomaterials in hip joint arthroplasty. A review on polymer and ceramics composites as alternative bearings. *Composites Part B: Engineering, 83*, 276–283.

8. Gómez-Barrena, E., Medel, F., & Puértolas, J. A. (2009). Polyethylene oxidation in total hip arthroplasty: evolution and new advances. *The Open Orthopaedics Journal*, *3*, 115.
9. Affatato, S., Colic, K., Hut, I., Mirjanić, D., Pelemiš, S., & Mitrovic, A. (2018). Short history of biomaterials used in hip arthroplasty and their modern evolution. In Saverio Affatato, Katarina Colic, Igor Hut, D. Mirjanić, S. Pelemiš & Aleksandra Mitrovic (eds.), *Biomaterials in Clinical Practice* (pp. 1–21). Springer, Cham.
10. Goyal, S., Tandon, T., Sangoi, D., & Dawe, E. J. (2019). Total joint replacement. In Iyer, K. M. & Khan, W. S. (eds.), *General Principles of Orthopedics and Trauma* (pp. 429–489). Springer, Cham.
11. Salari, M., Mohseni Taromsari, S., Bagheri, R., & Faghihi Sani, M. A. (2019). Improved wear, mechanical, and biological behavior of UHMWPE-HAp-zirconia hybrid nanocomposites with a prospective application in total hip joint replacement. *Journal of Materials Science*, *54*(5), 4259–4276.
12. Aherwar, A., Singh, A. K., & Patnaik, A. (2015). Current and future biocompatibility aspects of biomaterials for hip prosthesis. *AIMS Bioeng*, *3*(1), 23–43.
13. Ait Moussa, A., Fischer, J., Yadav, R., & Khandaker, M. (2017). Minimizing stress shielding and cement damage in cemented femoral component of a hip prosthesis through computational design optimization. *Advances in Orthopaedics*, *2017*, 1–12.
14. Singh, S. & Harsha, A. P. (2015). Analysis of femoral components of cemented total hip arthroplasty. *Journal of the Institution of Engineers (India): Series D*, *97*, 113–120.
15. Ishihara, K. (2015). Highly lubricated polymer interfaces for advanced artificial hip joints through biomimetic design. *Polymer Journal*, *47*(9), 585–597.
16. Filho, L., Schmidt, S., Leifer, K., Engqvist, H., Högberg, H., & Persson, C. (2019). Towards functional silicon nitride coatings for joint replacements. *Coatings*, *9*(2), 73.
17. Pietrzak, W. S. (2021). Ultra-high molecular weight polyethylene for total hip acetabular liners: a brief review of current status. *Journal of Investigative Surgery*, *34*(3), 321–323.
18. Goswami, C., Bhat, I. K., Bathula, S., Singh, T., & Patnaik, A. (2019). Physicomechanical and surface wear assessment of magnesium oxide filled ceramic composites for hip implant application. *Silicon*, *11*(1), 39–49.
19. Vallés, G., & Vilaboa, N. (2019). Osteolysis after total hip arthroplasty: basic science. In Eduardo García-Rey & Eduardo García-Cimbrelo (eds.), *Acetabular Revision Surgery in Major Bone Defects* (pp. 1–31). Springer, Cham.
20. Takahashi, K., Onodera, S., Tohyama, H., Kwon, H. J., Honma, K. I., & Yasuda, K. (2011). In vivo imaging of particle-induced inflammation and osteolysis in the calvariae of NFκB/luciferase transgenic mice. *Journal of Biomedicine and Biotechnology*, *2011*, 1–2.
21. Suñer, S., Tipper, J. L., Emami, N., Tipper, J. L., & Emami, N. (2016). Biological effects of wear particles generated in total joint replacements: trends and future prospects, *Tribology – Materials, Surfaces & Interfaces*, 39–52.
22. Maji, P. K., Roychowdhury, A., & Datta, D. (2013). Minimizing stress shielding effect of femoral stem—A review. *Journal of Medical Imaging and Health Informatics*, *3*(2), 171–178.
23. Gross, S. T., & Abel, E. W. (2001). A finite element analysis of hollow stemmed hip prostheses as a means of reducing stress shielding of the femur. *Journal of Biomechanics*, *34*(8), 995–1003.
24. Ebramzadeh, E., Sangiorgio, S. N., Longjohn, D. B., Buhari, C. F., Morrison, B. J., & Dorr, L. D. (2003). Effects of total hip arthroplasty cemented femoral stem surface finish, collar and cement thickness on load transfer to the femur. *Journal of Applied Biomaterials and Biomechanics*, *1*(1), 76–83.
25. Evans, S. L., & Gregson, P. J. (1994). Numerical optimization of the design of a coated, cementless hip prosthesis. *Journal of Materials Science: Materials in Medicine*, *5*(8), 507–510.

26. Xu, W., Crocombe, A. D., & Hughes, S. C. (2000). Finite element analysis of bone stress and strain around a distal osseointegrated implant for prosthetic limb attachment. *Proceedings of the Institution of Mechanical Engineers, Part H: Journal of Engineering in Medicine, 214*(6), 595–602.

27. Gemmell Jr, K. D., & Meyer, D. M. L. (2018). Wear of ultra high molecular weight polyethylene against synthetic sapphire as bearing coating for total joint replacements. *Research & Development in Material Science, 6*, 560–567.

28. Capello, W. N., D'Antonio, J. A., Feinberg, J. R., Manley, M. T., & Naughton, M. (2008). Ceramic-on-ceramic total hip arthroplasty: update. *The Journal of Arthroplasty, 23*(7), 39–43.

29. Atrey, A., Wolfstadt, J. I., Hussain, N., Khoshbin, A., Ward, S., Shahid, M., ... & Waddell, J. P. (2018). The ideal total hip replacement bearing surface in the young patient: a prospective randomized trial comparing alumina ceramic-on-ceramic with ceramic-on-conventional polyethylene: 15-year follow-up. *The Journal of Arthroplasty, 33*(6), 1752–1756.

30. Wang, T., Sun, J. Y., Zhao, X. J., Liu, Y., & Yin, H. B. (2016). Ceramic-on-ceramic bearings total hip arthroplasty in young patients. *Arthroplasty Today, 2*(4), 205–209.

31. Paxton, E. W., Inacio, M., Namba, R. S., Love, R., & Kurtz, S. M. (2015). Metal-on-conventional polyethylene total hip arthroplasty bearing surfaces have a higher risk of revision than metal-on-highly crosslinked polyethylene: results from a US registry. *Clinical Orthopaedics and Related Research®, 473*(3), 1011–1021.

32. Langhorn, J., Borjali, A., Hippensteel, E., Nelson, W., & Raeymaekers, B. (2018). Microtextured CoCrMo alloy for use in metal-on-polyethylene prosthetic joint bearings: multi-directional wear and corrosion measurements. *Tribology International, 124*, 178–183.

33. Shah, S. M., Walter, W. L., Tai, S. M., Lorimer, M. F., & de Steiger, R. N. (2017). Late dislocations after total hip arthroplasty: is the bearing a factor? *The Journal of Arthroplasty, 32*(9), 2852–2856.

34. Nečas, D., Vrbka, M., Galandáková, A., Křupka, I., & Hartl, M. (2019). On the observation of lubrication mechanisms within hip joint replacements. Part I: hard-on-soft bearing pairs. *Journal of the Mechanical Behavior of Biomedical Materials, 89*, 237–248.

35. Abazari, M. F., Gholizadeh, S., Karizi, S. Z., Birgani, N. H., Abazari, D., Paknia, S., ... & Delattre, C. (2021). Recent advances in cellulose-based structures as the wound-healing biomaterials: a clinically oriented review. *Applied Sciences, 11*(17), 7769.

36. Lee, H. H., Lee, S., Park, J. K., & Yang, M. (2018). Friction and wear characteristics of surface-modified titanium alloy for metal-on-metal hip joint bearing. *International Journal of Precision Engineering and Manufacturing, 19*(6), 917–924.

37. Drummond, J., Tran, P., & Fary, C. (2015). Metal-on-metal hip arthroplasty: a review of adverse reactions and patient management. *Journal of functional biomaterials, 6*(3), 486–499.

38. Choudhury, D., Walker, R., Ingle, P., Cheah, K., & Dowell, J. (2009). Friction reduction in metal-on-metal hip joint. *Journal of Medical Devices, 3*(2), 027509-1.

39. Lalmohamed, A., MacGregor, A. J., de Vries, F., Leufkens, H. G., & van Staa, T. P. (2013). Patterns of risk of cancer in patients with metal-on-metal hip replacements versus other bearing surface types: a record linkage study between a prospective joint registry and general practice electronic health records in England. *PloS One, 8*(7), e65891.

40. Macdonald, N., & Bankes, M. (2014). Ceramic on ceramic hip prostheses: a review of past and modern materials. *Archives of Orthopaedic and Trauma Surgery, 134*(9), 1325–1333.

41. Oberbach, T., Ortmann, C., Begand, S., & Glien, W. (2006). Investigations of an alumina ceramic with zirconia gradient for the application as load bearing implant for joint prostheses. In Faisal Mahmuddin, Juraj Marek, Gregor Pobegen & Ulrike Grossner (eds.), *Key Engineering Materials* (Vol. 309, pp. 1247–1250). Trans Tech Publications Ltd. Bäch SZ, SCHWYZ, Switzerland.

42. Roy, T., Choudhury, D., Ghosh, S., Mamat, A. B., & Pingguan-Murphy, B. (2015). Improved friction and wear performance of micro dimpled ceramic-on-ceramic interface for hip joint arthroplasty. *Ceramics International*, *41*(1), 681–690.

43. Affatato, S., Jaber, S. A., & Taddei, P. (2018). Ceramics for hip joint replacement. In Fatima Zivic, Saverio Affatato, Miroslav Trajanovic, Matthias Schnabelrauch, Nenad Grujovic, & Kwang Leong Choy (eds.), *Biomaterials in Clinical Practice* (pp. 167–181). Springer, Cham.

44. Castagnini, F., Bordini, B., Tassinari, E., Stea, S., Ancarani, C., & Traina, F. (2019). Delta-on-delta ceramic bearing surfaces in revision hip arthroplasty. *The Journal of Arthroplasty*, *34*(9), 2065–2071.

45. Meng, Q., Wang, J., Yang, P., Jin, Z., & Fisher, J. (2015). The lubrication performance of the ceramic-on-ceramic hip implant under starved conditions. *Journal of the Mechanical Behavior of Biomedical Materials*, *50*, 70–76.

46. Hu, D., Tie, K., Yang, X., Tan, Y., Alaidaros, M., & Chen, L. (2015). Comparison of ceramic-on-ceramic to metal-on-polyethylene bearing surfaces in total hip arthroplasty: a meta-analysis of randomized controlled trials. *Journal of Orthopaedic Surgery and Research*, *10*(1), 1–8.

47. Pitto, R. P., Garland, M., & Sedel, L. (2015). Are ceramic-on-ceramic bearings in total hip arthroplasty associated with reduced revision risk for late dislocation? *Clinical Orthopaedics and Related Research®*, *473*(12), 3790–3795.

48. Gallo, J., Barry Goodman, S., Lostak, J., & Janout, M. (2012). Advantages and disadvantages of ceramic on ceramic total hip arthroplasty: a review. *Biomedical Papers*, *156*(3), 204–212.

49. Howard, D. P., Wall, P. D. H., Fernandez, M. A., Parsons, H., & Howard, P. W. (2017). Ceramic-on-ceramic bearing fractures in total hip arthroplasty: an analysis of data from the National Joint Registry. *The Bone & Joint Journal*, *99*(8), 1012–1019.

50. Choudhury, D., Roy, T., Krupka, I., Hartl, M., & Mootanah, R. (2015). Tribological investigation of ultra-high molecular weight polyethylene against advanced ceramic surfaces in total hip joint replacement. *Proceedings of the Institution of Mechanical Engineers, Part J: Journal of Engineering Tribology*, *229*(4), 410–419.

51. Bandopadhyay, S., Bandyopadhyay, N., Ahmed, S., Yadav, V., & Tekade, R. K. (2019). Current research perspectives of orthopedic implant materials. *Biomaterials and Bionanotechnology*, *1*, 337–374.

52. Wang, S., Song, J., Liao, Z., Liu, Y., Zhang, C., & Liu, W. (2015). Study on the wettability and tribological behavior of different polymers as bearing materials for cervical prosthesis. *Journal of Materials Engineering and Performance*, *24*(6), 2481–2493.

53. Cash, D. J., & Khanduja, V. (2014). The case for ceramic-on-polyethylene as the preferred bearing for a young adult hip replacement. *Hip International*, *24*(5), 421–427.

54. Dong, Y. L., Li, T., Xiao, K., Bian, Y. Y., & Weng, X. S. (2015). Ceramic on ceramic or ceramic-on-polyethylene for total hip arthroplasty: a systemic review and meta-analysis of prospective randomized studies. *Chinese Medical Journal*, *128*(09), 1223–1231.

55. Pezzotti, G., & Yamamoto, K. (2014). Artificial hip joints: the biomaterials challenge. *Journal of the Mechanical Behavior of Biomedical Materials*, *31*, 3–20.

56. Traina, F., De Fine, M., Di Martino, A., & Faldini, C. (2013). Fracture of ceramic bearing surfaces following total hip replacement: a systematic review. *BioMed Research International*, 1–8.

57. Callaghan, J. J., & Liu, S. S. (2009). Ceramic on crosslinked polyethylene in total hip replacement: any better than metal on crosslinked polyethylene? *The Iowa Orthopaedic Journal*, *29*, 1.

58. Banoriya, D., Purohit, R., & Dwivedi, R. K. (2017). Advanced application of polymer based biomaterials. *Materials Today: Proceedings*, *4*(2), 3534–3541.

59. Tathe, A., Ghodke, M., & Nikalje, A. P. (2010). A brief review: biomaterials and their application. *International Journal of Pharmacy and Pharmaceutical Sciences*, *2*(4), 19–23.

60. Trommer, R. M., Maru, M. M., Oliveira Filho, W. L., Nykanen, V. P. S., Gouvea, C. P., Archanjo, B. S., ... & Achete, C. A. (2015). Multi-scale evaluation of wear in UHMWPE-metal hip implants tested in a hip joint simulator. *Biotribology*, 4, 1–11.
61. Pawelec, K. M., White, A. A., & Best, S. M. (2019). Properties and characterization of bone repair materials. In Kendell M. Pawelec and Josep A. Planell (eds.), *Bone Repair Biomaterials* (pp. 65–102). Woodhead Publishing, Abington Hall, Abington Cambridge, United Kingdom, CB21 6AH.
62. Gao, Y., & Jin, Z. M. (2019). Biomechanics and biotribology of UHMWPE artificial hip joints. In Jun Fu, Zhong-Min Jin, & Jin-Wu Wang (eds.), *UHMWPE Biomaterials for Joint Implants* (pp. 241–286). Springer, Singapore.
63. Chowdhury, S. R., Mishra, A., Pradhan, B., & Saha, D. (2004). Wear characteristic and biocompatibility of some polymer composite acetabular cups. *Wear*, 256(11–12), 1026–1036.
64. Steinbeck, M. J., Jablonowski, L. J., Parvizi, J., & Freeman, T. A. (2014). The role of oxidative stress in aseptic loosening of total hip arthroplasties. *The Journal of Arthroplasty*, 29(4), 843–849.
65. Dayyoub, T., Maksimkin, A. V., Kaloshkin, S., Kolesnikov, E., Chukov, D., Dyachkova, T. Y. P., & Gutnik, I. (2018). The structure and mechanical properties of the UHMWPE films modified by the mixture of graphene nanoplates with polyaniline. *Polymers*, 11(1), 23.
66. Garbuz, D. S., Hargreaves, B. A., Duncan, C. P., Masri, B. A., Wilson, D. R., & Forster, B. B. (2014). The John Charnley Award: diagnostic accuracy of MRI versus ultrasound for detecting pseudotumors in asymptomatic metal-on-metal THA. *Clinical Orthopaedics and Related Research®*, 472(2), 417–423.
67. Ermis, K., & Unal, H. (2018). Friction and wear performance of medical grade UHMWPE polymer with numerical analysis. *MOJ Polymer Science*, 2(2), 60–66.
68. McKellop, H., Shen, F. W., Lu, B., Campbell, P., & Salovey, R. (1999). Development of an extremely wear-resistant ultra high molecular weight polythylene for total hip replacements. *Journal of Orthopaedic Research*, 17(2), 157–167.
69. Sobieraj, M. C., & Rimnac, C. M. (2009). Ultra high molecular weight polyethylene: mechanics, morphology, and clinical behavior. *Journal of the Mechanical Behavior of Biomedical Materials*, 2(5), 433–443.
70. Sreekanth, P. R., & Kanagaraj, S. (2013). Assessment of bulk and surface properties of medical grade UHMWPE based nanocomposites using Nanoindentation and microtensile testing. *Journal of the Mechanical Behavior of Biomedical Materials*, 18, 140–151.
71. Panin, S. V., Kornienko, L. A., Alexenko, V. O., Buslovich, D. G., Bochkareva, S. A., & Lyukshin, B. A. (2020). Increasing wear resistance of UHMWPE by loading enforcing carbon fibers: effect of irreversible and elastic deformation, friction heating, and filler size. *Materials*, 13(2), 338.
72. Affatato, S., Jaber, S. A., & Taddei, P. (2018). Polyethylene based polymer for joint replacement. In Fatima Zivic, Saverio Affatato, Miroslav Trajanovic, Matthias Schnabelrauch, Nenad Grujovic, & Kwang Leong Choy (eds.), *Biomaterials in Clinical Practice* (pp. 149–165). Springer, Cham.
73. Williams, S., Butterfield, M., Stewart, T., Ingham, E., Stone, M., & Fisher, J. (2003). Wear and deformation of ceramic-on-polyethylene total hip replacements with joint laxity and swing phase microseparation. *Proceedings of the Institution of Mechanical Engineers, Part H: Journal of Engineering in Medicine*, 217(2), 147–153.
74. Baxter, R. M., MacDonald, D. W., Kurtz, S. M., & Steinbeck, M. J. (2013). Characteristics of highly cross-linked polyethylene wear debris in vivo. *Journal of Biomedical Materials Research Part B: Applied Biomaterials*, 101(3), 467–475.
75. Shimel, M., Gouzman, I., Grossman, E., Barkay, Z., Katz, S., Bolker, A., ... & Verker, R. (2018). Enhancement of wetting and mechanical properties of UHMWPE-based composites through alumina atomic layer deposition. *Advanced Materials Interfaces*, 5(14), 1800295.

76. Chen, S., Li, J., Jin, Y., Xiao, J., Khosla, T., Hua, M., ... & Duan, H. (2018). Fabrication of polyimide-modified UHMWPE composites and enhancement effect on tribological properties. *Polymer-Plastics Technology and Engineering, 57*(7), 700–707.
77. Kurtz, S. M. (2016). The origins of UHMWPE in total hip arthroplasty. In Steven M. Kurtz (ed.), *UHMWPE Biomaterials Handbook* (pp. 33–44). William Andrew Publishing, Pennsylvania.
78. Affatato, S. (2018). Towards wear testing of high demanding daily activities on total hip replacement: preliminary results. *Journal of the Brazilian Society of Mechanical Sciences and Engineering, 40*(5), 1–6.
79. Ravishanker Baliga, B. A., Sharath Rao, K. B., Raghuvir Pai, B. C., & Satish Shenoy, B. D., (2015). Current trends in mechanical property enhancement of UHMWPE for use in joint arthroplasty-a review. *International Conference on Computational Methods in Engineering and Health Sciences*, Universiti Putra, Malaysia.
80. Tenison, N., Baena, J. C., Yu, J., & Peng, Z. X. (2017). Development of mixing methods of UHMWPE/carbon nanotubes (CNT) composites for use in artificial joints. In Yunn lin hwang and Jeng Huar Horn (eds.), *Key Engineering Materials* (Vol. 739, pp. 81–86). Trans Tech Publications Ltd., Bäch SZ, SCHWYZ, Switzerland.
81. Puértolas, J. A., Castro, M., Morris, J. A., Ríos, R., & Ansón-Casaos, A. (2019). Tribological and mechanical properties of graphene nanoplatelet/PEEK composites. *Carbon, 141*, 107–122.
82. Shi, X., Bin, Y., Hou, D., & Matsuo, M. (2013). Surface characterization for ultrahigh molecular weight polyethylene/hydroxyapatite gradient composites prepared by the gelation/crystallization method. *ACS Applied Materials & Interfaces, 5*(5), 1768–1780.
83. Macuvele, D. L. P., Nones, J., Matsinhe, J. V., Lima, M. M., Soares, C., Fiori, M. A., & Riella, H. G. (2017). Advances in ultra high molecular weight polyethylene/hydroxy-apatite composites for biomedical applications: a brief review. *Materials Science and Engineering: C, 76*, 1248–1262.
84. Macuvele, D. L. P., Colla, G., Cesca, K., Ribeiro, L. F., da Costa, C. E., Nones, J., ... & Riella, H. G. (2019). UHMWPE/HA biocomposite compatibilized by organo-philic montmorillonite: an evaluation of the mechanical-tribological properties and its hemocompatibility and performance in simulated blood fluid. *Materials Science and Engineering: C, 100*, 411–423.
85. Fang, L., Leng, Y., & Gao, P. (2005). Processing of hydroxyapatite reinforced ultra-high molecular weight polyethylene for biomedical applications. *Biomaterials, 26*(17), 3471–3478.
86. Fang, L., Leng, Y., & Gao, P. (2006). Processing and mechanical properties of HA/UHMWPE nanocomposites. *Biomaterials, 27*(20), 3701–3707.
87. Kane, R. J., Converse, G. L., & Roeder, R. K. (2008). Effects of the reinforcement mor-phology on the fatigue properties of hydroxyapatite reinforced polymers. *Journal of the Mechanical Behavior of Biomedical Materials, 1*(3), 261–268.
88. Alothman, O. Y., Fouad, H., Al-Zahrani, S. M., Eshra, A., Al Rez, M. F., & Ansari, S. G. (2014). Thermal, creep-recovery and viscoelastic behavior of high density polyeth-ylene/hydroxyapatite nano particles for bone substitutes: effects of gamma radiation. *Biomedical Engineering Online, 13*(1), 1–15.
89. Hussain, M., Naqvi, R. A., Abbas, N., Khan, S. M., Nawaz, S., Hussain, A., ... & Khalid, M. W. (2020). Ultra-high-molecular-weight-polyethylene (UHMWPE) as a promising polymer material for biomedical applications: a concise review. *Polymers, 12*(2), 323.
90. Bracco, P., & Oral, E. (2011). Vitamin E-stabilized UHMWPE for total joint implants: a review. *Clinical Orthopaedics and Related Research®, 469*(8), 2286–2293.
91. Huang, Y. F., Xu, J. Z., Li, J. S., He, B. X., Xu, L., & Li, Z. M. (2014). Mechanical properties and biocompatibility of melt processed self-reinforced ultrahigh molecular weight polyethylene. *Biomaterials, 35*(25), 6687–6697.

92. Xiong, L., Xiong, D., Yang, Y., & Jin, J. (2011). Friction, wear, and tensile properties of vacuum hot pressing crosslinked UHMWPE/nano-HAP composites. *Journal of Biomedical Materials Research Part B: Applied Biomaterials, 98*(1), 127–138.

93. Zhang, M., Pare, P., King, R., & James, S. P. (2007). A novel ultra high molecular weight polyethylene–hyaluronan microcomposite for use in total joint replacements. II. Mechanical and tribological property evaluation. *Journal of Biomedical Materials Research Part A, 82*(1), 18–26.

94. Zhang, M., King, R., Hanes, M., & James, S. P. (2006). A novel ultra high molecular weight polyethylene–hyaluronan microcomposite for use in total joint replacements. I. Synthesis and physical/chemical characterization. *Journal of Biomedical Materials Research Part A: An Official Journal of The Society for Biomaterials, The Japanese Society for Biomaterials, and The Australian Society for Biomaterials and the Korean Society for Biomaterials, 78*(1), 86–96.

95. Crowley, J., & Chalivendra, V. B. (2008). Mechanical characterization of ultra-high molecular weight polyethylene–hydroxyapatite nanocomposites. *Bio-Medical Materials and Engineering, 18*(3), 149–160.

96. Maksimkin, A. V., Kaloshkin, S. D., Tcherdyntsev, V. V., Senatov, F. S., & Danilov, V. D. (2012). Structure and properties of ultra-high molecular weight polyethylene filled with disperse hydroxyapatite. *Inorganic Materials: Applied Research, 3*(4), 288–295.

97. Lusitâneo, D., et al. (2019). PT technology and management of the innovation, communitary university of the NU SC. *Materials Science and Engineering.*

98. Ganguly, D., Shahbazian-Yassar, R., & Shokuhfar, T. (2014). Recent advances in nanotubes for orthopedic implants. *Journal of Nanotechnology and Smart Materials, 1*, 201.

99. Nien, Y. H. (2011). The application of carbon nanotube to bone cement. *Carbon Nanotubes-Polymer Nanocomposites, 1*, 367–379.

100 Kang, X., Zhang, W., & Yang, C. (2016). Mechanical properties study of micro-and nano-hydroxyapatite reinforced ultrahigh molecular weight polyethylene composites. *Journal of Applied Polymer Science, 133*(3), 42869.

101 Kumar, R. M., Sharma, S. K., Kumar, B. M., & Lahiri, D. (2015). Effects of carbon nanotube aspect ratio on strengthening and tribological behavior of ultra high molecular weight polyethylene composite. *Composites Part A: Applied Science and Manufacturing, 76*, 62–72.

102 Oleiwi, J. K., Anaee, R. A., & Radhi, S. H. (2019). Compression and hardness with FTIR characterization of UHMWPE nanocomposites as ace tabular cup in hip joint replacement. *International Journal of Plastic and Polymer Technology, 8*(1), 1–10.

103 Oleiwi, J. K., Anaee, R. A., & Radhi, S. H. (2018). CNTS and NHA as reinforcement to improve flexural and impact properties of UHMWPE nanocomposites for hip joint applications. *Composites, 6*, 7.

104 Oleiwi, J. K., Anaee, R. A., & Radhi, S. H. (2018). Roughness wear and thermal analysis of UHMWPE nanocomposites as acetabular cup in hip joint replacement. *International Journal of Mechanical and Production Engineering Research and Development, 8*(6), 855–864.

105 Tai, Z., Chen, Y., An, Y., Yan, X., & Xue, Q. (2012). Tribological behavior of UHMWPE reinforced with graphene oxide nanosheets. *Tribology Letters, 46*(1), 55–63.

106 An, Y., Tai, Z., Qi, Y., Yan, X., Liu, B., Xue, Q., & Pei, J. (2014). Friction and wear properties of graphene oxide/ultrahigh-molecular-weight polyethylene composites under the lubrication of deionized water and normal saline solution. *Journal of Applied Polymer Science, 131*(1), 39640.

107 Taromsari, S. M., Salari, M., Bagheri, R., & Sani, M. A. F. (2019). Optimizing tribological, tensile & in-vitro biofunctional properties of UHMWPE based nanocomposites with simultaneous incorporation of graphene nanoplatelets (GNP) & hydroxyapatite (HAp) via a facile approach for biomedical applications. *Composites Part B: Engineering, 175*, 107181.

108 Sharma, M., Sharma, H., & Shannigrahi, S. (2017). Tribology of advanced composites/biocomposites materials. In Luigi Ambrosio (ed.), *Biomedical Composites* (pp. 413–429). Woodhead Publishing.

109 Massin, P., & Achour, S. (2017). Wear products of total hip arthroplasty: the case of polyethylene. *Morphologie*, *101*(332), 1–8.

110 Galli, R., Soares, M., Domingos, L. P., Batiston, E. B., Silva, L. L., de Mello, J. M. M., ... & Fiori, M. A. (2018). Biocomposite of ultra-high molecular weight polyethylene and hydroxyapatite with antibacterial properties by the incorporation of zinc oxide nanoparticles. In Clodomiro Alves Junior (ed.), *Materials Science Forum* (Vol. 930, pp. 258–263). Trans Tech Publications Ltd, Stafa-Zurich.

111 Gupta, A., Tripathi, G., Lahiri, D., & Balani, K. (2013). Compression molded ultra high molecular weight polyethylene–hydroxyapatite–aluminum oxide–carbon nanotube hybrid composites for hard tissue replacement. *Journal of Materials Science & Technology*, *29*(6), 514–522.

112 Roy, B. R., Nevelös, A. B., Ingham, E., Shaw, D. L., & Fisher, J. (2001). Comparison of ceramic on ceramic to ceramic on polyethylene total hip replacement. In Faisal Mahmuddin, Juraj Marek, Gregor Pobegen and Ulrike Grossner (eds.), *Key Engineering Materials* (Vol. 192, pp. 991–994). Trans Tech Publications Ltd., Bäch SZ, SCHWYZ, Switzerland.

Index

3D printing 156
3D tissue 94

additive manufacturing 155
aerosol jet 3D printing 162
alginate 23
alkaline phosphate 21
ANSYS 99
antibacterial molecules 108
antibiotics 102
anti-microbial 101
ASTM standards 158

bearing surface 184
binder jet printing 160
bio-based natural polymers 8
biocidal polymer 101
biocompatibility 13
biodegradable 13
bioerosion 44
bioimplants 158
biological ligands 61
biomarker 62
biomaterials 123, 128
biomedical 14
biomedical engineering 125
bio-polyethylene 7
biosensors 65

CAD model 99
carbon nanotube (CNT) 39
carboxymethyl chitin nanoparticles 21
cardiology 129
cell imaging 64
ceramic 37
chemotherapeutics 40
chitin and chitosan 9
collagen 15
composites 127
covalent binding 56
creep 148
curing behaviour 148
cytotoxicity 36

dental restoration 108
diffusion 43
diffusivities 80
discrete damage mechanism 96
drug delivery systems 60, 73
dynamic mechanical analysis 140

elasticity 25
electrochemical sensors 65
electrospinning 36
electrostatically 83
enzyme degradation 41
extrusion-based bioprinting 161

fibers 25
fibrils 128
fibrin 18
fibroblasts 46
fossil fuels 10
frequency sweep 143
fused deposition modelling 159

gel electrophoresis 45
gelatin 17
genotoxicity 45
glass transition 146
glucosamine and N-acetyl glucosamine 20

high density polyethylene 3
hip joint 181
humidity sweep 144
hyaluronic acid 19
hydrophilic 80

implants 34
inhalation 77
inkjet bio printing 161
interfacial interaction 145
intramuscular 76

laminated object manufacturing 161
laser-assisted bioprinting 162
liposomes 42
liquid crystal polymer (LCP) 39
loss modulus 141
low density polyethylene 3

mechanical properties 25
medical waste 98
metal-on-metal 185
metal-on-polyethylene (MOP) 184
metals 126
methacryloyloxydodecylpyridinium bromide
    (MDPB) 110
methacryloyloxyethyl phosphorylcholine
    (MPC) 109
microemulsion 105

micromechanics 96
microspheres 42
microwave irradiation 105
molecular imprinting 55, 58
molecular weight 41

nanocomposite 35
nanofillers 146
natural polymers 27
non-toxic 131
nylon 4

optimization 140
orthopaedic implants 129
osmotic control 81
osseointegration 131

permeability 26
pharmaceuticals 78
pharmacodynamics 75
pharmacokinetics 75
plasticizer 149
pluronic acid 172
poly (acrylic acid) 2
poly (alkylene oxide) 2
poly (vinyl alcohol) 2
poly-alcohols 80
poly vinyl chloride 4
polyacrylamide 2
polyamide (PA) 39
polybutylene succinate 7
polycaprolactone 17
polyhydroxyalkanoates (PHAs) 113
polyhydroxyalkanoates 6
polylactic acid 6
polylactic-co-glycolic acid (PLGA) 172
polymer blends 149
polymer-drug conjugate 86
polymeric materials 1
polymeric micelles 86
polymer-protein conjugate 86
polymethylmethacrylate (PMMA) 39
polypropylene 4

polystyrene 4
polytetrafluoroethylene 103
precipitation 105
proliferation 21
proliferation assay 46
prosthesis 182

quaternary ammonium methacrylates
      (QAMs) 109

redox-responsive polymers 84
rheological model 97

selective laser sintering 159
semi-crystalline 25
semi-crystalline polymers 2
shelf life 108
silk 24
sol gel 105
starch and cellulose 6
stereolithography 160
stiffness 146
storage modulus 141
stress sweep 143
subcutaneous 76
surgical implants 106
swelling control 81

Teflon 4
thermal stability 35
thermoplastics 3
time sweep 143
tissue engineering 157
tissue scaffolds 57
toxicology 33
tribological performance 121

ultra-high molecular weight polyethylene
      (UHMWPE) 133, 134

viscoelastic 96

wear 128

For Product Safety Concerns and Information please contact our EU
representative GPSR@taylorandfrancis.com
Taylor & Francis Verlag GmbH, Kaufingerstraße 24, 80331 München, Germany